Quick Look Nursing:

Pharmacology

Second Edition

MARILYN J. HERBERT-ASHTON, MS, RN, BC
Associate Professor
Coordinator of Grants Development,
   Special Projects, and Community Relations
Virginia Western Community College
Roanoke, Virginia

Adjunct Faculty
Department of Nursing
Finger Lakes Community College
Canandaigua, New York

NANCY ELAINE CLARKSON, MEd, RN, BC
Chairperson and Professor of Nursing
Department of Nursing
Finger Lakes Community College
Canandaigua, New York

World Headquarters
Jones and Bartlett Publishers
40 Tall Pine Drive
Sudbury, MA 01776
978-443-5000
info@jbpub.com
www.jbpub.com

Jones and Bartlett Publishers
Canada
6339 Ormindale Way
Mississauga, Ontario L5V 1J2
CANADA

Jones and Bartlett Publishers
International
Barb House, Barb Mews
London W6 7PA
UK

Jones and Bartlett's books and products are available through most bookstores and online booksellers. To contact Jones and Bartlett Publishers directly, call 800-832-0034, fax 978-443-8000, or visit our website, www.jbpub.com.

Substantial discounts on bulk quantities of Jones and Bartlett's publications are available to corporations, professional associations, and other qualified organizations. For details and specific discount information, contact the special sales department at Jones and Bartlett via the above contact information or send an email to specialsales@jbpub.com.

The authors, editor, and publisher have made every effort to provide accurate information. However, they are not responsible for errors, omissions, or for any outcomes related to the use of the contents of this book and take no responsibility for the use of the products and procedures described. Treatments and side effects described in this book may not be applicable to all people; likewise, some people may require a dose or experience a side effect that is not described herein. Drugs and medical devices are discussed that may have limited availability controlled by the Food and Drug Administration (FDA) for use only in a research study or clinical trial. Research, clinical practice, and government regulations often change the accepted standard in this field. When consideration is being given to use of any drug in the clinical setting, the health care provider or reader is responsible for determining FDA status of the drug, reading the package insert, and reviewing prescribing information for the most up-to-date recommendations on dose, precautions, and contraindications, and determining the appropriate usage for the product. This is especially important in the case of drugs that are new or seldom used.

Library of Congress Cataloging-in-Publication Data
Herbert-Ashton, Marilyn J.
  Pharmacology / Marilyn Herbert-Ashton, Nancy Clarkson. — 2nd ed.
      p. ; cm. — (Quick look nursing)
  Includes bibliographical references and index.
  ISBN-13: 978-0-7637-5128-9 (alk. paper)
  ISBN-10: 0-7637-5128-6 (alk. paper)
  1. Pharmacology. 2. Nursing.   I. Clarkson, Nancy Elaine.   II. Title.   III. Series.
  [DNLM: 1. Pharmacology—Nurses' Instruction. QV 4 H536p 2008]
  RM300.H465 2008
  615'.1—dc22

                              2007024685

6048

Production Credits
Executive Editor: Kevin Sullivan
Aquisitions Editor: Emily Ekle
Associate Editor: Amy Sibley
Production Director: Amy Rose
Editorial Assistant: Patricia Donnelly
Associate Production Editor: Amanda Clerkin
Senior Marketing Manager: Katrina Gosek
Associate Marketing Manager: Rebecca Wasley
Manufacturing and Inventory Control Supervisor: Amy Bacus
Composition: Auburn Associates, Inc.
Cover Layout Artist: Tim Dziewit
Cover Illustrator: Cara Judd
Printing and Binding: Malloy, Inc
Cover Printing: Malloy, Inc.

Printed in the United States of America
11 10 09 08 07   10 9 8 7 6 5 4 3 2 1

DEDICATION

In honor of my husband, Steve, my mother, Madeleine, and in memory of my father, Robert, who was a wonderful advocate for nursing.

Marilyn J. Herbert-Ashton

To the three most important people in my life—Stan, Jeff, and Lindsey. Your love and support sustain me every day.

Nancy Elaine Clarkson

CONTENTS

PART VII: ENDOCRINE SYSTEM DRUGS 399
Marilyn J. Herbert-Ashton, MS, RN, BC

PART VIII: FEMALE REPRODUCTIVE SYSTEM DRUGS 457
Marilyn J. Herbert-Ashton, MS, RN, BC

PART IX: MALE REPRODUCTIVE SYSTEM DRUGS 515
Marilyn J. Herbert-Ashton, MS, RN, BC

PART X: GASTROINTESTINAL SYSTEM DRUGS 527
Nancy Elaine Clarkson, MEd, RN, BC

PART XI: DRUGS ACTING ON THE IMMUNE SYSTEM AND ANTINEOPLASTIC AGENTS 563

Nancy Elaine Clarkson, MEd, RN, BC

PART XII: HERBAL REMEDIES 607

Marilyn J. Herbert-Ashton, MS, RN, BC

ABOUT THE AUTHORS

Marilyn J. Herbert-Ashton, MS, RN, BC, has over 25 years of teaching experience in nursing education and staff development. She is currently an Associate Professor and Coordinator of Grants Development, Special Projects and Community Relations at Virginia Western Community College, Roanoke, Virginia, and is also an Adjunct Nursing Instructor at Finger Lakes Community College, Canandaigua, New York, where she teaches a distance learning pharmacology course. She is published in the area of pharmacology and has taught pharmacology for over 20 years.

Nancy Elaine Clarkson, MEd, RN, BC, received her Bachelor of Science degree in Nursing from Keuka College, Keuka Park, New York, and her master's in Nursing Education from Teacher's College, Columbia University, New York, New York. She currently is Chairperson and Professor of Nursing in the Nursing Department at Finger Lakes Community College in Canandaigua, New York. During her extensive career in nursing education, Nancy has taught students in diploma, baccalaureate, and associate degree programs. She has focused her teaching in the subjects of medical-surgical nursing and pharmacology. She is previously published in the area of pharmacology. For many years, she has taught pharmacology in the classroom and more recently online via computer.

PREFACE

The study of pharmacology can be overwhelming to even the most seasoned healthcare professional. It is a daunting task to familiarize oneself with the volumes of information concerning medications available today. It is the goal of *Quick Look Nursing: Pharmacology, Second Edition* to simplify the drug data and organize it in such a way that the reader is provided with exactly the material needed for professional practice.

Quick Look Nursing: Pharmacology, Second Edition provides an overview of medications using a systems approach. Each unit in the book is organized around drugs that affect a particular body system or a condition that interferes with a client's overall health. The individual chapters within every unit contain a drug chart that lists prototype drugs for each classification in the unit. The prototype approach allows for easier organization and retention of drug knowledge. Drugs related to each prototype are also identified.

All chapters focus on prototype and related drugs and include drug action, use, pregnancy category, adverse and side effects, interactions, contraindications, nursing implications, and client teaching. At the end of each unit, there are a number of multiple choice questions with correct answers identified and rationale stated for each correct answer.

The authors have many years of collaboratively teaching pharmacology to registered nursing students in the classroom and online. They are both published in the area of pharmacology and have presented nationally on this topic.

This text is geared toward registered nursing students and practicing professional nurses. It is meant to serve as a concise synopsis of key information, a supplement to nursing course work, and a study aid. As with other texts in the *Quick Look Nursing Series*, *Quick Look Nursing: Pharmacology, Second Edition* offers a large amount of information presented in a succinct manner.

The authors are delighted to share the contents of this text with both students and practicing professional nurses. It is their hope that all who use the information presented here will enhance their knowledge of pharmacology, improve their practice, and provide preeminent care to their clients.

Marilyn J. Herbert-Ashton
Nancy Elaine Clarkson

I

Anti-Infectives

Nancy Elaine Clarkson, MEd, RN, BC

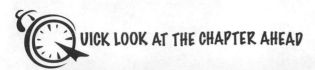 **QUICK LOOK AT THE CHAPTER AHEAD**

Bacteria, fungi, and viruses are found everywhere in our environment and resistant strains keep developing all the time. Anti-infective drugs have existed since the middle 1900s and new drugs in this group are continually being introduced. This chapter presents fundamental information that applies to the entire anti-infectives group.

1

Introductory Concepts

GENERAL CLIENT TEACHING FOR ANTI-INFECTIVES

- Take around the clock at evenly spaced time intervals to maintain blood levels.
- All doses must be taken so infection will not recur and resistant organisms will not develop.
- Most oral agents should be taken on an empty stomach as food decreases absorption.

 All doses must be taken so infection will not recur and resistant organisms will not develop.

 TERMINOLOGY

There are several terms associated with the anti-infectives with which one should be familiar. *Anti-infectives* include antibacterial, antifungal, and antiviral medications. *Antibacterial* and *antibiotic* typically mean a medication that treats a bacterial infection. A *broad spectrum* antibiotic is effective against many strains of microorganisms, and a *narrow spectrum* antibiotic is effective against only a few strains. If an antibiotic is *bactericidal,* it can kill microorganisms. An antibiotic that is *bacteriostatic* inhibits the growth of microorganisms without actually killing them.

 IDENTIFYING THE PATHOGEN

Once it has been determined that a client has an infection, the next step is to collect a sample of the pathogen for analysis. A culture and sensitivity test is usually performed to identify the offending pathogen and to determine which drug will be effective against the microorganism responsible for the infection. The test report will indicate whether the microorganism is susceptible (S) or resistant (R) to the tested drugs. It is important to collect the culture before the first dose of antibiotic is given as even one dose of medication could affect the test results.

 MECHANISMS OF DRUG ACTION

Six different modes of action used by anti-infective agents are:

1. Inhibition of bacterial cell wall synthesis. Examples of drugs that act this way are cephalosporins, penicillins, and vancomycin.

2. Inhibition of protein synthesis. Examples of drugs that act this way are aminoglycosides, erythromycin, and tetracyclines.
3. Interference with nucleic acid synthesis. Examples of drugs that act this way are fluoroquinolones and rifampin.
4. Inhibition of cell metabolism. Examples of drugs that act this way are sulfonamides and trimethoprim.
5. Disruption of cell membrane permeability. An example of drugs that act this way are antifungals.
6. Interruption of viral enzymes. An example of a drug that acts this way is acyclovir.

 ## HOST FACTORS

There are a number of factors concerning the client that will play a major role in the effectiveness or ineffectiveness of an antibiotic. Some of these factors are client age, pregnancy status, genetic characteristics, drug allergy history, site of the infection, state of the client's immune system, and status of liver and kidneys. All of these factors must be taken into consideration when considering which antibiotic is appropriate for the infected client.

 ## ANTI-INFECTIVE COMBINATION THERAPY

There are instances when more than one antibiotic may be needed to eradicate an infection. Appropriate situations for this therapy are infections caused by numerous microorganisms, treatment of serious infection, treatment of tuberculosis to prevent drug resistance, suppressed immune systems, reduction of drug toxicity in the client, and infections that require drugs whose actions enhance each other. It is important to note that combination therapy needs to be reserved for only those situations where it is clearly necessary.

 ## RESISTANCE

A current major health care concern is the increasing number of bacteria that are resistant to antibiotic treatment. Antibiotic-resistant microorganisms develop for a number of reasons that include: state of the client (host), type of infection and bacteria, environment where client is located, use of broad-spectrum agents, and insufficient antibiotic treatment of infections. Currently in the United States the major resistant strains of bacteria are methicillin-resistant staphylococcus aureus (MRSA), methicillin-resistant staphylococcus epidermides (MRSE), penicillin-resistant streptococcus pneumoniae, and vancomycin-resistant enterococci (VRE).

SUPERINFECTION

Superinfection is the development of a new infection that arises during antimicrobial management of a primary infection. Superinfections are common and typically occur when broad-spectrum antibiotics are being used. Broad-spectrum antibiotics suppress the growth of normal microbial flora of the gastrointestinal, genitourinary, and respiratory tracts, allowing other bacteria and fungi to grow and multiply. Signs and symptoms of superinfections include: the return of fever, stomatitis, diarrhea, vaginal discharge, and anal pruritus.

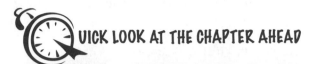
Penicillin, introduced in the 1940s, was the first antibiotic for clinical use. Since that time, a variety of penicillins have been developed. The penicillins are also known as the beta-lactam antibiotics because they contain a beta-lactam ring that is necessary for their anti-microbial activity. They are bactericidal and destroy numerous gram-positive and some gram-negative bacteria. The penicillins have been placed in four groups depending on their chemical structure and the type of bacteria they are able to kill: **natural penicillins, penicillinase-resistant penicillins, aminopenicillins, and extended-spectrum penicillins.** It should be noted that there is a group of combination drugs that contain penicillins and beta-lactamase inhibitors. The beta-lactamase inhibitors prevent destruction of penicillin from enzymes and enlarge the spectrum of antimicrobial activity of penicillin. These combination drugs are listed in the drug table on page 7. Penicillins in general have few adverse effects and are well tolerated. They are well distributed to most body tissues and fluids and are eliminated by the kidneys.

2

Penicillins

TERMS
- ☐ penicillin G potassium
- ☐ nafcillin (Unipen)
- ☐ ampicillin (Omnipen)
- ☐ ticarcillin (Ticar)
- ☐ ampicillin/sulbactam (Unasyn)

Table 2-1 Penicillins

Prototype Drug	Related Drugs	Drug Classification
penicillin G potassium	penicillin G benzathine penicillin G procaine (Wycillin) penicillin V (PenVee K)	Natural penicillins
nafcillin (Unipen)	cloxacillin (Tegopen) diclocacillin (Dynapen) oxicillin (Prostaphlin)	Penicillinase-resistant penicillins
ampicillin (Omnipen)	amoxicillin (Amoxil) bacampicillin (Spectrobid)	Aminopenicillins
ticarcillin (Ticar)	carbenicillin (Geocillan) meziocillin (Mezlin) piperacillin (Pipracil)	Extended-spectrum penicillins
ampicillin/sulbactam (Unasyn)	amoxicillin clavulanate (Augmentin) piperacillin/tazobactam (Zosyn) ticarcillin/clavulanate (Timentin)	Penicillin/beta-latamase inhibitor combinations

PENICILLIN CLIENT TEACHING

- Oral penicillin should be taken with 6 to 8 ounces of water. Do not take with acidic fluids as these will destroy the drug.
- Oral penicillin should be taken on an empty stomach for best absorption. The following can be taken with or without food: penicillin V (PenVee K), amoxicillin (Amoxil), amoxicillin clavulanate (Augmentin), and bicampicillin (Spectrobid).
- Take full course of medication.
- Take at evenly spaced intervals around the clock to maintain blood levels.
- Penicillin should not be taken if a previous allergic reaction has been experienced.
- Liquid penicillin should be shaken well before taken.

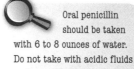
Oral penicillin should be taken with 6 to 8 ounces of water. Do not take with acidic fluids as these will destroy the drug.

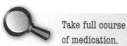
Take full course of medication.

Take at evenly spaced intervals around the clock to maintain blood levels.

- Liquid penicillin should be discarded after the expiration date and not taken past that date.
- Wear MedicAlert bracelet, necklace, or tag if allergic to penicillin.
- Report the following symptoms to the physician: skin rash, itching, hives, fever, or severe diarrhea.

 ## ACTION

The mechanism of action that the penicillins use is the inhibition of bacterial cell wall synthesis. Penicillin enters through the bacterial cell wall and finds its binding site (which is called the penicillin-binding protein). After attaching to this protein, the penicillin then interrupts normal cell wall synthesis, which in turn leads to the development of bacterial cell walls that are weak and easily destroyed. The bacteria usually die from lysis.

 ## USE

The penicillins are most commonly used to kill gram-positive bacteria: *Staphylococcus, Enterococcus,* and *Streptococcus.* The Aminopenicillins have activity against gram-negative bacteria.

Natural Penicillins

Penicillin G

- Drug of choice for pneumonia and meningitis caused by *Streptococcus pneumoniae*; pharyngitis caused by *Streptococcus pyogenes*; infectious endocarditis caused by *Streptococcus viridans*; meningitis caused by *N. meningitidis,* and syphilis caused by *T. pallidum*
- Also used for anthrax, tetanus, gas gangrene, and prophylactically for rheumatic fever and bacterial endocarditis in individuals with mitral valve prolapse, congenital heart disease, and prosthetic heart valves

Penicillinase-Resistant Penicillins

Nafcillin (Unipen)

- Used mainly for infections that are caused by penicillinase-producing Staphylococci

Aminopenicillins

Ampicillin (Omnipen)

- Useful for same infections as Penicillin G and also active against the following gram-negative bacteria: *Haemophilus influenzae, Escherichia coli (E. coli)*, Salmonella, and Shigella
- Used in bacterial meningitis, otitis media, septicemia, gonorrhea, and sinusitis

Extended-Spectrum Penicillins

Ticarcillin (Ticar)

- Mainly used for infections of *Pseudomonas aeruginosa*
- Usually given in combination with an aminoglycoside (such as gentamicin [Garamycin]) antibiotic to help increase the killing of the *Pseudomonas* bacteria

Penicillin-beta latamase Inhibitor Combinations

Amphicillin-sulbactan (Unasyn)

- Used in infections that are caused by bacteria that are resistant to beta-lactam antibiotics

ADVERSE EFFECTS AND SIDE EFFECTS

The penicillins are considered to be the safest of all the antibiotics.

- *The penicillins are classified as pregnancy category B agents with the exception of ticarcillin (Ticar), which is classified as pregnancy category C.*

- *CNS:* Anxiety, hallucinations, convulsions, lethargy, depression, coma
- *GI:* Nausea, vomiting, diarrhea, colitis
- *Hematologic:* Anemia, bone marrow depression, increased bleeding time
- *Other:* Rash, hives, hyper or hypokalemia, and taste alterations. Congestive heart failure (CHF) can be seen with ticarcillin (Ticar).
- *Allergic reactions:* An allergic response to the penicillins is seen in 1 to 10% of clients. The response can range from a skin rash to anaphylaxis. The response of greatest concern is anaphylaxis (bronchoconstriction, laryngeal edema, severe hypotension) as this can be fatal. There is cross-sensitivity among the penicillins so a client allergic to one penicillin is considered allergic to all of them. There is also a cross-sensitivity to the Cephalosporins in 5 to 10% of clients allergic to penicillins.

 ## INTERACTIONS

- Penicillin decreases the effectiveness of oral contraceptives and warfarin (Coumadin).
- Rifampin (Rifadin) and tetracyclines interfere with the bactericidal activity of penicillin.
- Nonsteroidal anti-inflammatory drugs (NSAIDs) compete with penicillin for protein binding sites and cause more free penicillin to circulate in the body.
- Probenecid (Benemid) extends the effectiveness of penicillin.
- Food interferes with the absorption of penicillin.

 ## CONTRAINDICATIONS

The penicillins are contraindicated in clients with history of severe allergic reaction to them and to the Cephalosporins.

 ## NURSING IMPLICATIONS

- Review history of any penicillin reactions with client.
- Give PO, IM, and IV.

- Doses for Penicillin G are ordered in units (1 unit = 0.6 μg).
- Monitor client for decreasing signs of infection.
- Monitor kidney function studies and I & O in clients with decreased kidney function.
- Monitor client for 30 minutes after parenteral dose of any penicillin for signs of allergic reaction.
- Dilute IM doses in diluent recommended by drug manufacturer and rotate sites.
- Monitor IV sites closely for irritation.
- Monitor clients on sodium restrictions closely who are receiving high doses of sodium Penicillin G, carbenicillin (Geocillin), and ticarcillin (Ticar) for signs of sodium overloading. Check serum sodium level and cardiac status.
- Monitor clients receiving high doses of potassium penicillin G for hyperkalemia. Check potassium serum level.
- Do not mix penicillins with Aminoglycosides in same IV solutions as penicillins can inactivate Aminoglycosides.
- Do not give a bacteriostatic drug with a penicillin as this could decrease the effectiveness of the penicillin. Give the penicillin first and then the bacteriostatic drug a few hours later.

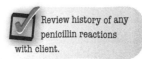
Review history of any penicillin reactions with client.

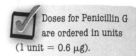
Doses for Penicillin G are ordered in units (1 unit = 0.6 μg).

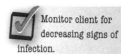
Monitor client for decreasing signs of infection.

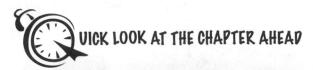

The cephalosporins have been employed in the treatment of infections since the 1960s. They have grown in popularity and are the most commonly used antibiotics today. Due to this, the number of bacteria resistant to this group is rising. Their structure and function are similar to penicillin and they are considered to be beta-lactam antibiotics. Cephalosporins are bactericidal and possess low toxicity. They have been divided into four generations and as progression is made from the first generation to the fourth generation: activity against gram-negative bacteria increases, ability to penetrate cerebrospinal fluid increases, cost increases, and there is greater resistance to beta-lactamases. The cephalosporins are well-distributed to most body tissues and fluids and are eliminated by the kidney.

3

Cephalosporins

TERMS
- [ ] cefazolin sodium (Ancef)
- [ ] cefoxitin (Mefoxin)
- [ ] ceftazidime (Fortaz)
- [ ] cefepime (Maxipime)

Table 3-1 Cephalosporins

Prototype Drug	Related Drugs	Drug Classification
cefazolin sodium (Ancef)	cefadroxil (Duricef) cephalexin (Keflex) cephapirin (Cefadyl) cephradine (Velosef)	First generation
cefoxitin (Mefoxin)	cefaclor (Ceclor) cefamandole (Mandol) cefmetazole (Zefazone) cefonicid (Monocid) cefotetan (Cefotan) cefprozil (Cefzil) cefuroxime (Zinacef) loracarbef (Lorabid)	Second generation
ceftazidime (Fortaz)	cefdinir (Omnicef) cefixime (Suprax) cefoperazone (Cefobid) cefotaxime (Claforan) cefpodoxime (Vantin) ceftibuten (Cedax) ceftizoxime (Cefizox) ceftriaxone (Rocephin)	Third generation
cefepime (Maxipime)	cefditoren (Spectracef)	Fourth generation

CEPHALOSPORIN CLIENT TEACHING

- Due to the similarities with penicillin, follow the same client teaching for penicillin found on page 7.
- Do not drink alcohol if taking cefmetazole (Zefazone), cefoperazone (Cefobid), or cefotetan (Cefotan) as this can cause a disulfiram-like (Antabuse) reaction.
- Do not drink alcohol for the first 72 hours after therapy is over.

Due to the similarities with penicillin, follow the same client teaching for penicillin found on page 7.

Do not drink alcohol if taking cefmetazole (Zefazone), cefoperazone (Cefobid), or cefotetan (Cefotan) as this can cause a disulfiram-like (Antabuse) reaction.

- Take on an empty stomach if possible, but okay to take with food if gastric problems occur.
- Aspirin and aspirin-containing products should be avoided while taking cefazolin (Kefzol), cefmetazole (Zefazone), cefoperazone (Cefobid), and cefotetan (Cefotan).

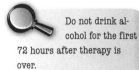
Do not drink alcohol for the first 72 hours after therapy is over.

ACTION

Cephalosporins inhibit bacterial cell wall synthesis, as do the penicillins. The reader is referred to the discussion of action of the penicillins found on page 8 for more detail.

USE

The cephalosporins are considered to be broad-spectrum and are used to kill both gram-positive and gram-negative bacteria.

First Generation

Cefazolin Sodium (Ancef)

- Effective against *Streptococci* and *Staphylococci.* Used for infections of soft tissue, bone, skin, urinary and biliary tracts, bacteremia, and endocarditis
- Also used for surgical prophylaxis

Second Generation

- Increased activity against gram-negative bacteria

Cefoxitin Sodium (Mefoxin)

- Effective against *Hemophilus influenzae, Enterobacter, Klebsiella, E. Coli,* and a few strains of *Proteus*
- Used for infections of urinary tract, skin, bone, joints, lower respiratory tract, septicemia

- Also used for surgical prophylaxis in orthopedic and cardiovascular surgery and in gynecological infections

Third Generation

- Greater activity against gram-negative bacteria

Ceftazidime (Fortaz)

- Effective against *Citrobacter, Serratia, Providencia, Enterobacter, Hemophilus influenzae, Neisseria meningitidis,* and *Streptococcus aeruginosa*
- Used for infections of bones, joints, skin, and lower respiratory tract
- Also used to treat meningitis bacteremia and gynecological infections

Fourth Generation

Cefepine (Maxipime)

- Effective against *Staphylococci* (except methicillin-resistant staphylococci), *Streptococci, E. coli,* and *Pseudomonas aeruginosa*
- Used for infections of the skin and urinary tract, and in pneumonia

ADVERSE EFFECTS AND SIDE EFFECTS

Cephalosporins are considered to be very safe. Their side effects and adverse effects are similar to the penicillins. Refer to page 9 for a detailed listing of these.

- *The cephalosporins are classified as pregnancy category B agents.*
- *Allergic reactions:* The most common reaction is a skin rash that appears a few days after treatment is begun. Anaphylaxis is rare. There is a cross-sensitivity to the penicillins in 5 to 10% of clients allergic to cephalosporins.
- *Hematological:* Cefazolin (Kefzol), cefmetazole (Zefazone), cefoperazone (Cefobid), and cefotetan (Cefotan) can cause bleeding by decreasing prothrombin levels.
- *Parenteral administration concerns:* Pain at IM injection site and thrombophlebitis at IV site.

INTERACTIONS

- Probenecid (Benemid) extends the effectiveness of cephalosporins.
- Alcohol combined with cefmetazole (Zefazone), cefoperazone (Cefobid), and cefotetan (Cefotan) causes a disulfiram-like (Antabuse) reaction (eg, nausea, vomiting, headache).
- Nonsteroidal anti-inflammatory drugs, anticoagulants, and thrombolytics should be used cautiously with cefazolin (Kefzol), cefmetazole (Zefazone), cefoperazone (Cefobid), and cefotetan (Cefotan), which cause bleeding tendencies.
- There is an increased risk of nephrotoxicity when Aminoglycoside antibiotics are taken with cefazolin.
- Loop diuretics combined with cephalosporins can increase renal toxicity.
- Tetracyclines decrease the effectiveness of cephalosporins.

 CONTRAINDICATIONS

The cephalosporins are contraindicated in clients with history of severe allergic reaction to them and to the penicillins. Cautious use in renal failure.

 NURSING IMPLICATIONS

- Give PO, IM, and IV.
- Review history of any cephalosporin reactions with client.
- IM injection should be given deeply into a large muscle mass.
- Monitor IV site for signs of redness, tenderness, and swelling.
- IV forms should be well-diluted.
- Monitor client for signs of decreasing infection.

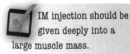
IM injection should be given deeply into a large muscle mass.

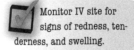
Monitor IV site for signs of redness, tenderness, and swelling.

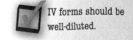
IV forms should be well-diluted.

- Check prothrombin time for clients taking cefazolin (Kefzol), cefmetazole (Zefazone), cefoperazone (Cefobid), and cefotetan (Cefabid).
- Monitor for pseudomembranous colitis.
- Oral suspensions should be refrigerated.
- Check blood urea nitrogen and creatinine levels if also taking aminoglycosides.
- Oral forms should be given with milk or food.

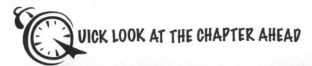

The aminoglycosides are natural, as well as semi-synthetic, bactericidal antibiotics. They are considered to be narrow-spectrum as they are usually used against gram-negative bacteria, but they are also effective against some gram-positive strains. Parenteral administration of these drugs provides good absorption, but they have poor oral absorption. If they are given orally, they are poorly absorbed from the gastrointestinal tract and thus are used to cleanse the tract before bowel surgery. The aminoglycosides are reserved to treat serious infections as they can produce powerful side effects. Serum drug levels must be checked frequently as there is a small difference between toxic and safe levels. Their distribution is mostly to extracellular fluid, and they are eliminated by the kidney.

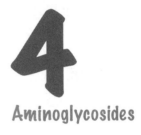

Aminoglycosides

TERM
☐ gentamycin (Garamycin)

Table 4-1 Aminoglycosides

Prototype Drug	Related Drugs	Drug Classification
gentamycin (Garamycin)	amikacin (Amikin) kanamycin (Kantrex) neomycin netilmicin (Netromycin) paromomycin (Humatin) streptomycin tobramycin (Nebcin)	Aminoglycosides

 ## AMINOGLYCOSIDE CLIENT TEACHING

- Aminoglycosides should not be taken if a previous allergic reaction has been experienced.
- Oral form should be taken on an empty stomach.
- Take full course of medication.

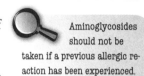
Aminoglycosides should not be taken if a previous allergic reaction has been experienced.

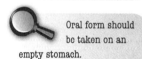
Oral form should be taken on an empty stomach.

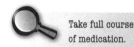
Take full course of medication.

 ## ACTION

The aminoglycosides interfere with protein synthesis in bacteria. They enter bacterial cell walls and bind to 30S and 50S ribosomes. These structures are necessary for protein synthesis to occur. As this process is disturbed, the bacterial cells cannot live and ultimately perish.

 ## USE

The main use of the aminoglycosides is in the parenteral form to combat serious infections that are caused by aerobic gram-negative organisms. The major bacteria that can be found in this category are: *Klebsiella,*

Proteus mirabilis, E. coli, Serratia, and *Pseudomonas aeurginosa.* A number of hospital-acquired infections that affect the blood, skin, bowel, wounds, and respiratory and urinary tracts can be treated with aminoglycosides. Streptomycin is used to treat tuberculosis that is resistant to other medications. The oral preparations of neomycin and kanamycin (Kantrex) are used to cleanse the bowel before surgery and to treat hepatic coma. Aminoglycosides are also given topically for ear, eye, and skin infections.

ADVERSE EFFECTS AND SIDE EFFECTS

- *The following aminoglycosides are classified as pregnancy category C agents: amikacin (Amikin), gentamycin (Garamycin), paromomycin (Humatin), and streptomycin. Those in pregnancy category D are: kanamycin (Kantrex), neomycin, netilmicin (Netromycin), and tobramycin (Nebcin).*
- *CNS:* Weakness, depression, confusion, numbness, tingling, and neuromuscular blockade
- *CV:* Hypertension, hypotension, and palpitations
- *EENT:* Ototoxicity
- *GI:* Nausea, vomiting, diarrhea, stomatitis, and weight loss
- *GU:* Nephrotoxicity
- *Hematologic:* Bone marrow depression
- *Other:* Hypersensitivity, joint pain, superinfection, apnea

INTERACTIONS

- Administering an aminoglycoside with a nephrotoxic drug increases the risk for kidney damage.
- The concurrent use of ethacrynic acid (a loop diuretic) with an aminoglycoside can increase damage to the inner ear.
- If an aminoglycoside is taken with a skeletal muscle relaxant, the neuromuscular blockade effect is increased.
- The extended-spectrum penicillins (ticarcillin [Ticar]) inactivate the aminoglycosides while the rest of the penicillins produce a synergistic effect when combined with the aminoglycosides.

- Aminoglycosides increase anticoagulant activity when taken with an anticoagulant.

CONTRAINDICATIONS

- The aminoglycosides are contraindicated in clients who are allergic to them. They must be used cautiously in clients with Parkinson's disease, dehydration, liver or kidney disease, myasthenia gravis, and hearing loss.

NURSING IMPLICATIONS

- Give PO, topically, IM, and IV.
- Review history of any aminoglycoside reactions with client.
- Do not mix penicillins with aminoglycosides in same IV solutions, as penicillins can deactivate aminoglycosides.
- IV doses should be administered slowly, at least over 30 minutes or more.
- Peak and trough levels must be monitored. Peak levels above 12.0 g/mL and trough levels above 2.0 g/mL are associated with toxicity.
- Client's hearing should be monitored.
- Monitor BUN, creatinine clearance, and I & O.
- Client needs to be well-hydrated while taking aminoglycosides.
- IV calcium gluconate can reverse neuromuscular blockade caused by aminoglycosides.
- Use caution if administering ototoxic and/or nephrotoxic drugs with aminoglycosides.
- If client is also receiving an extended-spectrum penicillin, administer aminoglycosides at least 2 hours apart.

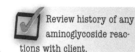

Review history of any aminoglycoside reactions with client.

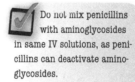

Do not mix penicillins with aminoglycosides in same IV solutions, as penicillins can deactivate aminoglycosides.

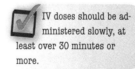

IV doses should be administered slowly, at least over 30 minutes or more.

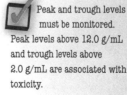

Peak and trough levels must be monitored. Peak levels above 12.0 g/mL and trough levels above 2.0 g/mL are associated with toxicity.

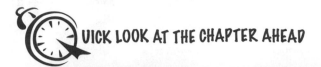

5

Tetracyclines

The tetracycline group of anti-infectives is composed of three drugs, which are derived from the common soil mold, Streptomyces (**demeclocycline** [Declomycin], **oxytetracycline** [Terramycin], and **tetracycline** [Acromycin]), as well as two other drugs that are semi-synthetically derived (**doxycycline** [Vibramycin] and **minocycline** [Minocin]). This group of medications is bacteriostatic, broad-spectrum, and needs the body's defense mechanisms to actually kill bacteria. All tetracyclines can bind to divalent and trivalent metallic ions such as aluminum, calcium, and magnesium. Thus, they should not be administered with substances that contain these ions as this results in decreased absorption of tetracycline. A great deal of microbial resistance has developed against this group over the years, and newer medications have been developed that are less toxic and more effective. However, the tetracyclines are still the drug of choice for a number of specific infections. They are well distributed to most body fluids and tissues except for cerebral spinal fluid and are excreted by the kidney and liver.

TERM
☐ **tetracycline (Acromycin)**

Table 5-1 Tetracyclines

Prototype Drug	Related Drugs	Drug Classification
tetracycline (Acromycin)	demeclocycline (Declomycin) doxycyline (Vibramycin) minocycline (Minocin) oxytetracycline (Terramycin)	Tetracyclines

TETRACYCLINE CLIENT TEACHING

- Each dose should be taken with 8 ounces of water.
- Take on an empty stomach. Doxycycline (Vibramycin) and minocycline (Minocin) can be taken with food.
- Cannot be taken with or within 2 hours of antacids, iron preparations, or dairy products
- Avoid exposure to sun. If one must be outside in sunlight, be sure to wear SPF 15 sunscreen, a hat, and cover any exposed skin.
- Report diarrhea, vaginal itching, or anal itching; report black, furry tongue immediately to physician.
- Do not take medication after the expiration date.
- Do not expose drug to light, heat, or humidity.

Cannot be taken with or within 2 hours of antacids, iron preparations, or dairy products

Avoid exposure to sun. If one must be outside in sunlight, be sure to wear SPF 15 sunscreen, a hat, and cover any exposed skin.

Do not take medication after the expiration date.

ACTION

The tetracyclines act by inhibiting protein synthesis in bacteria. They do this by attaching to the 30S ribosome unit, which in turn prevents the binding of transfer RNA to messenger RNA. This process impedes a number of necessary functions in the bacteria and thus the bacteria are unable to grow and eventually die.

USE

Tetracyclines are used to combat gram-positive and gram-negative micro-organisms. They are the drug of choice for treatment of Rocky Mountain spotted fever, cholera, typhus, granuloma inguinal, psittacosis, chancroid, Lyme Disease, trachoma, and gastric infections of *Helicobacter pylori (H. pylori)*. Other diseases in which they are used include endocervical, rectal, and urethral infections caused by Chlamydia; acne; combination therapy with other anti-infectives to treat pelvic inflammatory disease and sexually transmitted diseases; traveler's diarrhea caused by *E. coli*; and mycoplasma pneumonia. Demeclocycline (Declomycin) is used to treat the syndrome of inappropriate secretion of antidiuretic hormone.

ADVERSE EFFECTS AND SIDE EFFECTS

- *Tetracyclines are pregnancy category D agents.*
- *CNS:* Lightheadedness, dizziness, unsteadiness
- *GI:* Nausea, vomiting, diarrhea, hepatotoxicity, dysphagia
- *GU:* Nephrotoxicity

INTERACTIONS

- Oral absorption of tetracyclines is decreased if taken with dairy products, antacids, antidiarrheals, and iron preparations.
- Tetracyclines decrease the effectiveness of Penicillin G and oral contraceptives if taken together.
- Methoxyflurane taken with a tetracycline causes an increased risk of nephrotoxicity.
- Tetracycline and digoxin taken together can increase digoxin levels.

CONTRAINDICATIONS

- The tetracyclines are contraindicated in clients with a history of severe allergic reaction to them and during pregnancy and lactation. They should not be given to children under the age of 8 and should be used with caution in clients with kidney and/or liver dysfunction.

NURSING IMPLICATIONS

- Given orally, IM, and IV. Oral route preferred.
- Review history of any tetracycline reactions with client.
- Administer oral doses on an empty stomach.
- Offer small, frequent meals if nausea and vomiting occur.

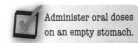
Administer oral doses on an empty stomach.

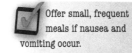
Offer small, frequent meals if nausea and vomiting occur.

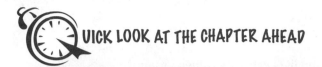

The macrolides were introduced in the early 1950s; the first member of the group was erythromycin. Erythromycin is considered to be among the safest of all antibiotics that are currently available. Today however, there is less use of erythromycin because this drug has many drug interactions, microbial resistance has developed to erythromycin, and newer macrolides have been created. Currently there are six members of this group with azithromycin (Zithromax). clarithromycin (Biaxin) and telithromycin (Ketek) being the newest members. The macrolides can be bacteriostatic or bactericidal depending on their concentration in susceptible bacteria and they are also considered to be broad-spectrum. Erythromycin has a spectrum of use similar to penicillin and is often used with clients who are allergic to penicillin. There are a number of bacterial infections in which the macrolides are the first line of treatment. The macrolides are well distributed to most body tissues and fluids except for cerebral spinal fluid (CSF) and they do cross the placenta. They are excreted by the liver.

6

Macrolides

TERM

☐ **erythromycin (E-Mycin, Ilosone, EES, Erythrocin stearate)**

Table 6-1 Macrolides

Prototype Drug	Related Drugs	Drug Classification
erythromycin (E-Mycin, Ilosone, EES, Erythrocin stearate)	azithromycin (Zithromax) clarithromycin (Biaxin) dirithromycin (Dynabac) telithromycin (Ketek) troleandomycin (Tao)	Macrolides

 ## MACROLIDE CLIENT TEACHING

- Each dose should be taken with 8 ounces of water only. Do not take with fruit juices.
- Food interferes with the absorption of some Macrolides so ask your health care provider about whether your prescription can be taken with or without food.
- Report the following symptoms to the physician: diarrhea, vomiting, abdominal pain, jaundice, dark-colored urine, light-colored stools, or lethargy as these are signs of liver damage. Also report the following signs of ototoxicity: nausea, tinnitus, dizziness, and vertigo.
- Do not breast-feed while taking a Macrolide antibiotic.

 Each dose should be taken with 8 ounces of water only. Do not take with fruit juices.

 Report the following symptoms to the physician: diarrhea, vomiting, abdominal pain, jaundice, dark-colored urine, light-colored stools, or lethargy as these are signs of liver damage. Also report the following signs of ototoxicity: nausea, tinnitus, dizziness, and vertigo.

 ## ACTION

The macrolides inhibit protein synthesis in the bacterial cell. They attach themselves to the 50S ribosomal subunit inside the bacterial cell, which stops the production of protein that the bacterial cell needs for growth. Ultimately bacteria die, and they will sometimes die immediately if the concentration of the drug is high enough.

USE

The macrolides are used primarily for gram-positive bacterial infections. They aren't as effective for gram-negative organisms. Erythromycin is the drug of choice to treat *Bordetella pertussis,* which is the microbe that causes whooping cough and also the drug of choice against *Coryne-bacterium diphtheriae,* which is the agent that causes acute diphtheria. When it is combined with rifampin (Rifadin), it is considered to be the treatment of choice for Legionnaires' disease (pneumonia caused by *Legionella pneumophila*). Further, it is the drug of choice for the chlamy-dial infections of urethritis and cervicitis and *M. pneumoniae,* which causes pneumonia. Erythromycin is a good substitute for clients who are allergic to penicillin and is used to treat respiratory tract infections caused by *Streptococcus pneumoniae* and group A *Streptococcus pyogenes*; bacterial endocarditis, rheumatic fever, and syphilis.

 ## ADVERSE EFFECTS AND SIDE EFFECTS

Macrolides, like penicillins, are considered to be among the safest of all the antibiotics.

- *Macrolides are considered pregnancy category C agents.*
- *CNS:* Dizziness, headache, vertigo, somnolence
- *CV:* Chest pain, palpitations
- *Derm:* Rash, urticaria, pruritus
- *EENT:* Hearing loss, tinnitus
- *GI:* Nausea, vomiting, diarrhea (these are the most common adverse effects of the macrolides), heartburn, anorexia, stomatitis, cholestatic hepatitis (considered the most serious adverse effect)
- *Other:* Thrombophlebitis at IV site

 ## INTERACTIONS

- Macrolides decrease the metabolism of carbamazepine (Tegretol) and cyclosporine (Sandimmune) and can cause toxicity of these medications in the body.

- Macrolides decrease the metabolism of benzodiazepines and increase the CNS depression of these drugs.
- The effects of corticosteroids are increased when taken with macrolides.
- The concurrent use of macrolides and digoxin can cause digitalis toxicity.
- Oral anticoagulants and macrolides can cause increased bleeding.
- If theophylline (Theo-Dur) and macrolides are taken together, the effectiveness of the theophylline is increased and the effectiveness of the macrolide is decreased.
- Food will decrease absorption of nonenteric-coated erythromycin tablets.

CONTRAINDICATIONS

- The macrolides are contraindicated in clients who are allergic to them. They should be used cautiously in clients with liver disease, GI disease, impaired hearing, and cardiac arrhythmias. The ophthalmic preparation is contraindicated in fungal, viral, and mycobacterial eye infections.

NURSING IMPLICATIONS

- Give PO, IV, and topically.
- Review history of any macrolide reactions with client.
- Give erythromycin stearate on an empty stomach. Other oral forms of erythromycin can be given with or without food.
- Use sterile water to reconstitute parenteral erythromycin.
- Erythromycin solutions must be used within 8 hours if stored at room temperature. Solutions stored in the refrigerator must be used within 24 hours.

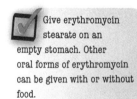
Give erythromycin stearate on an empty stomach. Other oral forms of erythromycin can be given with or without food.

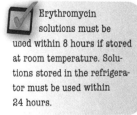
Erythromycin solutions must be used within 8 hours if stored at room temperature. Solutions stored in the refrigerator must be used within 24 hours.

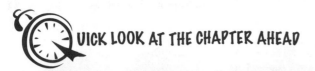

The fluoroquinolones are a fairly new group of antibiotics that are both broad-spectrum and synthetic. They are considered to be very powerful in their range of activity and are bactericidal while having few adverse reactions. Even though this group of medications is new, there is a great deal of microbial resistance that has developed due to the misuse of these drugs. The fluoroquinolones can be given orally, parenterally, and topically, although many are given only in the oral form as they have excellent absorption. Due to this, many infections that required hospitalization for intravenous medication treatment can now be treated on an outpatient basis with these oral drugs. They are absorbed by the GI tract and well distributed in the body. The principal organ for excretion is the kidneys. These drugs are found in breast milk, and they cross the placenta.

7

Fluoroquinolones

TERM

☐ ciprofloxacin (Cipro)

Table 7-1 Fluroquinolones

Prototype Drug	Related Drugs	Drug Classification
ciprofloxacin (Cipro)	alatrofloxacin (Trovan IV)	Fluoroquinolones
	enoxacin (Penetrex)	
	gatifloxacin (Tequin)	
	levofloxacin (Levaquin)	
	lomefloxacin (Maxaquin)	
	moxifloxacin (Avelox)	
	norfloxacin (Noroxin)	
	ofloxacin (Floxin)	
	sparfloxacin (Zagam)	
	trovafloxacin (Trovan)	

 ## FLUOROQUINOLONE CLIENT TEACHING

- Any sudden joint pain should be reported.
- Stop use of caffeine.
- No breast-feeding
- No driving or performing activities that require close attention until reaction to drug is known.

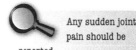

Any sudden joint pain should be reported.

 ## ACTION

The fluoroquinolones kill bacteria by changing their DNA. The drugs interfere with DNA gyrase, which is an enzyme needed to synthesize bacterial DNA. When bacteria are unable to produce DNA, they cannot live.

 ## USE

The fluoroquinolones are used to treat infections in the following areas: respiratory, genitourinary, and GI systems; soft tissues; skin; bones; and joints. They are also useful in the treatment of multidrug-resistant tuberculosis, gonorrhea, mycobacterium avium complex (MAC) infections in clients with Acquired Immune Deficiency Syndrome (AIDS), and fever in clients with cancer who have neutropenia. Fluoroquinolones are active against most aerobic gram-negative bacteria and a few gram-positive strains. They are effective against: *E. coli*, *Klebsiella*, Salmonella, Shigella, *Campylobacter jejuni*, *Pseudomonas aeruginosa*, *Haemophilus influenzae*, *meningococci*, and numerous *Streptococci*. They are resistant to *Clostridium difficile (C. difficle)* and have little effect against anaerobes.

ADVERSE EFFECTS AND SIDE EFFECTS

- *Fluoroquinolones are pregnancy category C agents.*
- *CNS:* Dizziness, fatigue, headache, restlessness, insomnia, depression, seizures
- *Derm:* Rash, pruritus, urticaria, flushing
- *EENT:* Tinnitus, blurred vision
- *GI:* Nausea, vomiting, diarrhea, constipation, heartburn, oral candidiasis, dysphagia, pseudomembranous colitis, flatulence, increased liver function tests
- *Hematologic:* Bone marrow depression
- *Other:* Fever, chills, photosensitivity (in lomefloxacin [Maxaquin]). In rare instances, tendon rupture, usually of the Achille's tendon, has occurred.

INTERACTIONS

- Concurrent administration of a fluoroquinolone with sucralfate (Carafate); antacids; didanosine (Videx); salts of aluminum, magnesium, calcium, zinc, and iron; and food decreases absorption of the fluoroquinolone.
- Theophyllines taken with fluoroquinolones can cause theophylline toxicity.
- Fluoroquinolones can decrease blood levels of the hydantoins and increase the incidence of a seizure occuring.
- Fluoroquinolones interfere with liver metabolism of caffeine.
- Fluoroquinolones decrease the effectiveness of birth control pills.
- St. John's wort taken with fluoroquinolones can cause photosensitivity reactions.

CONTRAINDICATIONS

- The fluoroquinolones are contraindicated in clients who are allergic to them, pregnant and lactating women, and children under the age of 18.
- They should be used cautiously in clients with liver disease, kidney disease, GI disease, and dehydration.
- Ciprofloxacin (Cipro) stimulates the CNS and must be used cautiously in clients with CNS and cerebrovascular disease.

 NURSING IMPLICATIONS

- Give PO, parenterally, and topically.
- Intravenous preparations should be given over 1 hour via a large vein.
- Antacids shouldn't be given within 4 hours of an oral fluoroquinolone.
- Check urine pH and keep below 6.8 to decrease crystalluria.
- Monitor I & O.
- Increase fluid intake to 2 to 3 L/day.
- Offer small frequent meals to clients with GI upset.

 Intravenous preparations should be given over 1 hour via a large vein.

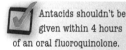 Antacids shouldn't be given within 4 hours of an oral fluoroquinolone.

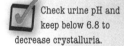 Check urine pH and keep below 6.8 to decrease crystalluria.

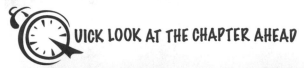

The vancomycins currently have only one member of the group, which is the prototype vancomycin (Vancocin). This drug is a naturally occurring antibiotic and it is bactericidal. It is used in the treatment of severe infections, but because it produces very severe toxic effects, its use is limited. Initially, vancomycin (Vancocin) had very widespread use in the treatment of **Staphylococcus aureus** infections. The Centers for Disease Control and Prevention have recommended a decreased use of vancomycin (Vancocin) to limit the spread of vancomycin-resistant organisms. Vancomycin (Vancocin) is usually given intravenously as the absorption from the gastrointestinal (GI) tract is unsatisfactory. The oral route is used for some GI infections. It is distributed into almost all body fluids and tissues and has a serum half-life of 4 to 6 hours in clients with normal kidney function. In those with impaired kidney function and in the elderly, the half-life can last up to 146 hours. The intravenous form of the drug is excreted mainly through the kidney, while the oral form is excreted in the feces.

8

Vancomycins

TERM
☐ vancomycin (Vancocin, Vancoled)

Table 8-1 Vancomycins

Prototype Drug	Related Drugs	Drug Classification
vancomycin (Vancocin, Vancoled)	There are no related drugs at this time	Glycopeptide

VANCOMYCINS CLIENT TEACHING

- Take according to physician directions.
- Must take entire prescription
- Take at evenly spaced intervals around the clock to keep blood levels even.
- Report hearing abnormalities to physician immediately.
- Advise physician of skin rash, fever, or sore throat.
- Report for ordered blood work: complete blood count, (CBC), peak, and trough levels.
- Develop awareness of I & O.

Report hearing abnormalities to physician immediately.

Advise physician of skin rash, fever, or sore throat.

ACTION

Vancomycin (Vancocin) prevents cell wall synthesis in bacteria by attaching to molecules in the cell wall that are necessary for biosynthesis. This, in turn, leads to death of the bacteria.

USE

Parenteral Preparation

- Serious infections not responsive to other anti-infective medications
- Drug of choice for methicillin-resistant *Staphalococcus aureus* or *Staphalococcus epidermides*

Oral Preparation

- Drug of choice for pseudomembraneous colitis caused by *C. difficle*

ADVERSE EFFECTS AND SIDE EFFECTS

- *Vancomycins are pregnancy category C drugs.*
- *CNS:* Vertigo, ataxia
- *EENT:* Ototoxicity causing tinnitis, hearing loss (considered most serious effect)
- *GI:* Nausea
- *GU:* Nephrotoxicity, uremia
- *Hematologic:* Thrombocytopenia, esinophilia, leukopenia
- *Other:* "Red neck" or "red man" syndrome associated with rapid IV infusion and caused by histamine release. Symptoms include: redness of face, neck, and upper body; hypotension; fever; chills; tachycardia; pruritus; and paresthesias. Thrombophlebitis at IV injection site

INTERACTIONS

- Concurrent use with antihyperlipidemic agents cholestyramine and colestipol interferes with absorption of oral vancomycin (Vancocin)
- Increased risk of ototoxicity with concurrent use of other known ototoxic drugs: aminoglycosides, furosemide (Lasix), ethacrynic acid (Edecrin), and salicylates
- Increased risk of nephrotoxicity with concurrent use of other known nephrotoxic drugs: polymixin B (Aerosporin), aminogylcosides, cisplatin (Platinol), cyclosporine (Sandimmune), and amphotericin B (Fungizone)
- Concurrent use with metformin (Glucophage) may cause lactic acidosis.
- Concurrent use with nondepolarizing muscle relaxants (eg, atracurium [Tracrim], metocurine) can cause an increase in neuromuscular blockade.

CONTRAINDICATIONS

- Hypersensitivity
- Pregnancy
- Lactating women need to have breast-fed neonates and infants monitored for toxic levels of drug.
- Renal disease requires cautious use.
- IM administration
- Hearing loss
- Any ototoxic or nephrotoxic drug
- Cautious use of oral preparation in inflammatory bowel disease (increases drug absorption, thus increasing possibility of drug toxicity)
- Cautious use in elderly clients

 ## NURSING IMPLICATIONS

- IV preparation should be infused over 60 minutes or longer. NEVER infuse quickly.
- Use sterile water for reconstitution.
- Compatible with D5W and NS
- Follow manufacturer's directions for reconstitution.
- Assess IV site frequently for extravasation as serious skin complications (necrosis, tissue sloughing) may occur.
- May need to administer antihistamine before intravenous dosing
- Assess blood pressure (BP) and pulse during IV administration.
- Assess following lab studies: CBC, liver, and kidney function.
- Assess peak and trough levels in clients with renal disease, clients above 60 years of age, neonates, and infants. Levels of 60 to 80 mcg/mL may cause ototoxicity.
- Monitor hearing and I & O.

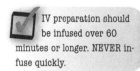 IV preparation should be infused over 60 minutes or longer. NEVER infuse quickly.

 Use sterile water for reconstitution.

 Compatible with D5W and NS

 Follow manufacturer's directions for reconstitution.

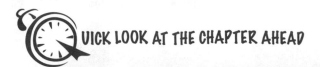

UICK LOOK AT THE CHAPTER AHEAD

The newest class of anti-infectives contains drugs that are used against resistant strains of bacteria. The first group of drugs in this class are the Streptogramins which were introduced in 1999.[1] There are two drugs in this group, quinupristin and dalfopristin. They have a synergistic effect and are sold in the United States as a combined drug called Synercid. Quinupristin/dalfopristin (Synercid) is bactericidal and is used to treat infections caused by methicillin-resistant and vancomycin-resistant bacteria as well as **Staphylococcus aureus** and epidermides. This drug must be used very discriminately so that other new resistant strains of bacteria don't develop. Quinupristin/dalfopristin (Synercid) is given intravenously. It is well distributed to the skin and soft tissues and excreted through bile via feces.

The Oxazolidinones were introduced in 2000 when the first and only member of the group, linezolid (Zyvox), was approved for use in the United States. Linezolid (Zyvox) is a synthetic drug that was developed to treat serious infections caused by methicillin-resistant and vancomycin-resistant bacteria. It is bactericidal when used against anaerobic, gram-positive, and gram-negative bacteria. This drug must be used cautiously, and numerous health care facilities require their Infectious Disease Committee to approve its use.[2] Linezolid (Zyvox) can be given orally and intravenously. It is distributed all over the body after quick absorption from the gastrointentinal tract and is excreted via the urine.

9

Drugs for Resistant Bacterial Strains

TERMS
- ☐ linezolid (Zyvox)
- ☐ quinupristin/dalfopristin (Synercid)

Table 9-1 Drugs for Resistant Bacterial Strains

Prototype Drug	Related Drugs	Drug Classification
linezolid (Zyvox)	There are no related drugs at this time.	Oxazolidinone
quinupristin/dalfopristin (Synercid)	There are no related drugs at this time.	Streptogramin

DRUGS FOR RESISTANT BACTERIAL STRAINS CLIENT TEACHING

Linezolid (Zyvox)

* Oral form can be taken with or without food.
* Tryamine containing foods need to be limited to <100.0 mg/meal.
* Do not breast-feed.
* Avoid caffeine and alcohol.
* Consult with physician before taking any over-the-counter drug as there are many interactions.

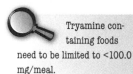

Tryamine containing foods need to be limited to <100.0 mg/meal.

Avoid caffeine and alcohol.

ACTION

Linezoid (Zyvox) prevents protein synthesis in the bacteria by impeding an early step in the protein-making process. It is believed that this action may slow down the bacteria's ability to become resistant.

Quinupristin/dalfopristin (Synercid) suppresses protein synthesis in bacteria by permanently stopping the function of the ribosomes.

USE

Linezolid (Zyvox)

* Nosocomial or community-acquired pneumonia caused by *Streptococcus pneumoniae*

- Nosocomial or community-acquired pneumonia and complicated skin infections caused by Methicillin-Resistant *Staphylococcus aureus* (MRSA)
- Bacteremia caused by Vancoycin-Resistant *Enterococcus faecium* (VREF)

Quinupristin/Dalfopristin (Synercid)

- Life-threatening infections caused by VREF and MRSA
- Complicated skin and skin structure infections from *Streptococcus pyogenes*

ADVERSE EFFECTS AND SIDE EFFECTS

Linezolid (Zyvox)

- *Pregnancy category C*
- *CNS:* Insomnia, headache, dizziness
- *CV:* Hypertension

Quinupristin/Dalfopristin (Synercid)

- *Considered pregnancy category C*
- *CNS:* Headache
- *Derm:* Itching, rash

INTERACTIONS

Linezolid (Zyvox)

- Concurrent use with monoamine oxidase inhibitors   or levodopa (Dopar) can cause hypertensive crisis.
- Concurrent use with sympathomimetics may elevate blood pressure.
- Concurrent use with selective seratonin reuptake inhibitors can cause serotonin syndrome.
- Food, which contains Tyramine, can increase blood pressure.

- Ephedra, ginseng, and ma-huang can cause nervousness, headache, and/or increased blood pressure.

Quinupristin/Dalfopristin (Synercid)

- Increases the levels of alprazolam (Xanax), cyclosporine (Sandimmune), diazepam (Valium), Erythromycin (E-Mycin), lidocaine (Xylocaine), nifedipine (Procardia), verapamil (Calan), vinca alkaloids

CONTRAINDICATIONS

Linezolid (Zyvox)

- Hypersensitivity
- Cautious use in the following: oral suspension when given to phenylketonurics, as it contains aspartame; and in clients with blood dyscrasias, as it may cause bone marrow suppression

Quinupristin/Dalfopristin (Synercid)

- Hypersensitivity
- Lactation
- Cautious use in clients with decreased liver function
- Not approved for use in children

NURSING IMPLICATIONS

Linezolid (Zyvox)

- Give PO and IV.
- Mixed oral suspension should not be shaken.

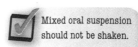

Mixed oral suspension should not be shaken.

Quinupristin/Dalfopristin (Synercid)

- Given IV.
- Monitor liver function tests.
- Do not shake IV solution when reconstituting.

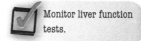

Monitor liver function tests.

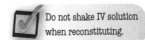

Do not shake IV solution when reconstituting.

- Flush IV line with D5W before and after administration. Do not flush with saline or heparin.

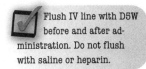

Flush IV line with D5W before and after administration. Do not flush with saline or heparin.

REFERENCES

1. Karch A. *Focus on Nursing Pharmacology*. Philadelphia, PA: Lippincott, Williams & Wilkins; 2008:100.

2. Aschenbrenner D, Cleveland L, Venable S. *Drug Therapy in Nursing*. Philadelphia, PA: Lippincott, Williams & Wilkins; 2006:707.

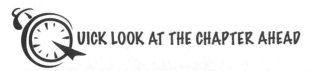

Urinary tract infection (UTI) and other urinary problems are treated with various medications. Four classes of drugs that are used for UTI will be discussed in this chapter: **sulfonamides, urinary tract antiseptics, urinary tract analgesics**, and a miscellaneous anti-infective that is used specifically for UTI. Urinary antispasmodics will also be discussed.

The sulfonamides are synthetic and are all derived from sulfanilamide, the first sulfonamide that was discovered. Because they achieve high concentrations in the kidneys, which are the organs that eliminate them from the body, they are a good choice for the treatment of UTI. The sulfonamides have a broad spectrum of activity and are given orally. They are considered to be bacteriostatic.

The urinary tract antiseptics are unable to reach therapeutic levels in the tissues or blood and are not used to treat systemic infections. They are used specifically for the treatment of UTI. They concentrate in the urine and are used successfully against common bacteria found in the urinary tract. They are considered to be second-line treatment for UTI.[1] There is no prototype for this group, so each drug will be discussed individually. They are all given orally.

Phenazopyridine (Pyridium) is used as a urinary tract analgesic. It doesn't have any anti-infective action but is used to relieve the symptoms of UTI. It is given orally.

Fosfomycin (Monurol) is a synthetic, broad-spectrum antibiotic. It is bactericidal and given orally as a one-time dose. Improvements in symptoms of UTI are seen in 2 to 3 days after administration.

10

Drugs That Act on the Urinary Tract

TERMS
- ☐ **sulfamethoxazole-trimethoprim (Bactrim)**
- ☐ **phenazopyridine (Pyridium)**
- ☐ **Qxybutnin (Ditropan)**

Spasms of the urinary tract can be caused by various problems. The urinary antispasmodics are used to stop the spasms.

Table 10-1 Drugs That Act on the Urinary Tract

Prototype Drug	Related Drugs	Drug Classification
sulfamethoxazole-trimethoprim (Bactrim)	sulfasalazine (Azulfidine) sulfisoxazole (Gantrisin)	Sulfonamides
There is no prototype for this classification	cinoxacin (Cinobac) methenamine (Hiprex) nalidixic acid (NegGram) nitrofurantoin (Macrodantin)	Urinary tract antiseptics
phenazopyridine (Pyridium)		Urinary tract analgesic
There is no prototype for his classification	fosfomycin (Monurol)	Miscellaneous anti-infective
Oxybutnin (Ditropan)	darifenacin (Enablex) solifenacin (VESIcare) tolteradine (Detrol)	Urinary antispasmodics

DRUGS THAT ACT ON THE URINARY TRACT CLIENT TEACHING

Sulfonamides

- Take with 8 ounces of water on an empty stomach.
- Take all of medication.
- Stop drug if skin rash appears.
- Stay out of sun and wear sunscreen and protective clothing if you have to be exposed.
- Drink 8 to 10 glasses of water per day.

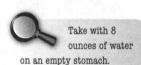

Take with 8 ounces of water on an empty stomach.

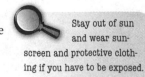

Stay out of sun and wear sunscreen and protective clothing if you have to be exposed.

Urinary Tract Antiseptics

Cinoxacin (Cinobac)

- Take all of medication.
- Take drug around the clock.
- Notify physician if symptoms worsen or tinnitus occurs.
- No driving or hazardous activities until reaction to drug is known
- Do not breast-feed.

 Notify physician if symptoms worsen or tinnitus occurs.

 Do not breast-feed.

Methenamine (Hiprex)

- Take with food.
- Do not breast-feed.
- Do not take OTC antacids containing sodium bicarbonate or sodium carbonate.
- Increase foods that will acidify urine (proteins, pruncs, plums, cranberry juice).

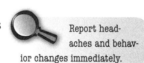 Do not take OTC antacids containing sodium bicarbonate or sodium carbonate.

Nalidixic Acid (NegGram)

- Take all of drug exactly as prescribed.
- Report headaches and behavior changes immediately.
- Increase fluid intake to 2 to 3 L/day.
- Stay out of sun for 3 months after drug is discontinued.
- Report vision problems in initial days of therapy.
- Do not breast-feed.

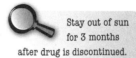 Report headaches and behavior changes immediately.

Stay out of sun for 3 months after drug is discontinued.

Nitrofurantoin (Macrodantin)

- IM injection is painful.
- Urine may turn brown.
- Do not force fluids.
- Do not breast-feed.

Urinary Tract Analgesic

Phenazopyridine (Pyridium)

- Urine will turn red-orange and will stain clothes.
- Report yellow color of skin or sclera immediately.
- Stop drug when discomfort is gone.
- Breast-feed only after discussing with physician.

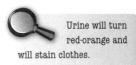

Urine will turn red-orange and will stain clothes.

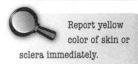

Report yellow color of skin or sclera immediately.

Urinary Antispasmodics

- Do not breast-feed.
- Do not get overheated as fever and heat stroke can develop.
- No driving or hazardous activities until reaction to drug is known

Do not get overheated as fever and heat stroke can develop.

Miscellaneous Anti-Infective

Fosfomycin (Monurol)
- Drug must be mixed with 3 to 4 ounces of water and taken immediately. Cannot be taken dry.
- Do not breast-feed.

℞ ACTION

Sulfonamides

Subdue the growth of bacteria by interfering with the synthesis of folic acid that is required for the biosynthesis of protein, DNA, and RNA.

Urinary Tract Antiseptics

Cinoxacin (Cinobac)

- Interferes with protein synthesis and DNA replication in the bacterial cell

Methenamine (Hiprex)

- Breaks down into formaldehyde and ammonia in acid urine
  Formaldehyde causes death of bacteria by denaturing bacterial proteins.

Nalidixic Acid (NegGram)

- Causes bacterial cell to die by interfering with replication of DNA

Nitrofurantoin (Macrodantin)

- Disrupts enzyme systems of bacterial cell leading to its death

Urinary Tract Analgesic

Phenazopyridine (Pyridium)

- Mechanism of action is unknown.

Urinary Antispasmodics

- Relax urinary muscles to relieve spasms

Miscellaneous Anti-Infective

Fosfomycin (Monurol)
- Interferes with the enzyme pyruvyl transferase, which is important in bacterial cell wall synthesis

 USE

Sulfonamides

- Acute UTI, especially if caused by *E. coli*
- Trachoma
- Nocardiosis
- Sexually transmitted diseases
- Ulcerative colitis (Sulfasalazine [Azulfidine])

Urinary Tract Antiseptics

Cinoxacin (Cinobac)

- Acute and recurrent UTI caused by gram-negative bacteria

Methenamine (Hiprex)

- Chronic UTI. Not indicated for UTI of the upper urinary tract as formaldehyde cannot form as drug passes through kidney.

Nalidixic Acid (NegGram)

- Acute and recurrent UTI only

Nitrofurantoin (Macrodantin)

- Acute and recurrent UTI of lower urinary tract

Urinary Tract Analgesic

Phenazopyridine (Pyridium)

- Relief of pain, burning, urgency, and frequency caused from irritation to the urinary tract

Urinary Antispasmodics

- Relieve bladder spasm
- Treat signs of overactive bladder

Miscellaneous Anti-Infective

Fosfomycin (Monurol)

- Acute UTI

ADVERSE EFFECTS AND SIDE EFFECTS

Sulfonamides

- *Pregnancy category C*
- *CNS:* Headache, dizziness, vertigo, depression, ataxia, convulsions

- *Derm:* Rash
- *GI:* Nausea, vomiting, diarrhea, stomatitis, anorexia, abdominal pain
- *GU:* Crystalluria, proteinuria, hematuria
- *Hematologic:* Thrombocytopenia, aplastic anemia, hemolytic anemia, agranulocytosis
- *Other:* Hypersensitivity reactions, photosensitivity

Urinary Tract Antiseptics

Cinoxacin (Cinobac)

- *Pregnancy category B*
- *CNS:* Dizziness, headache, insomnia, anxiety
- *CV:* Edema
- *Derm:* Rash
- *EENT:* Tinnitus
- *GI:* Nausea, anorexia, rectal itching, metallic taste, abdominal pain
- *Other:* Photophobia

Methenamine (Hiprex)

- *Pregnancy category C*
- *GI:* Nausea, vomiting, anorexia
- *GU:* Crystalluria, hematuria, albuminuria

Nalidixic Acid (NegGram)

- *Pregnancy category B during second and third trimesters*
- *CNS:* Headache, vertigo, seizures
- *EENT:* Blurred vision, diplopia
- *GI:* Nausea, vomiting
- *Hematologic:* Hemolytic anemia, eosinophilia
- *Other:* Hypersensitivity, photosensitivity

Nitrofurantoin (Macrodantin)

- *Pregnancy category B*
- *CNS:* Peripheral neuropathy
- *Derm:* Pruritus, urticaria
- *GI:* Nausea, vomiting, diarrhea, anorexia
- *GU:* Crystalluria, brown or dark yellow urine
- *Resp:* Asthma attack, allergic pneumonitis

Urinary Tract Analgesic

Phenazopyridine (Pyridium)

- *Pregnancy category B*
- *CNS:* Vertigo, headache
- *GU:* Kidney stones
- *Hematologic:* Hemolytic anemia

Urinary Antipasmodics

- *Pregnancy category C except for oxybutnin (Ditropan), which is category B*
- *CNS:* Drowsiness
- *Derm:* Pruritis
- *EENT:* Blurred vision
- *GI:* Dry mouth

Miscellaneous Anti-Infective

Fosfomycin (Monurol)
- *Pregnancy category B*
- *CNS:* Headache
- *GI:* Diarrhea
- *GU:* Vaginitis
- *Resp:* Pharyngitis, rhinitis

INTERACTIONS

Sulfonamides

- Increases the effects of oral hypoglycemics (eg, tolbutamide [Orinase], glyburide [DiaBeta], glipizide [Glucotrol], etc), phenytoin (Dilantin), and warfarin (Coumadin)
- Concurrent use with cyclosporine (Sandimmune) increases risk for nephrotoxicity

Urinary Tract Antiseptics

Cinoxacin (Cinobac)

- Concurrent use with probenecid (Benemid) decreases elimination of cinoxacin (Cinobac) through the kidney.

Methenamine (Hiprex)

- Concurrent use with sulfamethoxazole causes precipitate in acid urine.
- Concurrent use with sodium bicarbonate and/or acetazolamide (Diamax) can stop hydrolysis to formaldehyde.

Nalidixic Acid (NegGram)

- Multivitamins containing zinc or iron, antacids, calcium, magnesium, sucralfate (Carafate), and dida-nosine (Videx) interfere with absorption.
- Can elevate hypoprothrombinemic effects of warfarin (Coumadin)

Nitrofurantoin (Macrodantin)

- Concurrent use with antacids decreases absorption.
- Concurrent use with fluoroquinolones and/or nalidixic acid (NegGram) reduces antimicrobial effects.
- Elevated drug toxicity if taken with probenecid (Benemid) or sulfinpyrazone (Anturane)

Urinary Tract Analgesic

Phenazopyridine (Pyridium)

- No interactions

Urinary Antispasmodics

- Concurrent use of oxybutnin (Ditropan) with haloperidol (Haldol) and the phenothiazines will decrease effectiveness of haloperidol (Haldol) and the phenothiazines.

Miscellaneous Anti-Infectives

Fosfomycin (Monurol)

- Concurrent use with metoclopramide (Reglan) diminishes urinary excretion.

 ## CONTRAINDICATIONS

Sulfonamides

- Hypersensitivity to these drugs, to sulfonylureas or thiazide diuretics, which have a cross-sensitivity
- Pregnancy
- Lactation
- Cautious use in clients with kidney disease or kidney stone history

Urinary Tract Antiseptics

Cinoxacin (Cinobac)

- Hypersensitivity
- Anuria
- Dehydration
- Lactation
- Pregnancy
- Children under 18 years of age

Methenamine (Hiprex)

- Kidney and/or liver disease
- Dehydration
- Gout
- Use with sulfonamides

Nalidixic Acid (NegGram)

- Seizure history
- Infants less 3 months of age
- First trimester of pregnancy

Nitrofurantoin (Macrodantin)

- Renal impairment
- Infants less than 3 months of age

Urinary Tract Analgesic

Phenazopyridine (Pyridium)

- Renal impairment
- Hepatitis

Urinary Antispasmodics

- Obstruction of urinary tract
- Glaucoma
- Myasthenia gravis
- Obstruction of GI tract

Miscellaneous Anti-Infective

Fosfomycin (Monurol)

- Hypersensitivity
- Lactation

NURSING IMPLICATIONS

Sulfonamides

- Give PO. Sulfamethoxazole-trimethoprim (Bactrim) is also given IV.
- Give cautiously to clients with kidney impairment.
- IV administration should be slow or via drip.
- Do not administer to clients with allergy to sulfonylureas, loop or thiazide diuretics.
- Monitor complete blood count.
- Assess for hemolysis.

> Do not administer to clients with allergy to sulfonylureas, loop or thiazide diuretics.

- Increase fluid intake in client to 1200 mL/day.
- Alkalize urine.

Urinary Tract Antiseptics

Cinoxacin (Cinobac)

- Give PO.
- Maintain consistent urinary level by administering at evenly spaced intervals over each 24-hour period.
- Assess ambulation.
- Repeat culture and sensitivity if drug response is inadequate.

> Maintain consistent urinary level by administering at evenly spaced intervals over each 24-hour period.

Methenamine (Hiprex)

- Give PO.
- Administer with food.
- Oral suspension has an oil base and should be carefully administered to elderly and debilitated clients to prevent aspiration pneumonia.
- Assess urine pH and keep at 5.5 or less. Give ascorbic acid or food to keep urine acid.
- Assess I & O. Do not force fluids.

> Oral suspension has an oil base and should be carefully administered to elderly and debilitated clients to prevent aspiration pneumonia.

Nalidixic Acid (NegGram)

- Give PO.
- Administer on empty stomach. Can give with food or milk if GI distress occurs.
- Assess renal and hepatic function tests.
- Assess for central nervous system reactions which can happen 30 minutes after initial dose or after second or third dose. The elderly, infants, and children are susceptible.

> Assess for central nervous system reactions which can happen 30 minutes after initial dose or after second or third dose. The elderly, infants, and children are susceptible.

Nitrofurantoin (Macrodantin)

- Give PO.
- Assess I & O.

- Do not crush tablets. Dilute oral suspension and rinse mouth after administration.
- Assess for urinary superinfections.
- Monitor for nausea, which is common.
- Assess for pulmonary sensitivity reaction, which typically occurs in first week of therapy and, seen more frequently in elderly.
- Assess for pulmonary sensitivity in extended therapy.
- Assess for peripheral neuropathy, which can be irreversible.

> Assess for pulmonary sensitivity reaction, which typically occurs in first week of therapy and, seen more frequently in elderly.

Urinary Tract Analgesic

Phenazopyridine (Pyridium)

- Give PO.
- Food has no effect on drug.
- Assess kidney function tests in clients with impaired kidney function.

> Assess kidney function tests in clients with impaired kidney function.

Urinary Antispasmodics

- Give PO and topically.
- Do not chew or crush pills if in sustained-release form.
- Tolerance to drug can develop.
- Keep doctor aware of drug effects.

> Do not chew or crush pills if in sustained-release form.

Miscellaneous Anti-Infective

Fosfomycin (Monurol)

- Give PO.
- Mix dose with 3 to 4 ounces of water, dissolve, and give immediately.

REFERENCE

1. Lehne R. *Pharmacology for Nursing Care*. Philadelphia, PA: WB Saunders; 2007:1012.

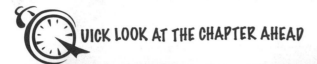
Tuberculosis (TB) is an ancient disease but it continues to be found worldwide. It is estimated that there are 8 million new cases of TB found per year in the world and most happen in developing countries.[1] Reasons for the continuing presence of TB include the development of multidrug-resistant mycobacteria and AIDS.[1]

The antitubercular drugs are divided into two groups, the first- and second-line drugs. First-line drugs will be discussed individually. Isoniazid (INH) is the prototype drug for TB, because it is included in all treatment regimens except one, INH-resistant TB.[2] The drugs used for treatment of TB are used in combination as this allows for the drugs to act on the bacteria at different phases of their life cycle as well as to reduce development of resistant strains.[3]

11

Antitubercular Drugs

TERM
☐ isoniazid (INH)

Table 11-1 Antitubercular Drugs

Prototype Drug	Related Drugs	Drug Classification
isoniazid (INH)	ethambutol (Myambutol) ethionamide (Trecator SC) pyrazinamide (PZA) rifampin (Rifadin)	Antitubercular agents
	streptomycin	Aminoglycoside

 ## ANTITUBERCULAR DRUGS CLIENT TEACHING

Isoniazid (INH)

- Do not drink alcohol.
- Do not eat foods that contain histamine or tyramine.
- Do not breast-feed.
- Stop drug if any of these symptoms occur: jaundice, dark urine, clay-colored stools, chills, fever, skin rash.
- Report numbness or tingling in hands and feet to physician.

Stop drug if any of these symptoms occur: jaundice, dark urine, clay-colored stools, chills, fever, skin rash.

Report numbness or tingling in hands and feet to physician.

Ethambutol (Myambutol)

- Do not breast-feed.
- Report any eye problems.

Report any eye problems.

Ethionamide (Trecator SC)

- Do not drink alcohol.
- Do not breast-feed.
- Change position slowly.

Change position slowly.

Pyrazinamide (PZA)

- Do not breast-feed.
- Tell physician of any urination problems.
- Increase fluids.

Tell physician of any urination problems.

Rifampin (Rifadin)

- Do not breast-feed.
- Do not stop and restart drug as flu-like syndrome may occur.
- Body secretions will be red-orange colored.
- Contact lenses may be permanently stained red-orange.
- Additional birth control necessary if taking oral contraceptives.

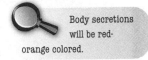

Body secretions will be red-orange colored.

Streptomycin

- See "Client Teaching" for Aminoglycosides in Chapter 4.

 ## ACTION

Isoniazid (INH)

- Prevents synthesis of mycolic acid, which is an integral part of the mycobacteria cell wall

Ethambutol (Myambutol)

- Prevents RNA synthesis in the mycobacteria cell wall, thus stopping growth.

Ethionamide (Trecator SC)

- Action is unknown but it is hypothesized that drug hinders protein synthesis in the bacteria.

Pyazinamide (PZA)

- Action unknown

Rifampin (Rifadin)

- Hinders DNA-dependent RNA polymerase which stops RNA synthesis and ultimately, protein synthesis.

Streptomycin

- See "Action" of Aminoglycosides in Chapter 4.

USE

Isoniazid (INH)

- Given for treatment and/or prophylaxis of TB
- Given alone if used for prophylaxis and given in combination with other antitubercular agents if used for treatment of TB

Ethambutol (Myambutol)

- Used in combination with other antitubercular agents to treat pulmonary TB

Ethionamide (Trecator SC)

- Given to treat active TB after primary drugs have not worked
- Must be given in combination with other antituberculosis drugs.

Pyrazinamide (PZA)

- Given to treat TB after primary drugs have not worked. Appears to work best in early stages of treatment

Rifampin (Rifidin)

- Drug of choice for pulmonary TB
- Used in combination with other antitubercular agents
- Also used in treatment of leprosy

Streptomycin

- See "Use" of Aminoglycosides in Chapter 4.

 ADVERSE EFFECTS AND SIDE EFFECTS

Isoniazid (INH)

- *Pregnancy category C*
- *CNS:* Peripheral neuropathy, paresthesias
- *EENT:* Visual disturbances, optic neuritis
- *Fluids and electrolytes (F & E):* Hyperkalemia, hypocalcemia, hypophosphatemia

- *GI:* Elevated liver enzymes, hepatitis, decreased pyridoxine (Vitamin B$_6$)
- *GU:* Urinary retention in males
- *Hematologic:* Aplastic or hemolytic anemia
- *Resp:* Dyspnea
- *Other:* Hypersensitivity

Ethambutol (Myambutol)

- *Pregnancy category B*
- *CNS:* Dizziness, hallucinations, confusion, paresthesias
- *EENT:* Retrobulbar optic neuritis, loss of red-green color spectrum, photophobia, eye pain
- *GI:* Abdominal pain, anorexia
- *Other:* Hypersensitivity

Ethionamide (Trecator SC)

- *Pregnancy category D*
- *CNS:* Peripheral neuritis, restlessness, hallucinations, convulsions
- *CV:* Postural hypotension
- *Endocrine:* Hypothyroidism, menorrhagia
- *GI:* Nausea, vomiting, anorexia, diarrhea, metallic taste, hepatitis
- *Other:* Impotence

Pyrazinamide (PZA)

- *Pregnancy category C*
- *CNS:* Headache
- *Derm:* Urticaria
- *GI:* Liver toxicity
- *GU:* Urination problems
- *Hematologic:* Hemolytic anemia
- *Other:* Photosensitivity, elevated uric acid, gout, arthralgia

Rifampin (Rifadin)

- *Pregnancy category C*
- *CNS:* Fatigue, drowsiness, confusion, dizziness, extremity pain
- *EENT:* Visual impairments
- *GI:* Nausea, vomiting, abdominal cramps, diarrhea, liver injury, hepatitis
- *GU:* Hematuria, renal failure
- *Hematologic:* Anemia, thrombocytopenia

- *Other:* Red-orange color of body secretions, hypersensitivity, flu-like syndrome

Streptomycin

- *Pregnancy category C*
- See "Adverse Effects and Side Effects" of Aminoglycosides in Chapter 4.

INTERACTIONS

Isoniazid (INH)

- Drinking alcohol or taking drug with rifampin (Rifadin) or PZA increases chance of liver damage.
- Concurrent use with phenytoin (Dilantin) causes phenytoin toxicity.
- Food interferes with absorption.

Ethambutol (Myambutol)

- Antacids containing aluminum interfere with absorption.

Ethionamide (Trecator SC)

- Concurrent use with INH or cycloserine (Seromycin) raises risk for nerve damage.

Pyrazinamide (PZA)

- Concurrent use with rifampin (Rifadin) raises risk for liver damage.

Rifampin (Rifidin)

- Drinking alcohol or taking drug with INH or PZA increases chance of liver damage.
- Decreases effects of numerous drugs. Major concern of this with corticosteroids, oral contraceptives, thyroid hormones, oral sulfonylureas, warfarin (Coumadin), phenytoin (Dilantin), digoxin (Lanoxin)

Streptomycin

- See "Interactions" of Aminoglycosides in Chapter 4.

CONTRAINDICATIONS

Isoniazid (INH)

- Acute liver disease
- Hypersensitivity
- Use cautiously in lactation, chronic alcoholism, individuals over 35 years of age, chronic liver disease, seizure disorder.

Ethambutol (Myambutol)

- Hypersensitivity
- Lactation
- Children less than 13 years of age
- Optic neuritis

Ethionamide (Trecator SC)

- Hypersensitivity
- Use cautiously in liver disease and diabetes mellitus.

Pyrazinamide (PZA)

- Liver disease

Rifampin (Rifidin)

- Hypersensitivity
- Lactation
- Diseases caused by meningococci
- Use cautiously with alcoholics and in liver disease.

Streptomycin

- See "Contraindications" of Aminoglycosides in Chapter 4.

 NURSING IMPLICATIONS

For All Antitubercular Drugs

- Treatment of TB involves a combination of drugs.
- Compliance tends to be a problem as treatment is long.

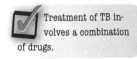
Treatment of TB involves a combination of drugs.

- Client education is very important for compliance.
- Baseline tests of sputum culture and sensitivity and chest x-ray are generally ordered.

Isoniazid (INH)

- Give PO and IM.
- Monitor liver function tests.
- Assess eye function.
- Assess blood pressure during initial therapy as orthostatic hypotension may occur.
- Ensure client is taking supplemental pyridoxine (Vitamin B_6).
- Administer on empty stomach. Can be given with food if GI upset occurs.
- Administer IM deeply in large muscle.
- IM injection can be painful.
- IM solution should be at room temperature to dissolve any crystals that have formed.

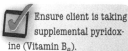
Ensure client is taking supplemental pyridoxine (Vitamin B_6).

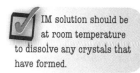
IM solution should be at room temperature to dissolve any crystals that have formed.

Ethambutol (Myambutol)

- Give PO.
- Can give with food
- Monitor I & O.
- Assess eyes using ophthalmoscope for baseline data and then monthly.

Assess eyes using ophthalmoscope for baseline data and then monthly.

Ethionamide (Trecator SC)

- Give PO.
- Can give with food
- Can be given in one dose
- Client should take supplemental pyridoxine (Vitamin B_6).
- Monitor the following tests: complete blood count, urinalysis, kidney and liver function.

Client should take supplemental pyridoxine (Vitamin B_6).

Pyrazinamide (PZA)

- Give PO.
- Assess for liver toxicity and bleeding tendencies.

- Stop drug if gout or liver reactions occur.
- Assess uric acid levels.

> ✓ Assess for liver toxicity and bleeding tendencies.

Rifampin (Rifadin)

- Give PO and IV.
- Give on empty stomach.
- Open capsule and mix with food or fluid if client is unable to swallow.
- Assess liver function tests.
- Daily Prothrombin Time (PT) if client receiving anticoagulant
- IV administration should be slow (3 hours).

> ✓ Open capsule and mix with food or fluid if client is unable to swallow

Streptomycin

- See "Nursing Implications" for Aminoglycosides in Chapter 4.

REFERENCES

1. Lehne R. *Pharmacology for Nursing Care.* Philadelphia, PA: WB Saunders; 2007:1014.

2. Aschenbrenner D, Cleveland L, Venable S. *Drug Therapy in Nursing.* Philadelphia, PA: Lippincott, Williams & Wilkins; 2006:747.

3. Karch A. *Focus on Nursing Pharmacology.* Philadelphia, PA: Lippincott, Williams & Wilkins; 2008:129.

A virus is a speck of RNA or DNA covered by protein that lives by placing its own RNA or DNA into a healthy cell and then gains control of the cell.[1] Viruses cause a wide range of diseases from the "flu" to AIDS. They are difficult to kill because they are able to live in human cells.[2]

The antiviral drugs prevent viruses from reproducing, and this allows the body's immune system to kill them.[3] At present there are a limited number of viruses for which antiviral drugs can have an effect. These include Influenza viruses, Herpes viruses, Cytomegalovirus (CMV), Human immunodeficiency virus (HIV), Respiratory syncytial virus (RSV), and hepatitis viruses.[3] This chapter will discuss five major drug classes that are used in the treatment of viruses: **drugs for influenza; drugs for CMV and Herpes, protease inhibitors, nucleoside reverse transcriptase inhibitors,** and **non-nucleoside reverse transcriptase inhibitors**—all of which are used in the fight against HIV and AIDS.

12

Antivirals

TERMS
- ☐ **rimantadine (Flumadine)**
- ☐ **acyclovir (Zovirax)**
- ☐ **saquinavir (Fortovase)**
- ☐ **zidovudine (Retrovir)**
- ☐ **nevirapine (Viramune)**

Table 12-1 Antivirals

Prototype Drug	Related Drugs	Drug Classification
rimantadine (Flumadine)	amantadine (Symmetrel) oseltamivir (Tamiflu) ribavirin (Virazole) zanamivir (Relenza)	Drugs for Influenza
acyclovir (Zovirax)	cidofovir (Vistide) famciclovir (Famvir) foscarnet (Foscavir) ganciclovir (Cytovene) valacyclovir (Valtrex) valganciclovir (Valcyte)	Drugs for CMV and Herpes
saquinavir (Fortovase)	amprenavir (Agenerase) indinavir (Crixivan) lopinavir (Kaletra) nelfinavir (Viracept) ritonavir (Norvir)	Protease inhibitors
zidovudine (Retrovir)	abacavir (Ziagen) didanosine (Videx) lamivudine (Epivir) stavudine (Zerit) tenofovir (Viread) zalcitabine (Hivid)	Nucleoside reverse transcriptase inhibitors
nevirapine (Viramune)	delaviridine (Rescriptor) efavirenz (Sustiva) emitricitabine (Emtriva)	Non-nucleoside reverse transcriptase inhibitors

ANTIVIRAL DRUG CLIENT TEACHING

Drugs for Influenza

Rimantadine (Flumadine)

- Do not breast-feed.
- No activities that require concentration until drug reaction known
- Tell physician of side effects of chest palpitations, leg edema, or breathing problems.

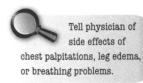

Tell physician of side effects of chest palpitations, leg edema, or breathing problems.

Drugs for CMV and Herpes

Acyclovir (Zovirax)

- Drug is not a cure.
- Wash affected area three to four times a day with soap, and dry well.
- No sexual contact when lesions present
- Always wear a condom.
- Begin treatment as soon as symptoms appear.
- Do not get ointment in eyes.
- No breast-feeding

Wash affected area three to four times a day with soap, and dry well.

No sexual contact when lesions present

Always wear a condom.

Protease Inhibitors

Saquinavir (Fortovase)

- Take exactly as ordered.
- Body fat will be redistributed.
- Tell physician of diabetes symptoms: polyuria, polyphagia, polydipsia.
- Increase fluid intake to 1.5 L/day.
- Avoid transferring HIV to others.
- Do not breast-feed.
- Drug is not a cure.

Increase fluid intake to 1.5 L/day.

Nucleoside Reverse Transcriptase Inhibitors

Zidovudine (Retrovir)

- Take exactly as ordered.
- Tell physician of symptoms of lactic acidosis immediately: fatigue, nausea, vomiting, anorexia, hyperventilation.
- Drug is not a cure.
- Do not breast-feed.
- Avoid transferring HIV to others.

Tell physician of symptoms of lactic acidosis immediately: fatigue, nausea, vomiting, anorexia, hyperventilation.

Non-Nucleoside Reverse Transcriptase Inhibitors

Nevirapine (Viramune)

- Stop drug if skin rash develops.
- No activities that require concentration until drug reaction is known
- Do not breast-feed.
- Use additional birth control if taking oral contraceptives.

> Stop drug if skin rash develops.

℞ ACTION

Drugs for Influenza

Rimantadine (Flumadine)

- Has an inhibitory effect that works early in the viral replication cycle of Influenza A virus
- Also prevents viral uncoating

Drugs for CMV and Herpes

Acyclovir (Zovirax)

- Enters cells where virus is found and prevents viral DNA replication through the work of an enzyme

Protease Inhibitors

Saquinavir (Fortovase)

- Protease is an enzyme that is necessary for the HIV virus to grow. These drugs prevent protease from acting.

Nucleoside Reverse Transcriptase Inhibitors

Zidovudine (Retrovir)

- Prevents protein synthesis in the viral cell, which in turn stops reproduction of HIV

Non-Nucleoside Reverse Transcriptase Inhibitors

Nevirapine (Virmune)

* Hinders the shift of information that the virus needs to reproduce by attaching to HIV reverse transcriptase and impeding DNA and RNA activities

 USE

Drugs for Influenza

Rimantidine (Flumadine)

* Treatment and prevention of Influenza A. Amantadine (Symmetrel) is used to treat Parkinson's disease, and ribavirin (Virazole) is used in the treatment of Herpes and RSV.

Drugs for CMV and Herpes

Acyclovir (Zovirax)

* Used specifically for treatment of Herpes simplex type 1 and 2 infections
* Cidofovir (Vistide), foscarnet (Foscavir), ganciclovir (Cytovene), and valganciclovir (Valcyte) are used for CMV.

Protease Inhibitors

Saquinavir (Fortovase)

* Given to adults and children with HIV in combination with other antiviral drugs

Nucleoside Reverse Transcriptase Inhibitors

Zidovudine (Retrovir)

* Given to adults and children with HIV. Used to stop maternal transmission of HIV

- Lamivudine (Epivir) is used to treat chronic Hepatitis B.
- These drugs can be given in combination with other antiviral drugs.

Non-Nucleoside Transcriptase Inhibitors

Nevirapine (Viramune)

- Used in combination with other antiviral drugs to treat HIV in adults and children

ADVERSE EFFECTS AND SIDE EFFECTS

Drugs for Influenza

Rimantadine (Flumadine)

- *Pregnancy category C*
- *CNS*: Headache, dizziness, sleep disturbance, fatigue
- *GI*: Abdominal pain, anorexia, dry mouth

Drugs for CMV and Herpes

Acyclovir (Zovirax)

- *Pregnancy category C*
- *CNS:* Headache
- *Derm:* Rash, itching, stinging, burning
- *GI:* Nausea, vomiting, diarrhea
- *GU:* Kidney damage
- *Hematologic:* Hemolytic uremic syndrome, thrombocytopenic purpura

Protease Inhibitors

Saquinavir (Fortovase)

- *Pregnancy category B*
- *CNS:* Paresthesias, confusion, seizures, tremors, anxiety, depression
- *CV:* Hypo- or hypertension, chest pain
- *Derm:* Rash, itching, seborrhea, photosensitivity
- *EENT:* Tinnitis, visual disturbance

- *Endocrine:* Hyperglycemia
- *GI:* Diarrhea, vomiting, abdominal pain
- *Hematologic:* Splenomegaly, anemia
- *Resp:* Rhinitis, laryngitis, bronchitis, dyspnea
- *Other:* Hypersensitivity, myalgia

Nucleoside Reverse Transcriptase Inhibitors

Zidovudine (Retrovir)

- *Pregnancy category C*
- *CNS:* Headache
- *Derm:* Rash
- *F & E:* Lactic acidosis
- *GI:* Anorexia, nausea, vomiting
- *Hematologic:* Bone marrow depression
- *Resp:* Wheezing, cough
- *Other:* Fever, malaise, myalgia

Non-Nucleoside Reverse Transcriptase Inhibitors

Nevirapine (Viramune)

- *Pregnancy category C except for emtricitabine (Emtriva), which is category B*
- *CNS:* Headache
- *Derm:* Rash
- *GI:* Hepatitis, diarrhea, nausea
- *Hematologic:* Anemia, neutropenia
- *Other:* Myalgia, paresthesias, fever

INTERACTIONS

Drugs for Influenza

Rimantadine (Flumadine)

- Concurrent use with anticholinergic drugs increases the anticholinergic effects.

Drugs for CMV and Herpes

Acyclovir (Zovirax)

- There are additive antiviral effects if given with interferon.
- Concurrent use with probenecid (Benemid) slows elimination of acyclovir.
- Zidovudine (Retrovir) increases lethargy and neurotoxicity.

Protease Inhibitors

Saquinavir (Fortovase)

- The following decrease levels of saquinavir (Fortovase): phenobarbital, phenytoin (Dilantin), carbamazepine (Tegretol), dexamethasone (Decadron), rifabutin (Ansamycin), and rifampin (Rifadin).
- The following increase levels of saquinavir (Fortovase): indinavir (Crixivan), clarithromycin (Biaxin), ritonavir (Norovir), ketoconazole (Nixoral), and delavirdine (Rescriptor).
- Saquinavir (Fortovase) elevates levels of the following: sildenafil (Viagra), nelfinavir (Viracept), ergot derivatives, midazolam (Versed), and triazolam (Halicion).
- Concurrent use with St. John's wort can lower antiretroviral activity.

Nucleoside Reverse Transcriptase Inhibitors

Zidovudine (Retrovir)

- Ganciclovir and acetaminophen increase bone marrow depression.
- Acyclovir increases neurotoxicity.
- Levels increase with beta-interferon.
- Hematologic toxicity increases with cytotoxic drugs.
- Additive effect against HIV with didanosine and zalcitabrine.

Non-Nucleoside Reverse Transcriptase Inhibitors

Nevirapine (Viramune)

- Decreased levels of oral contraceptives
- Lowered levels of nevirapine with rifabutin and rifampin

- Lowered levels of protease inhibitors
- Elevated metabolism of drugs metabolized by CYP3A4 hepatic microsomal enzyme system

CONTRAINDICATIONS

Drugs for Influenza

Rimantadine (Flumadine)

- Hypersensitivity
- Lactation
- Pregnancy
- Kidney or liver disease
- Cautious use in seizure disorder
- Drugs for CMV and Hepatitis

Acyclovir (Zovirax)

- Hypersensitivity
- Lactation
- Pregnancy
- Kidney or CNS disease

Protease Inhibitors

Saquinavir (Fortovase)

- Lactation
- Hypersensitivity
- Nucleoside reverse transcriptase inhibitors
- Zidovudine (Retrovir)
- Hypersensitivity
- Caution in pregnancy

Non-Nucleoside Reverse Transcriptase Inhibitors

Nevirapine (Viramune)

- Hypersensitivity
- Lactation

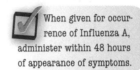

NURSING IMPLICATIONS

Drugs for Influenza

Rimantadine (Flumadine)

- Give PO. Give Ribavirin (Virazole) PO and by inhalation. Give Zanamivir (Relenza) by inhalation only.
- Stop drug if seizures occur.
- Assess for dyspnea, elevated blood pressure, palpitations, pedal edema.
- When given for occurrence of Influenza A, administer within 48 hours of appearance of symptoms.

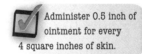
When given for occurrence of Influenza A, administer within 48 hours of appearance of symptoms.

Drugs for CMV and Herpes

Acyclovir (Zovirax)

- Give PO, IV, and topically.
- Shake suspension before administration.
- Use finger cot or glove for topical application.
- Administer 0.5 inch of ointment for every 4 square inches of skin.
- Lesions must be totally covered.
- Give IV dose slowly, over 1 hour at least.
- Do not give by IV bolus.
- Assess IV site for tissue damage.
- Assess I & O
- Assess creatinine and BUN with IV route.

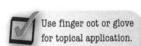
Use finger cot or glove for topical application.

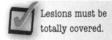
Administer 0.5 inch of ointment for every 4 square inches of skin.

Lesions must be totally covered.

Protease Inhibitors

Saquinavir (Fortovase)

- Give PO.
- All protease inhibitors can be given with food.

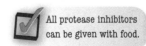
All protease inhibitors can be given with food.

- Amprenavir (Agenerase) and indinavir (Crixivan) should be taken with low-fat food and can also be taken on an empty stomach.
- Weigh client periodically.
- Assess CBC, electrolytes, blood glucose, and liver function studies.

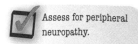

Assess for peripheral neuropathy.

- Assess for peripheral neuropathy.

Nucleoside Reverse Transcriptase Inhibitors

Zidovudine (Retrovir)

- Give PO and IV.
- Assess CBC and CD4 count often.
- Give IV slowly—at least over 1 hour.
- Blood transfusion may be needed if client becomes anemic.

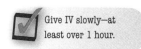

Give IV slowly—at least over 1 hour.

Non-Nucleoside Reverse Transcriptase Inhibitors

Nevirapine (Viramune)

- Give PO.
- Give with food or on empty stomach.
- Discontinue drug if rash occurs.
- Assess CBC, liver, and kidney function tests baseline and then periodically.

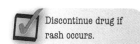

Discontinue drug if rash occurs.

REFERENCES

1. Karch A. Focus on *Nursing Pharmacology.* Philadelphia, PA: Lippincott, Williams & Wilkins; 2008:138.

2. Lilley L Harrington S Snyder J. *Pharmacology and the Nursing Process.* St. Louis, MO: Mosby; 2007:610.

3. Lilley L Harrington S Snyder J. *Pharmacology and the Nursing Process.* St. Louis, MO: Mosby; 2007:611.

Fungi can be found everywhere and are divided into two groups: **molds** and **yeasts**. A fungal infection can be systemic and very potent or superficial and weak.[1] The antifungal drugs discussed in this chapter are divided into three groups. The first group is composed of drugs that act systemically in the body. The second group, the Azoles, treat systemic fungal infections and are a newer class of drugs.[2] The third group is used topically to treat fungal infections of the mucous membranes and skin.

13

Antifungals

TERMS
- ☐ amphotericin B (Fungizone)
- ☐ fluconazole (Diflucan)

Table 13-1 Antifungals

Prototype Drug	Related Drugs	Drug Classification
amphotericin B (Fungizone)	caspofungin (Cancidas) flucytosine (Ancobon) griseofulvin (Fulvicin) micafungin (Mycamine) nystatin (Mycostatin)	Systemic antifungals (Polyenes)
fluconazole (Diflucan)	butoconazole (Femstat 3) clotrimazole (Lotrimin) econazole (Spectrazole) itraconazole (Sporanox) ketoconazole (Nizoral) miconazole (Monistat) oxiconazole (Oxistat) sertaconazole (Ertaczo)	Azoles
There is no prototype for this classification	butenafine (Mentax) ciclopirox (Loprox) haloprogin (Halotex) naftifine (Naftin) terbinafine (Lamisil) tolnaftate (Tinactin)	Topicals

ANTIFUNGAL CLIENT TEACHING

For Systemic Antifungals and Azoles

- Treatment may be for an extended time.
- Take all of medication.
- Take OTC preparations only after checking with physician.
- Report fever, chills, vomiting, abdominal pain, and skin rash.
- Do not breast-feed.
- All oral forms can be taken with food except ketoconozole (Nizoral) for GI upset.

Report fever, chills, vomiting, abdominal pain, and skin rash.

For All Topicals

- Wash affected skin with soap and water and dry thoroughly before applying drug.

Wash affected skin with soap and water and dry thoroughly before applying drug.

- Do not breast-feed.
- Discontinue if skin rash appears and report to physician.
- Dissolve troches slowly in mouth.
- Vaginal application must be placed high in vagina.
- Stay recumbent for at least 10 minutes after vaginal application.
- Avoid getting drug in the eyes.
- Do not apply occlusive dressing unless told to do so.
- Do not use near an open wound.

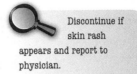

Discontinue if skin rash appears and report to physician.

 ## ACTION

For All Antifungals

Change the permeability of the fungal cell wall, causing death of the cell and failure of the cell to reproduce. For example, Amphotericin B (Fungizone) attaches to ergosterol in the fungal cell and opens pores in the cell wall.

 ## USE

For All Systemic Antifungals and Azoles

- Treatment of the following fungal infections: aspergillosis; blastomycosis; candidiasis; coccidiodomycosis; crytococcal meningitis; histoplasmosis; leishmaniasis; moniliasis; mucormycosis; onychomycosis; tinea barbae, tinea capitis, tinea corporis, tinea cruris, tinea pedis, and tinea unguium

For All Topicals

- Treatment of the following fungal infections: athlete's foot, topical mycosis, tinea infections, and vaginal *Candida* infections

ADVERSE EFFECTS AND SIDE EFFECTS

For All Systemic Antifungals and Azoles

- *Pregnancy category C for all, except amphotericin B (Fungizone), miconazole (Monistat), topical clotrimazole (Lotrimin), and oxiconazole (Oxistat) are category B*
- *CNS:* Headache, visual problems, peripheral neuritis, dizziness, seizures, insomnia
- *CV:* Arrhythmias, tachycardia, hypertension
- *Derm:* Rash, urticaria, photosensitivity, hives
- *Endocrine:* Hypothyroidism, hypoadrenalism
- *EENT:* Transient hearing loss, blurred vision
- *F & E:* Hypokalemia, hyponatremia
- *GI:* Nausea, vomiting, diarrhea, anorexia, cramps, liver toxicity
- *GU:* Impotence, vaginal burning and itching, renal dysfunction
- *Hematologic:* Anemia, bone marrow suppression, thrombocytopenia, leukopenia
- *Other:* Fever, chills, malaise, arthralgias

For All Topicals

- *Pregnancy category B, except for tolnaftate (Tinactin), which is category C*
- *Derm:* Burning, rash, irritation, swelling
- *GI:* Nausea, vomiting, liver dysfunction
- *GU:* Urinary burning and frequency

 ## INTERACTIONS

For All Systemic Antifungals and Azoles

- Elevated risk of renal toxicity if amphotericin B (Fungizone) is taken with corticosteroids or nephrotoxic drugs
- Concurrent use of the azoles with the following results in elevated blood levels of these drugs: warfarin (Coumadin), phenytoin

(Dilantin), oral hypoglycemics, digoxin (Lanoxin), and cyclo-sporine (Sandimmune).

- Life-threatening cardiovascular episodes if Azoles taken concurrently with midazolam (Versed), lovastatin (Mevacor), triazolam (Halcion), and simvastatin (Zocor).

For All Topicals

- As topicals are not being absorbed systemically, there are no interactions.

CONTRAINDICATIONS

For All Systemic Antifungals and Azoles

- Hypersensitivity
- Lactation
- Pregnancy
- Liver or kidney disease

For All Topicals

- Hypersensitivity

NURSING IMPLICATIONS

For All Systemic Antifungals and Azoles

- Give PO and IV.
- Baseline culture and sensitivity (C & S)
- Assess IV site for phlebitis.
- Infuse IV medication slowly (2 to 4 hours).
- Monitor liver and kidney lab studies.
- Monitor I & O
- Monitor nutrition and offer frequent small meals if GI symptoms are present.

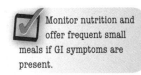

Monitor nutrition and offer frequent small meals if GI symptoms are present.

- Oral forms may be taken with food if GI symptoms are present.
- Ketoconozole (Nizoral) must be taken on empty stomach.
- Administer analgesics and antipyretics to assist in controlling fever, headache, and chills.

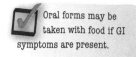
Oral forms may be taken with food if GI symptoms are present.

For All Topicals

- Baseline C & S
- Assess lesions for effects of drug.

REFERENCES

1. Lilley L, Harrington S, Snyder J. *Pharmacology and the Nursing Process.* St. Louis, MO: Mosby; 2007:643.

2. Karch A. *Focus on Nursing Pharmacology*. Philadelphia, PA: Lippincott, Williams & Wilkins; 2008:162.

UICK LOOK AT THE CHAPTER AHEAD

Protozoa cause numerous infections that are found worldwide. Common infections that occur are malaria, leishmaniasis, giardiasis, trichomomiasis, trypanosomiasis, and amebiasis. These infections are a real health concern as billions of individuals are affected.[1] Fortunately, these infections are uncommon in the United States, but there is an increased rate found in individuals with compromised immune systems.[1] Protozoa thrive in humid and warm environments. Thus, they are found frequently in tropical climates. This chapter will discuss the drugs used to treat protozoal infections caused by insect bites, specifically malaria, and those that are caused by contact or ingestion of the organism.

14

Antiprotozoals

TERMS
☐ chloroquine (Aralen)
☐ metronidazole (Flagyl)

Table 14-1 Antiprotozoals

Prototype Drug	Related Drugs	Drug Classification
chloroquine (Aralen)	hydroxychloroquine (Plaquenil) mefloquine (Lariam) primaquine pyrimethamine (Daraprim) quinine	Antimalarials
metronidazole (Flagyl)	atovaquone (Mepron) nitazoxanide (Alinia) pentamidine (Pentam 300) tinidazole (Tindamax)	Other antiprotozoals

ANTIPROTOZOALS CLIENT TEACHING

Antimalarials

Chloroquine (Aralen)

- Do not breast-feed.
- Urine may discolor to brown or rusty yellow.
- No activities requiring concentration until drug reaction is known
- If experiencing any of the following, report immediately: muscle weakness, ear or eye problems, loss of balance, and blood dyscrasia problems (eg, sore throat, fatigue, and/or bruising/ bleeding).
- Wear dark glasses in bright light.

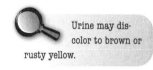
Urine may discolor to brown or rusty yellow.

Wear dark glasses in bright light.

Other Antiprotozoals

Metronidazole (Flagyl)

- Do not breast-feed.
- Urine may discolor to reddish or dark brown.
- No alcohol or products containing alcohol until 48 hours after therapy finished

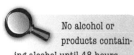
No alcohol or products containing alcohol until 48 hours after therapy finished

- Sexual partners need concurrent treatment.
- Symptoms of candidiasis must be reported.
- No intercourse unless male wears a condom

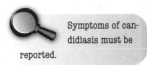

Symptoms of candidiasis must be reported.

 ## ACTION

Antimalarials

The actions of the antimalarials depend on the family of chemical agents with which they are associated. The prototype, chloroquine (Aralen), attaches to nucleoproteins and interrupts protein synthesis. It also prevents reproduction by interfering with DNA and RNA polymerase and interferes with the parasite's ability to use erythrocyte hemoglobin.

Other Antiprotozoals

These drugs interrupt DNA synthesis in susceptible protozoa, which prevents reproduction and causes death of the cell.

 ## USE

Antimalarials

- Utilized as prophylaxis, treatment, and prevention of relapse of malaria

Other Antiprotozoals

- Given to treat specific infections caused by individual protozoa. The prototype, metronidazole (Flagyl), is used to treat giardiasis, amebiasis, and trichomoniasis.

ADVERSE EFFECTS AND SIDE EFFECTS

Antimalarials

- *All are pregnancy category C, except quinine, which is category X.*
- *CNS:* Dizziness, headache
- *Derm:* Hair loss, pruritus, rash
- *EENT:* Possible blindness, ototoxicity
- *GI:* Anorexia, nausea, vomiting, dyspepsia, liver damage
- *Other:* Fever, chills, malaise, cinchonism (nausea, vomiting, tinnitus, vertigo) related to high doses of quinine

Other Antiprotozoals

- *All are pregnancy category C except metronidazole (Flagyl), which is category B, and tinidazole (Tindamax), which is category D in the first trimester and category C in the second and third trimesters.*
- *CNS:* Dizziness, headache, ataxia, peripheral neuropathy
- *GI:* Diarrhea, nausea, vomiting, abdominal cramps, unpleasant taste, liver toxicity

INTERACTIONS

Antimalarials

Chloroquine (Aralen)

- Antacids and laxatives containing aluminum and magnesium decrease absorption of chloroquine (Aralen).
- Can disrupt response to rabies vaccine
- Concurrent administration with valproic acid (Depakene) decreases serum levels of valproic acid (Depakene) and increases risk of seizures.

Other Antiprotozoals

Metronidazole (Flagyl)

- Can increase lithium (Eskalith) levels
- Elevated metronidazole (Flagyl) metabolism with Phenobarbital
- Acute psychosis seen with disulfiram
- The following can cause disulfiram (Antabuse) reaction: alcohol; IV administration of nitroglycerin (Nitro-Bid), sulfamethoxazole, or trimethoprim (Primsol); oral solutions of lopinavir/ritonavir (Kaletra), citalopram (Celexa), or ritonavir (Norvir).
- Transient neutropenia can occur with azathioprine (Imuran) and/or fluorouracil (Adrucil).
- Concurrent use with oral anticoagulants potentiates hypoprothrombinemia.

 ## CONTRAINDICATIONS

Antimalarials

Chloroquine (Aralen)

- Hypersensitivity
- Kidney disease
- Pregnancy
- Lactation
- Porphyria
- Retinal disease
- Use cautiously in liver disease, neurologic diseases, and alcoholism

Other Antiprotozoals

Metronidazole (Flagyl)

- First trimester of pregnancy
- Lactation
- Hypersensitivity

- Liver disease
- Kidney disease
- Blood dyscrasias
- CNS diseases

 ## NURSING IMPLICATIONS

Antimalarials

Chloroquine (Aralen)

- Give PO and IM.
- This group typically given in combination with other drugs in the group
- Can give with food to decrease GI problems
- Check child's dose as this group is highly susceptible to overdosage.
- Give IM deep into large muscle.
- Separate administration with magnesium and aluminum containing antacids by at least 4 hours.
- Perform baseline complete blood count and electrocardiogram.
- Assess vision changes.
- Assess deep tendon reflexes and muscle strength.

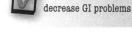
Can give with food to decrease GI problems

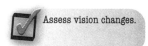
Assess vision changes.

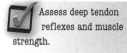
Assess deep tendon reflexes and muscle strength.

Other Antiprotozoals

Metronidazole (Flagyl)

- Give PO, topically (for rosacea), and IV.
- Topical application needs to be thin over affected area.
- Tablets can be crushed.
- Can give with food or milk
- Extended release form has to be swallowed whole on empty stomach.
- Give IV slowly—over 1 hour.

- Compatible solutions for IV reconstitution are normal saline (NS) or sterile water.

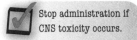

Compatible solutions for IV reconstitution are normal saline (NS) or sterile water.

- Can mix IV solution with ringers lactate (RL), NS, or D5W
- IV solution must be neutralized with sodium bicarbonate.
- No equipment containing aluminum when preparing IV dose
- Stop administration if CNS toxicity occurs.

Stop administration if CNS toxicity occurs.

- Assess white blood cell count and differential baseline during and after therapy.
- Check for increased lithium (Eskalith) levels if client is taking lithium (Eskalith).

Check for increased lithium (Eskalith) levels if client is taking lithium (Eskalith).

- If client has history of congestive heart failure or taking corticosteriods, assess for sodium retention.
- Assess for candidiasis and report to physician.

REFERENCE

1. Lilley L Harrington S Snyder J. *Pharmacology and the Nursing Process.* St. Louis, MO: Mosby; 2007:653.

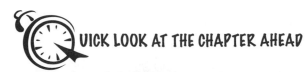

Worm or helmintic infections are a problem found all over the world. It is estimated that about one billion individuals have worms somewhere in their bodies.[1] The worms that are commonly found in human infections are tapeworms, flukes, and roundworms. As antihelmintic drugs destroy specific worms, it is very important to correctly identify the worm causing the infection so the appropriate drug can be prescribed.

15

Antihelmintics

TERM
☐ **mebendazole (Vermox)**

Table 15-1 Antihelmintics

Prototype Drug	Related Drugs	Drug Classification
mebendazole (Vermox)	albendazole (Albenza) ivermectin (Stromectol) oxamniquine (Vansil) praziquantel (Biltricide) pyrantel pamoate (Antiminth) thiabendazole (Mintezol)	Antihelmintics

ANTIHELMINTICS CLIENT TEACHING

- Do not breast-feed.
- Wash hands after touching contaminated articles.
- Infected individual needs to sleep alone.
- Shower often.
- Washcloths, towels, bedding, and underwear should be changed often.
- All medication must be taken.

Wash hands after touching contaminated articles.

Infected individual needs to sleep alone.

Shower often.

ACTION

The action of each antihelmintic differs as it works on various metabolic processes in the specific worm. The prototype drug, mebendazole (Vermox), prevents the uptake of glucose and other nutrients, which in turn prevents reproduction and leads to cell death.

USE

- The antihelmintics combat infections caused by flukes, tapeworms, and roundworms. Mebendazole (Vermox) is used to treat hookworms, pinworms, roundworms, and whipworms.

ADVERSE EFFECTS AND SIDE EFFECTS

- *All are pregnancy category C, except praziquental (Biltricide), which is category B.*

Mebendazole (Vermox)

- *CNS:* Dizziness
- *GI:* Diarrhea, transient abdominal pain
- *Other:* Fever

INTERACTIONS

Mebendazole (Vermox)

- Concurrent use with phenytoin (Dilantin) and/or cárbamazepine (Tegretol) raises metabolism of meb-endazole (Vermox).

CONTRAINDICATIONS

Mebendazole (Vermox)

- Children
- Pregnancy
- Lactation

NURSING IMPLICATIONS

Mebendazole (Vermox)

- Give PO.
- Can crush or chew tablets
- Can mix tablets with food

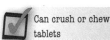
Can crush or chew tablets

Can mix tablets with food

- All family members should be treated.
- If infection is not gone in 3 weeks, a second course of drugs can be given.

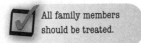

All family members should be treated.

REFERENCE

1. Karch A. *Focus on Nursing Pharmacology.* Philadelphia, PA: Lippincott, Williams & Wilkins; 2008:192.

PART I • QUESTIONS

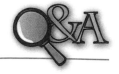

1. An antibiotic is ordered to be taken TID. Which of the following times would be appropriate for administration?
   a. 9 am, 3 pm, 6 pm
   b. 1 am, 9 am, 5 pm
   c. 8 am, Noon, 4 pm
   d. 6 am, Noon, 6 pm

2. Which group of anti-infectives acts by inhibiting protein synthesis in the bacterial cell?
   a. Fluoroquinolones
   b. Sulfonamides
   c. Aminoglycosides
   d. Penicillins

3. What should the nurse be assessing in a client receiving a high dose of ticarcillin (Ticar)?
   a. Serum sodium level
   b. Hemoglobin
   c. Serum blood glucose
   d. Serum potassium level

4. Which statement about the penicillins is FALSE? The penicillins:
   a. Are considered to be the safest of all the antibiotics.
   b. Decrease the effectiveness of oral contraceptives.
   c. Should be taken with citrus juices.
   d. Are bactericidal.

5. A third-generation cephalosporin is different from a first-generation cephalosporin in that the third-generation cephalosporin:
   a. Costs less.
   b. Has less resistance to beta-lactamases.
   c. Is unable to penetrate cerebral spinal fluid (CSF).
   d. Has increased activity against gram-negative bacteria.

6. A client is ordered to receive a cephalosporin. The client has an allergy to penicillin. The nurse's initial action in this situation is to:
   a. Give the cephalosporin as ordered.
   b. Ask the client to describe the penicillin allergy.
   c. Call the physician and report the allergy.
   d. Monitor the client for any adverse effects.

7. Which aminoglycoside is used to cleanse the bowel before surgery?
   a. Neomycin
   b. Gentamycin (Garamycin)
   c. Streptomycin
   d. Amikacin (Amikin)

8. A client receiving an aminoglycoside has the following peak and trough level results:
   Peak level: 15.0 g
   Trough level: 4.0 g
   How should the nurse interpret these results?
   a. The dose of the aminoglycoside needs to be increased.
   b. The client should be switched to a different antibiotic.
   c. The client is in the toxic range of the aminoglycoside.
   d. The client is ready to receive the aminoglycoside orally.

9. The nurse should instruct the client receiving an oral tetracycline to do which of the following:
   a. Take the medication with a full glass of milk.
   b. Stop the medication if you develop heart palpitations.
   c. Store the medication in a clear plastic bottle.
   d. Stay out of the sun while receiving the medication.

10. Which client should be given tetracycline?
    a. A 15-year-old boy with acne
    b. A 23-year-old pregnant woman with Lyme Disease
    c. A 6-year-old girl with Rocky Mountain Spotted Fever
    d. A 45-year-old man with tuberculosis

11. Which of the following is considered to be the most common adverse effects of the macrolide antibiotics?
    a. Nasal stuffiness
    b. Pink-tinged urine
    c. Nausea and vomiting
    d. Dysphagia

12. Erythromycin is often given to clients who are allergic to:
    a. Tetracyclines.
    b. Penicillin.
    c. Cephalosporins.
    d. Aminoglycosides.

13. A client taking a fluoroquinolone should restrict the intake of:
    a. Dairy products.
    b. Caffeine.
    c. Vitamin C.
    d. Green, leafy vegetables.

14. Which of the following statements about the fluoroquinolones is true? The fluoroquinolones are:
    a. Narrow-spectrum.
    b. Bacteriostatic.
    c. Excreted by the kidneys.
    d. Not found in breast milk.

15. Intravenous vancomycin (Vancocin) should be used cautiously in which of the following clients?
    a. An 18-year-old
    b. A 30-year-old
    c. A 50-year-old
    d. A 75-year-old

16. The "red neck" or "red man" syndrome associated with vancomycin (Vancocin) is caused by:
    a. An elevated red blood cell count.
    b. A release of histamine.
    c. An increased blood pressure.
    d. Exposure to the sun.

17. All of the following statements about intravenous quinupristin/dalfopristin (Synercid) are true EXCEPT:
    a. Infuse IV dose over 20 minutes.
    b. It is preferable to infuse IV dose via a central line.
    c. Do not shake intravenous solution when reconstituting.
    d. Flush IV line with D5W before and after administration.

18. The client who is taking linezolid (Zyvox) should limit the intake of which of the following food?
    a. Grapefruit
    b. Wheat flour
    c. Cheddar cheese
    d. Whole milk

19. Which of the following side effects is associated with the sulfonamides?
    a. Tinnitis
    b. Edema
    c. Diplopia
    d. Crystalluria

20. Which of the following statements, made by the client taking methenamine (Hiprex), indicates a need for more teaching by the nurse?
    a. "I will take the drug with food."
    b. "I will use sodium bicarbonate as my antacid."
    c. "I will eat more plums."
    d. "I will drink the usual amount of fluids and not increase them."

21. The antitubercular drugs are given in combination because they:
    a. Can act on different phases of the bacterial cell life cycle.
    b. Eradicate the mycobacterium more quickly.
    c. Are more cost-effective if given together.
    d. Cause fewer side effects.

22. Which of the following should the nurse teach the client about Rifampin (Rifadin)?
    a. Change position slowly.
    b. Report numbness or tingling in hands and feet.
    c. Do not stop and re-start taking drug.
    d. Tell physician of any eye problems.

23. All of the following are true about the topical application of acyclovir (Zovirax) EXCEPT:
    a. Keep out of the eyes.
    b. Totally cover lesions.
    c. Apply with fingers.
    d. Give 0.5 inch of ointment for every 4 square inches of skin.

24. The nurse needs to assess which of the following side effects in the client taking zidovudine (Retrovir)?
    a. Seizures
    b. Lactic acidosis
    c. Splenomegaly
    d. Hyperglycemia

25. Which one of the following oral antifungal drugs must be taken on an empty stomach?
    a. Fluconazole (Diflucan)
    b. Miconazole (Monistat)
    c. Ketoconazole (Nizoral)
    d. Clotrimazole (Lotrimin)

26. There is an increased risk of renal toxicity if amphotericin B (Fungizone) is taken with which of the following medications:
    a. Corticosteroid
    b. Digoxin (Lanoxin)
    c. Heparin
    d. Phenytoin (Dilantin)

27. A client taking metronidazole (Flagyl) should not ingest the following:
    a. Caffeine
    b. Nicotine
    c. Alcohol
    d. Dairy products

28. Chloroquine (Aralen) is contraindicated in which of the following:
    a. Liver disease
    b. Blood dyscrasias
    c. CNS diseases
    d. Retinal diseases

29. All of the following statements about mebendazole (Vermox) are true EXCEPT:
    a. Treats flukes
    b. Can cause abdominal pain and diarrhea
    c. Is contraindicated in children
    d. Can be crushed or chewed

PART I • ANSWERS

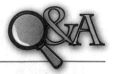

1. **The correct answer is b.** Antibiotics need to be taken around the clock at evenly spaced intervals so blood levels can be maintained. This is the only answer in which the drug would be given around the clock.

2. **The correct answer is c.** The aminoglycosides mechanism of drug action is to inhibit protein synthesis in the bacterial cell. Other anti-infectives that also act in this way are the macrolides and the tetracyclines.

3. **The correct answer is a.** Ticarcillin (Ticar) contains sodium. The client receiving high doses of this drug should be assessed for signs of sodium overload by the nurse as well as have the serum sodium level monitored.

4. **The correct answer is c.** Oral penicillins should be taken with 6 to 8 ounces of water. They should not be taken with acidic fluids as these will destroy the drugs.

5. **The correct answer is d.** All of the following happen as the cephalosporins progress from the first to the fourth generation: activity against gram-negative bacteria increases; the ability to penetrate CSF increases; cost increases; and there is greater resistance to beta-lactamases.

6. **The correct answer is b.** The nurse needs to first assess the penicillin allergy as there is cross sensitivity between the penicillins and cephalosporins. Once this has been done, the nurse should contact the physician with this information.

7. **The correct answer is a.** The aminoglycosides neomycin and kanamycin (Kantrex) are both used to cleanse the bowel before surgery.

8. **The correct answer is c.** Peak levels above 12.0 g/mL and trough levels above 2.0 g/mL are associated with toxicity of an aminoglycoside.

9. **The correct answer is d.** Tetracyclines cause photosensitivity, so the client should stay out of the sun while taking these medications. If the client has to be outside, then he or she should be instructed to use sunscreen with SPF 15 and cover any exposed skin.

10. **The correct answer is a.** Tetracyclines should not be given to pregnant women and children under the age of 8, as they can cause permanent discoloration of developing teeth. They are not used in the treatment of tuberculosis but are indicated in the treatment of acne.

11. **The correct answer is c.** Nausea, vomiting, and diarrhea are the most common adverse effects of the macrolides.

12. **The correct answer is b.** Erythromycin has a spectrum of use similar to the penicillins and is often used in clients who are allergic to penicillin.

13. **The correct answer is b.** Fluoroquinolones can interfere with the liver's metabolism of caffeine and this can cause excessive stimulation of the CNS. Thus, caffeine should be stopped when a client is taking a fluoroquinolone.

14. **The correct answer is c.** The principal organ for excretion of the fluoroquinolones is the kidney. The other statements are false.

15. **The correct answer is d.** Vancomycin (Vancocin) should be used cautiously in the elderly as this group has reduced kidney function and the drug is excreted via the kidney. The half-life can last as long as 146 hours in the elderly, and this can cause toxic effects of the drug to develop.

16. **The correct answer is b.** "Red neck" or "red man" syndrome associated with vancomycin (Vancocin) occurs with rapid intravenous administration of the drug, which causes a release of histamine.

17. **The correct answer is a.** Intravenous quinupristin/dalfopristin (Synercid) should be infused over 1 hour.

18. **The correct answer is c.** Foods containing tyramine should be avoided when the client is receiving linezolid (Zyvox). Aged cheeses, such as cheddar cheese, are high in tyramine and should not be eaten.

19. **The correct answer is d.** Crystalluria is a side effect associated with the Sulfonamides. Clients receiving these drugs should increase fluid intake to 1200 mL/day to avoid this problem. Also, these drugs should be given cautiously to clients with kidney impairment and history of kidney stones.

20. **The correct answer is b.** A client taking methenamine (Hiprex) needs to keep his/her urine acidic. Sodium bicarbonate will make the urine alkaline and should not be taken.

21. **The correct answer is a.** Antitubercular drugs are given in combination, because this allows for the drugs to work on different phases of the bacterial cell life cycle, as well as combination therapy reduces development of resistant strains of bacteria.

22. **The correct answer is c.** The client should not stop and then restart taking the drug as this can cause a flu-like syndrome to occur.

23. **The correct answer is c.** The ointment form of acyclovir (Zovirax) must be applied with a finger cot or glove to prevent transmission to other areas on the skin and to other people.

24. **The correct answer is b.** Lactic acidosis is a side effect that can occur with any nucleoside reverse transcriptase inhibitor. Symptoms include hyperventilation, nausea, vomiting, abdominal pain, anorexia, and fatigue.

25. **The correct answer is c.** Ketoconazole (Nizoral) must be taken on an empty stomach.

26. **The correct answer is a.** If amphotericin B (Fungizone) is taken with corticosteroids or nephrotoxic drugs, there is an increased risk for renal toxicity.

27. **The correct answer is c.** The ingestion of alcohol or alcohol-containing products while taking metronidazole (Flagyl) can cause a disulfiram (Antibuse) reaction.

28. **The correct answer is d.** Chloroquine (Aralen) should not be taken if the client has retinal disease or any changes in the visual field.

29. **The correct answer is a.** Mebendazole (Vermox) is used to treat whipworms, hookworms, pinworms, and roundworms.

II

Central Nervous System Drugs

Nancy Elaine Clarkson, MEd, RN, BC

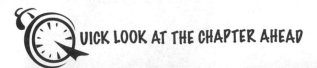

QUICK LOOK AT THE CHAPTER AHEAD

Pain is a very individual experience. It is related to actual or potential damage of tissue and includes displeasing emotions. Pain can be decreased or increased by many things. Analgesics are drugs that help to alleviate pain without loss of consciousness. Opioid analgesics were originally obtained from the opium plant. There are three groups of opioid analgesics that interact with opioid receptors to bring pain relief. The first group is the **opioid agonists**. These drugs stimulate the activity of opioid receptor sites in the body. The second group, the **opioid agonists-antagonists**, obstruct some receptor sites and stimulate others. These drugs are less addictive than the opioid agonists. The last group, the **opioid antagonists**, reverse the effects of the opioids and are given for opioid overdose. This chapter will also discuss the nonopioid analgesic, acetaminophen (Tylenol). This drug has both antipyretic and analgesic properties. It is often found in combination with opioid agonists.

16

Analgesics

TERMS
☐ morphine (Roxanol)
☐ pentazocine (Talwin)
☐ butorphanol (Stadol)
☐ naloxone (Narcan)
☐ acetaminophen (Tylenol)

Table 16-1 Analgesics

Prototype Drug	Related Drugs	Drug Classification
morphine (Roxanol)	alfentanil (Alfenta) codeine fentanyl (Duragesic) hydrocodone (Hycodan) hydromorphone (Dilaudid) levomethadyl (Orlaam) levorphanol (Levo-Dromoran) meperidine (Demerol) methadone (Dolophine) oxycodone (OxyContin) oxymorphone (Numorphan) propoxyphene (Darvon) remifentanil (Ultiva) sufentanil (Sufental)	Opioid agonists
pentazocine (Talwin) butorphanol (Stadol)	buprenorphine (Buprenex) dezocine (Dalgan) nalbuphine (Nubain)	Opioid agonists-antagonists
naloxone (Narcan)	nalmefene (Revex) naltrexone (ReVia)	Opioid antagonists
acetaminophen (Tylenol)	There are no related drugs at this time	Nonopioid analgesic

ANALGESICS CLIENT TEACHING

Opioid Agonists

Do not adjust dosage without talking to physician.

- Do not adjust dosage without talking to physician.
- Do not stop taking abruptly—taper drug with direction by physician.
- Do not breast-feed.
- No alcohol or other central nervous system (CNS) depressants while taking this drug
- No activities that require concentration

Do not stop taking abruptly—taper drug with direction by physician.

- Move slowly to sitting or standing positions to avoid or lessen hypotension.
- Cough regularly.
- No over-the-counter (OTC) drugs until consulting with physician

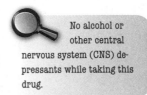

No alcohol or other central nervous system (CNS) depressants while taking this drug.

Opioid Agonists-Antagonists

- See client teaching for Opioid Agonists.

Opioid Antagonists

- After receiving drug, relate any postoperative pain to health care provider.

Nonopioid Analgesic

- Do not breast-feed.
- Take as directed and do not exceed dosing.
- Only take OTC drugs on advice of physician.
- Children can receive five doses in 24 hours. Consult physician for additional dosing.

ACTION

Opioid Agonists

- Stimulate Mu, Kappa, Epsilon, and possibly Delta receptor sites to bring about pain relief, euphoria, and sedation

Opioid Agonists-Antagonists

- Block and stimulate different opioid receptors to produce pain relief, sedation, and euphoria
- Can cause psychotic-type reactions and withdrawal in clients who have taken opioids for extended periods of time

Opioid Antagonists

- Attach to opioid receptors without stimulating them and reverse effects of opioids

Nonopioid Analgesic

- Interferes with pain impulse peripherally by inhibiting prostaglandin synthesis
- Also acts on hypothalamus to decrease body temperature

 USE

Opioid Agonists

- Relief of moderate to severe pain
- Adjunct to general anesthesia
- Relief of chronic pain
- Antitussive
- Preoperative medication
- Morphine is used to treat pain of myocardial infarction (MI) and dyspnea in pulmonary edema and acute left ventricular failure.

Opioid Agonists-Antagonists

- Pain relief during labor and delivery
- Relief of moderate to severe pain
- Adjunct to general anesthesia

Opioid Antagonists

- Narcotic overdose
- Reversal of respiratory depression from narcotics

Nonopioid Analgesic

- Fever reducer
- Relief of mild to moderate pain
- Aspirin substitute

ADVERSE EFFECTS AND SIDE EFFECTS

Opioid Agonists

- *Pregnancy category B for morphine, levorphanol (Levo-Dromoran), meperidine (Demerol), methadone (Dolophine), oxycodone (Oxy-Contin), and oxymorphone (Numorphan). The rest are category C.*
- *CNS:* Dizziness, drowsiness, insomnia, disorientation, seizures (infants and children)
- *CV:* Orthostatic hypotension, bradycardia, palpitations, cardiac arrest
- *Derm:* Pruritis, rash, urticaria, flushing of face, neck and upper thorax
- *EENT:* Visual disturbances, miosis
- *GI:* Nausea, vomiting, constipation, anorexia, dry mouth, biliary colic
- *GU:* Urinary retention or urgency, dysuria, oliguria
- *Resp:* Respiratory depression or arrest
- *Other:* Hypothermia, muscle flaccidity, cold, clammy skin sweating

Opioid Agonists-Antagonists

- *Pregnancy category C*
- *CNS:* Euphoria, dizziness, drowsiness, light-headedness, mood alterations, confusion
- *CV:* Tachycardia, palpitations, hypertension
- *Derm:* Rash, pruritis, reactions at injection site (induration, skin sloughing, nodule formation), flushing
- *EENT:* Visual problems
- *GI:* Dry mouth, nausea, vomiting, constipation, altered taste
- *GU:* Urinary retention
- *Resp:* Respiratory depression
- *Other:* Allergic reactions, shock

Opioid Antagonists

- *Pregnancy category B, although Naltrexone (ReVia) is category C*
- *CNS:* Tremors, drowsiness
- *CV:* Hypertension, tachycardia

- *Derm:* Sweating
- *GI:* Nausea, vomiting
- *Hematologic:* Elevated partial thromboplastin time (PTT)
- *Resp:* Hyperventilation
- *Other:* Reversal of analgesia

Nonopioid Analgesic

- *Pregnancy category B*
- *GI:* Hepatic necrosis

INTERACTIONS

Opioid Agonists

- Concurrent use with phenothiazines can antagonize analgesia.
- Monoamine oxidase inhibitors can cause a hypertensive crisis.
- The following potentiate CNS depressant effects: sedatives, alcohol, CNS depressants, barbiturates, tricyclic antidepressants, and benzodiazepines.
- Increased sedation with St. John's wort, kava-kava, and valerian.

Opioid Agonists-Antagonists

- CNS depressants and alcohol have additive CNS depressant effectives.
- Narcotic analgesics may initiate narcotic withdrawal.

Opioid Antagonists

- None

Nonopioid Analgesic

- Decreased absorption with concurrent use of cholestyramine (Questran)
- Excessive alcohol intake elevates risk of hepatotoxicity.

- Chronic use of the following elevates risk for chronic hepatotoxicity: rifampin (Rifadin), phenytoin (Dilantin), carbamazepine (Tegretol), and barbiturates.

 ## CONTRAINDICATIONS

Opioid Agonists

- Hypersensitivity
- Lactation
- Pregnancy
- Increased intracranial pressure
- Seizure disorder
- Respiratory depression
- Alcoholism
- Prostatic hypertrophy
- Diarrhea caused by poisoning
- Postoperative clients with biliary tract surgery and surgical anastomosis
- Pancreatitis
- Undiagnosed acute abdomen
- Acute ulcerative colitis
- Liver or kidney insufficiency
- Addison's disease
- Hypothyroidism

Opioid Agonists-Antagonists

- Increased intracranial pressure
- Head injury
- Drug abuse
- Pregnancy
- Lactation
- Cautious use in liver and kidney disease, respiratory depression, biliary surgery, clients with MI accompanied by nausea and vomiting

Opioid Antagonists

- Pregnancy
- Lactation
- Respiratory depression from non-opioid drugs
- Cautious use in infants and children, narcotic dependence, cardiac irritability

Nonopioid Analgesic

- Hypersensitivity

 # NURSING IMPLICATIONS

Opioid Agonists

- Give PO, SC, IM, IV, rectal, epidural, transdermal, transmucosa, and intrathecal.
- All are controlled substances.
- Assess vital signs before administration. Withhold drug and report to physician respirations less than 12 per minute, drastically lowered blood pressure, or pulse from baseline.
- IV push needs to be given slowly (4 to 5 minutes).

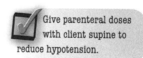
IV push needs to be given slowly (4 to 5 minutes).

- Give parenteral doses with client supine to reduce hypotension.
- Sustained release tablets must be taken whole.

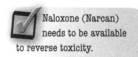
Give parenteral doses with client supine to reduce hypotension.

- Assess pain before and after administration.
- Naloxone (Narcan) needs to be available to reverse toxicity.

Naloxone (Narcan) needs to be available to reverse toxicity.

- No activities requiring concentration
- Assess for constipation and urinary retention.
- Monitor (I & O).
- Minimize miosis by keeping lights on.
- Encourage coughing.

Opioid Agonists-Antagonists

- Give PO, SC, IM, IV, and intranasal.
- Refer to nursing implications for opioid-agonists.

Opioid Antagonists

- Give SC, IM, and IV.
- IV can be given undiluted.
- Drug action lasts 40 minutes.
- Repeat dosing as necessary as some narcotic action lasts longer than naloxone.
- Assess vital signs.

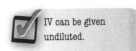

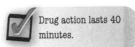

Nonopioid Analgesic

- Give PO and PR.
- Acetylcysteine (Mucomyst) is the antidote for overdose.
- High carbohydrate meals may slow absorption rate.
- Assess for liver damage.

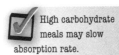

The first drugs used to treat depression were amphetamines. They activated the central nervous system and disguised the client's depressed behavior, but had the potential to be abused. Next came the first generation of antidepressants, which included the monoamine oxidase inhibitors (MAOIs), and the tricyclic antidepressants (TCAs). The second generation of antidepressants include the selective serotonin reuptake inhibitors (SSRIs) and other miscellaneous drugs. The antidepressants have a number of effects on the body besides relieving the signs of depression. They help to regulate sleep and appetite, enhance mental alertness and lessen suicidal thoughts.

17

Antidepressants

TERMS
- [ ] imipramine (Tofranil)
- [ ] phenelzine (Nardil)
- [ ] fluoxetine (Prozac)
- [ ] bupropion (Wellbutrin)

111

Table 17-1 Antidepressants

Prototype Drug	Related Drugs	Drug Classification
imipramine (Tofranil)	amitriptyline (Elavil) amoxapine (Asendin) clomipramine (Anafranil) desipramine (Norpramin) doxepin (Sinequan) maprotiline (Ludiomil) nortriptyline (Pamelor) protriptyline (Vivactil) trimipramine (Surmontil)	Tricyclic antidepressants (TCAs)
phenelzine (Nardil)	isocarboxazid (Marplan) tranylcypromine (Parnate)	Monoamine Oxidase Inhibitors (MAOIs)
fluoxetine (Prozac)	citalopram (Celexa) duloxetine (Cymbalta) escitalopram (Lexapro) fluvoxamine (Luvox) paroxetine (Paxil) sertraline (Zoloft)	Selective serotonin reuptake inhibitors (SSRIs)
bupropion (Wellbutrin)	mirtazapine (Remeron) nefazodone (Serzone) trazodone (Desyrel) venlafaxine (Effexor	Miscellaneous antidepressants

ANTIDEPRESSANTS CLIENT TEACHING

For All Antidepressants

- Drug can take up to 3 to 4 weeks to relieve depression.
- Take drug even if you feel symptom free.

TCAs

- Take drug as prescribed.
- Get up slowly when lying down and sitting up to avoid orthostatic hypotension.
- Tell physician if you develop fast heart rate, constipation, urinary retention, blurred vision, photophobia, or dry mouth.

Drug can take up to 3 to 4 weeks to relieve depression.

Get up slowly when lying down and sitting up to avoid orthostatic hypotension.

Tell physician if you develop fast heart rate, constipation, urinary retention, blurred vision, photophobia, or dry mouth.

- No activities requiring concentration until response to medication is known
- Do not breast-feed.
- No OTC drugs until discussing with physician
- Stay out of the sun.

No activities requiring concentration until response to medication is known

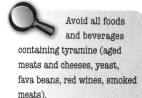

MAOIs

- Avoid all foods and beverages containing tyramine (aged meats and cheeses, yeast, fava beans, red wines, smoked meats).
- No OTC drugs until discussing with physician
- Report headache immediately.
- No caffeine
- Change positions slowly.
- Do not breast-feed.
- Weigh yourself 2 to 3 times per week.

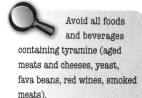
Stay out of the sun.

Avoid all foods and beverages containing tyramine (aged meats and cheeses, yeast, fava beans, red wines, smoked meats).

SSRIs

- Report skin rash.
- Do not breast-feed.
- No activities requiring concentration until drug effects are known
- Diabetics need to monitor blood glucose.

Report skin rash.

Miscellaneous Antidepressants

- Do not breast-feed.
- Drug must be taken at same time every day.
- Drug cannot be stopped abruptly.
- No activities requiring concentration until drug effects are known
- No alcohol
- Weekly weight

Drug must be taken at same time every day.

Drug cannot be stopped abruptly

ACTION

TCAs

- Prevent reuptake of the neurotransmitters serotonin (5HT) and norepinephrine (NE) and cause them to build up in the brain. It is thought that the amassing of these neurotransmitters in the brain diminishes depression.

MAOIs

- Stop the enzyme, monoamine oxidase, from dissolving the neurotransmitters of 5HT and NE in the brain.

SSRIs

- Prevent reuptake of 5HT, thus elevating its levels in the brain.

Miscellaneous Antidepressants

- Exert different effects on dopamine, 5HT and NE. The prototype, bupropion (Wellbutrin), weakly blocks reuptake of 5HT and NE.

 ## USE

TCAs

- Depression
- Sedative properties make these drugs work well in clients who have depression accompanied by insomnia and anxiety.
- Children less than 6 years of age who have enuresis
- Chronic, intractable pain
- Some are useful for obsessive-compulsive disorders (OCDs).

MAOIs

- Depression not responding to other antidepressants

SSRIs

- Depression
- Bulimia
- Panic attacks
- OCDs
- Post-traumatic stress syndrome
- Premenstrual dysphoric disorder
- Social phobias

Miscellaneous Antidepressants

- Depression
- Smoking cessation
- Anxiety disorders

ADVERSE EFFECTS AND SIDE EFFECTS

TCAs

- *All are pregnancy category C, except for maprotiline (Ludiomil), which is category B and nortriptyline (Pamelor), which is category D.*
- *CV:* Heart block, dysrhythmias, orthostatic hypotension, palpitations, tachycardia
- *CNS:* Drowsiness, sedation, extrapyramidal effects, dizziness, confusion, tremors, anxiety
- *Derm:* Rash, photosensitivity, hair loss
- *EENT:* Blurred vision, minimal mydriasis, tinnitus
- *Endocrine:* Impotence, testicular swelling, gynecomastia, galactorrhea, increased or decreased blood glucose, syndrome of inappropriate antidiuretic hormone
- *GI:* Increased appetite, dry mouth, constipation, abdominal cramps, heartburn
- *GU:* Urinary retention, nocturia
- *Hematologic:* Bone marrow depression
- *Resp:* Dyspnea
- *Other:* Hypersensitivity, increased perspiration, cold and heat tolerance changes

MAOIs

* *Pregnancy category C*
* *CNS:* Dizziness, restlessness, insomnia, headache, drowsiness, confusion, memory loss, seizures
* *CV:* Edema, palpitations, tachycardia, orthostatic hypotension, hypertensive crisis
* *Derm:* Rash, photosensitivity
* *EENT:* Blurred vision
* *Endocrine:* Impotence
* *GI:* Nausea, constipation, dry mouth, anorexia, abdominal cramps
* *Hematologic:* Leukopenia, normocytic and normochromic anemia
* *Resp:* Respiratory depression

SSRIs

* *Pregnancy category B, except for citalopram (Celexa), duloxetine (Cymbalta), escitalopram (Lexapro), and sertraline (Zoloft), which are category C.*
* *CNS:* Insomnia, nervousness, headache, anxiety, fatigue
* *CV:* Chest pain, palpitations
* *Derm:* Rash, pruritis, increased perspiration
* *EENT:* Blurred vision
* *F & E:* Hyponatremia
* *GI:* Dry mouth, constipation, diarrhea, nausea
* *GU:* Sexual dysfunction
* *Other:* Hypersensitivity

Miscellaneous Antidepressants

* *Pregnancy category C, except for bupropion (Wellbutrin), which is category B*
* *CNS:* Headache, tremors, dizziness, seizures, insomnia, agitation
* *CV:* Tachycardia
* *Derm:* Rash
* *EENT:* Blurred vision
* *GI:* Constipation, nausea, vomiting, dry mouth, weight gain, or weight loss

INTERACTIONS

TCAs

* Concurrent use with warfarin (Coumadin) increases anticoagulant effects.
* CNS depressants cause additive CNS depressant effects.
* Elevated stimulation of sympathetic nervous system if used concurrently with adrenergics
* Concurrent use with chlorpromazine (Thorazine) and anticholinergics elevates atropine-like effects.
* Concurrent use with rantidine (Zantac), fluoxetine (Prozac), and cimetidine (Tagament) elevates blood levels of TCAs.
* If given with MAOI, can cause hyperpyretic crisis leading to death.
* Concurrent use with sympathomimetics or clonidine (Catapres) elevates risk of hypertension and arrhythmias.
* St. John's wort can produce serotonin syndrome.
* Seizure threshold declines with ginkgo.

MAOIs

* Tyramine-containing foods cause hypertensive crisis.
* Concurrent use with sympathomimetics causes increased sympathomimetic effects.
* Concurrent use with oral antidiabetic agents and/or insulin causes increases hypoglycemic effects.
* Concurrent use with SSRIs can cause serotonin syndrome.
* Concurrent use with TCAs can cause seizures, coma, and hypertensive crisis.

SSRIs

* Concurrent use with MAOIs causes hypertensive crisis.
* Increases toxicity of TCAs
* Decreases carbamazepine (Tegretol) metabolism
* Increases effects of warfarin (Coumadin)
* Concurrent use with St. John's wort can cause serotonin syndrome.
* Concurrent use with alcohol increases liver function tests.

Miscellaneous Antidepressants

- Concurrent use with phenobarbitol, cimetidine (Tagamet), phenytoin (Dilantin), and carbamazepine (Tegretol) decreases their effects.
- Elevated adverse effects of MAOIs and levodopa (Dopar)

 CONTRAINDICATIONS

TCAs

- Drug allergy
- Recent myocardial infarction (MI)
- Concurrent use of MAOIs
- Pregnancy
- Lactation
- Cautious use in seizure disorder, schizophrenia, narrow-angle glaucoma, increased intraocular pressure, GI diseases, mania, client with suicide ideations

MAOIs

- Headache history
- Allergy
- Pheochromocytoma
- Cardiovascular disease
- Kidney or liver disease
- 24 hours after or 48 hours before myelography
- Cautious use in clients undergoing elective surgery, seizure disorder, hyperthyroidism, lactation, pregnancy

SSRIs

- Allergy
- Pregnancy
- Lactation
- Cautious use in diabetes, kidney, and liver disease
- MAOI therapy

Miscellaneous Antidepressants

- Recent MI
- Hypersensitivity
- Seizure disorder
- Bulimia
- Anorexia nervosa
- Concurrent administration of MAOI
- CNS tumor
- Head trauma
- Cautious use in liver and kidney disease and pregnancy

 ## NURSING IMPLICATIONS

For All Antidepressants

- Assess client's behavior, especially suicide potential.
- Check that each dose of medication is swallowed.
- Medication should continue 6 months to a year after symptoms are gone.
- Depressed clients need emotional support and other therapies.

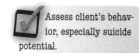 Assess client's behavior, especially suicide potential.

 Medication should continue 6 months to a year after symptoms are gone.

TCAs

- Give PO and IM.
- Perform base electrocardiogram.
- Give whole dose at HS.
- Take orthostatic blood pressure.
- Adolescents and elderly need reduced doses.
- Monitor liver and kidney studies and blood glucose.
- Weigh client.
- Report extrapyramidal symptoms.
- Assess urine and bowel function.

 Give whole dose at HS.

 Take orthostatic blood pressure.

MAOIs

- Give PO.
- Take orthostatic blood pressure.
- Assess for hypomania.
- Drug must be tapered slowly when being discontinued.
- Stop drug 10 days before elective surgery.
- Baseline liver function test and CBC
- Periodic eye exams

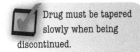

Assess for hypomania.

Drug must be tapered slowly when being discontinued.

SSRIs

- Give PO.
- Can give with food
- Administer in morning.
- Assess sodium level.
- Weigh weekly.
- Give entire daily dose by noon to prevent insomnia.
- Monitor for suicide ideation.

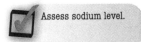

Administer in morning.

Assess sodium level.

Miscellaneous Antidepressants

- Give PO.
- Can give with food
- Assess liver and kidney function.
- Give cautiously to clients with seizure disorder and monitor for seizures.

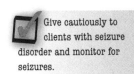

Give cautiously to clients with seizure disorder and monitor for seizures.

The antiseizure drugs are used to control seizures but not to cure the cause of the seizures.[1] These drugs come from many different chemical groups and are usually taken for very long periods of time. The first drug to treat tonic-clonic seizures effectively was phenobarbital (Luminal). Currently there are many drug choices to treat tonic-clonic seizures.

The objective of any antiseizure drug is to remove or decrease seizure activity while causing few side effects.[2] However, the drugs that are presently being used have a wide range of side effects and are not always successful in treating seizure activity. The current method of treatment is the use of one medication and there are many drugs from which to select.[2]

18
Antiseizure Drugs

TERMS
- ☐ phenytoin (Dilantin)
- ☐ phenobarbital (Luminal)
- ☐ diazepam (Valium)
- ☐ ethosuximide (Zarontin)
- ☐ carbamazepine (Tegretol)

121

Table 18-1 Antiseizure Drugs

Prototype Drug	Related Drugs	Drug Classification
phenytoin (Dilantin)	ethotoin (Peganone) fosphenytoin (Cerebyx) mephenytoin (Mesantoin)	Hydantoins
phenobarbital (Luminal)	mephobarbital (Mebaral) primidone (Mysoline)	Barbiturates and barbiturate-like drugs
diazepam (Valium)	clonazepam (Klonopin) clorazepate (Tranxene)	Benzodiazepines
ethosuximide (Zarontin)	methsuximide (Celontin) phensuximide (Milontin)	Succinimides
carbamazepine (Tegretol)	oxcarbazepine (Trileptal)	Miscellaneous anti-seizure drugs
There is no prototype for this classification	acetazolamide (Diamox) felbamate (Felbatol) gabapentin (Neurontin) lamotrigine (Lamictal) levetriacetam (Keppra) pregabalin (Lyrica) tiagabine (Gabitril) topiramate (Topamax) valporic acid (Depakene) zonisamide (Zonegran)	Adjunct antiseizure drugs

 ANTISEIZURE DRUGS CLIENT TEACHING

For All Antiseizure Drugs

* Must take drug exactly as ordered
* Record all seizure activity.
* Wear MedicAlert bracelet.
* Do not perform activities requiring concentration until drug response and seizure activity is known.
* Do not stop drug abruptly.
* Do not drink alcohol.

 Must take drug exactly as ordered.

 Record all seizure activity.

 Do not stop drug abruptly.

 Do not drink alcohol.

Hydantoins

- Take with food if have stomach upset.
- Shake oral suspension.
- Report excessive sedation.
- Report skin rash.
- Monitor gum growth, and perform good oral hygiene.
- Urine can become pink-red-brown tinged.
- Do not breast-feed.
- Flu vaccine can increase seizure activity.

Report excessive sedation.

Report skin rash.

Monitor gum growth, and perform good oral hygiene.

Urine can become pink-red-brown tinged.

Barbiturates and Barbiturate-Like Drugs

- Sedation occurs in early treatment.
- Children may become hyperactive and irritable.
- Drug can cause birth defects.
- Do not breast-feed.
- Do not get pregnant.
- Increase Vitamin D in diet.

Sedation occurs in early treatment.

Increase Vitamin D in diet.

Benzodiazepines

- Do not get pregnant.
- Tell physician of any OTC drugs before you take them.

Succinimides

- Weekly weight
- Do not breast-feed.

Miscellaneous Antiseizure Drugs

- Stay out of sun and use sunscreen.
- Do not breast-feed.
- Females may have break-through bleeding.

Stay out of sun and use sunscreen.

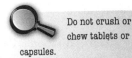

Adjunct Antiseizure Drugs

- Do not crush or chew tablets or capsules.
- Avoid pregnancy.
- Report jaundice, abdominal pain, nausea, malaise, or anorexia to physician.

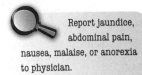

Do not crush or chew tablets or capsules.

Report jaundice, abdominal pain, nausea, malaise, or anorexia to physician.

℞ ACTION

Hydantoins

- Restrain neurons that are producing seizure activity by preventing sodium from re-entering them.

Barbiturates and Barbiturate-Like Drugs

- Attach to gamma-aminobutyric acid (GABA) receptors and suppress seizure activity.
- Also act directly to suppress the cerebellum, cortex, and reticular activating system and cause various levels of sedation all the way to coma.

Benzodiazepines

- See "Action" of barbiturates.

Succinimides

- Act directly on neurons in thalamus to suppress low-threshold calcium currents, which inhibit seizure activity.

Miscellaneous Antiseizure Drugs

- See "Action" of hydantoins.

Adjunct Antiseizure Drugs

- See action of hydantoins, barbiturates, and succinimides.

USE

Hydantoins

- All types of seizures except absence seizures. Phenytoin (Dilantin) is the drug most often prescribed for seizure activity and is also used to treat some cardiac arrhythmias.[1]

Barbiturates and Barbiturate-Like Drugs

- Tonic-clonic and partial seizures. Not used for absence seizures.
- Also used for inducing sleep and daytime sedation.

Benzodiazipines

- Diazepam (Valium) is the drug of choice for status epilepticus. It is also used to relieve anxiety in alcohol withdrawal and to relieve muscle spasms. These drugs are used in absence, atonic, and myoclonic seizures.

Succinimides

- Absence seizures

Miscellaneous Antiseizure Drugs

- Simple and complex partial seizures and tonic-clonic seizures
- Also used in trigeminal and glossopharyngeal neuralgias and bipolar disorder

Adjunct Antiseizure Drugs

- Used in combination with other antiseizure drugs to treat partial seizures, simple or complex absence seizures, and Lennox-Gastaut syndrome

ADVERSE EFFECTS AND SIDE EFFECTS

Hydantoins

- *Pregnancy category D*
- *CNS:* Ataxia, sedation, cognitive impairment
- *CV:* Hypotension, cardiac arrhythmias
- *Derm:* Rash, hirsutism
- *EENT:* Nystagmus, diplopia, photophobia
- *GI:* Gingival hyperplasia, constipation, weight loss
- *GU:* Acute renal failure
- *Hematologic:* Thrombocytopenia, leukopenia, anemia, bleeding tendencies in newborn
- *Resp:* Pulmonary fibrosis, pneumonitis
- *Other:* Rickets, osteomalacia, fetal hydantoin syndrome

Barbiturates and Barbiturate-Like Drugs

- *Pregnancy category D*
- *CNS:* Drowsiness, irritability, and hyperactivity in children; confusion and agitation in elderly
- *CV:* Hypotension, syncope, bradycardia
- *Derm:* Rash, Stevens-Johnson Syndrome
- *F & E:* Hypocalcemia
- *GI:* Diarrhea, constipation, epigastric pain, hepatic damage
- *Hematologic:* Thrombocytopenia, megaloblasic anemia, agranulocytosis, bleeding tendencies in newborns
- *Resp:* Respiratory depression
- *Other:* Physical dependence, acute intermittent porphyria, rickets, osteomalacia

Benzodiazepines

- *Pregnancy category D with the exception of clonazepam (Klonopin), which is category C*
- *CNS:* Drowsiness, confusion, ataxia, paradoxical excitement
- *CV:* Hypotension, edema, tachycardia, cardiovascular collapse
- *EENT:* Nystagmus, blurred vision, diplopia
- *GI:* Dry mouth, constipation, nausea, liver disease, hiccups

- *GU:* Urinary retention and/or incontinence
- *Resp:* Laryngospasm, coughing
- *Other:* Pain

Succinimides

- *Pregnancy category C except phensuximide (Milontin), which is category D*
- *CNS:* Dizziness, drowsiness, lethargy
- *CV:* Postural hypotension
- *Endocrine:* Hypothyroidism
- *GI:* Nausea, vomiting, diarrhea, epigastric pain, hepatitis
- *GU:* Impotence, menorrhagia

Miscellaneous Antiseizure Drugs

- *Carbamazepine (Tegretol) is pregnancy category D and oxcarbazepine (Trileptal) is category C.*
- *CNS:* Headache, ataxia, vertigo, unsteadiness
- *CV:* Heart block, edema, arrhythmias
- *Derm:* Rash, urticaria, Stevens-Johnson Syndrome, photosensitivity
- *EENT:* Nystagmus, blurred vision, diplopia, abnormal hearing
- *Endocrine:* syndrome of inappropriate antidiuretic hormone, hypothyroidism
- *GI:* Anorexia, dry mouth, diarrhea, constipation, liver disease, pancreatitis
- *GU:* Impotence, urinary retention, and/or frequency
- *Hematologic:* Anemia, leukopenia, thrombocytopenia, aplastic anemia
- *Other:* Arthralgia, myalgia

Adjunct Antiseizure Drugs

- *Pregnancy category C, except for valporic acid (Depakene), which is category D*
- *CNS:* Insomnia, headache, confusion, fatigue, weakness, drowsiness
- *GI:* Anorexia, nausea, vomiting, liver disease
- *Hematologic:* Bone marrow suppression
- *Resp:* Upper respiratory infection

INTERACTIONS

Hydantoins

- Concurrent use of the following with Hydantoins causes decreased effects of these drugs: glucocorticoids, warfarin (Coumadin), and oral contraceptives.
- The following elevate Hydantoin levels and can cause Hydantoin toxicity: valporic acid (Depakene), cimetidine (Tagamet), isoniazid (INH), diazepam (Valium), and alcohol.
- The following decrease Hydantoin levels and can cause increased risk of seizures: alcohol, phenobarbitol, and carbamazepine (Tegretol).
- There is an additive CNS depressant effect if the Hydantoins are given with these drugs: barbiturates, alcohol, any CNS depressant.
- Concurrent use with ginkgo may increase seizure activity.

Barbiturate and Barbiturate-Like Drugs

- Dose of barbiturate must be decreased if given with valproic acid (Depakene), as plasma level of barbiturate will be elevated by 40%.
- Additive CNS depressant effects if given with any known CNS depressant
- The following have decreased effects if given with barbiturates: oral contraceptives, warfarin (Coumadin).
- Concurrent use with kava-kava and valerian increases CNS depressant effects.

Benzodiazepines

- Additive CNS depressant effects if given with any known CNS depressant
- Do not combine with valproic acid (Depakene) as there is increased seizure activity.
- Concurrent use with kava-kava and valerian increases CNS depressant effects.
- Concurrent use with ginko may increase seizure activity.

Succinimides

- Concurrent use with phenobarbital can increase seizure activity.
- Concurrent use with INH increases levels of succinimides.
- Concurrent use with carbamazepine (Tegretol) decreases levels of succinimides.
- Concurrent use with ginkgo can increase seizure activity.

Miscellaneous Antiseizure Drugs

- Concurrent use with warfarin (Coumadin) and oral contraceptives decreases the effectiveness of the antiseizure drugs.
- Grapefruit juice increases levels of these drugs.
- Concurrent use with phenobarbital and phenytoin (Dilantin) decreases the effects of the antiseizure drugs.

Adjunct Antiseizure Drugs

- Concurrent use with alcohol or any CNS depressant drug causes further CNS depression.

CONTRAINDICATIONS

Hydantoins

- Hypersensitivity
- Adams-Stokes syndrome
- Pregnancy
- Lactation
- Complete/incomplete heart block
- Sinus bradycardia
- Seizure activity caused by hypoglycemia

Barbiturates and Barbiturate-Like Drugs

- Lactation
- Pregnancy

- Hypersensitivity
- Renal disease
- Respiratory disease
- Liver disease
- History of porphyria
- Uncontrolled pain

Benzodiazepines

- Pregnancy
- Lactation
- Within 14 days of monoamine oxidase inhibitor (MAOI) use
- Open or narrow-angle glaucoma
- Alcohol poisoning
- Shock
- Coma
- Decreased vital signs

Succinimides

- Lactation
- Pregnancy
- Hypersensitivity
- Hepatic disease
- Renal disease

Miscellaneous Antiseizure Drugs

- Children under 6 months
- Pregnancy
- Lactation
- Hypertension
- Cardiac disease
- Kidney disease
- Liver disease
- Increased intraocular pressure
- Systemic lupus erythematosus

Adjunct Antiseizure Drugs

- Liver disease
- Hypersensitivity
- Bone marrow suppression
- Cautious use in pregnancy, lactation, and renal disease

NURSING IMPLICATIONS

For All Antiseizure Drugs

- Noncompliance is a major problem.
- CNS depression is commonly seen at beginning of treatment.
- Drugs must be withdrawn slowly (weeks to months).

 Noncompliance is a major problem.

 Drugs must be withdrawn slowly (weeks to months).

Hydantoins

- Give PO, IM, and IV.
- Separate oral administration by 2 to 3 hours for antacids.
- Infuse IV slowly (50.0 mg/min).
- Assess IV site frequently.
- Flush IV catheter with normal saline after administration.
- Not compatible with dextrose solutions
- Therapeutic blood level is 10.0 to 20.0 mcg/mL.
- Monitor CBC, serum blood levels, glucose, magnesium, calcium, and liver function tests.
- Assess for gingival hyperplasia.
- Clients on long-term therapy need vitamin D and sun exposure.

 Separate oral administration by 2 to 3 hours for antacids.

 Not compatible with dextrose solution

 Monitor CBC, serum blood levels, glucose, magnesium, calcium, and liver function tests.

 Assess for gingival hyperplasia.

 Clients on long-term therapy need vitamin D and sun exposure.

Barbiturates and Barbiturate-Like Drugs

- Give PO, IM, and IV.
- IV infusion must be given within 30 minutes of preparation.
- Assess IV site for signs of necrosis.
- Give IM deeply in large muscle.
- Assess client for signs of sedation.
- Therapeutic blood level is 15.0 to 40.0 mcg/mL.
- If client is in pain, drug will cause restlessness.
- Observe for paradoxical reactions in children, the elderly, and debilitated clients.

 Assess IV site for signs of necrosis.

 Give IM deeply in large muscle.

 If client is in pain, drug will cause restlessness.

Benzodiazepines

- Give PO, IM, IV, and rectally.
- Sustained release form must be swallowed whole.
- Give IM in large muscle and inject slowly.
- Monitor CBC and liver function.
- Monitor I & O
- Physical dependence can occur.
- Assess client closely when drug given IV.
- Ensure client safety.

 Sustained release form must be swallowed whole.

Give IM in large muscle and inject slowly.

Succinimides

- Give PO.
- Can give with food
- Therapeutic blood level is 40.0 to 80.0 mcg/mL.
- Assess CBC, renal, and hepatic function.

 Assess CBC, renal, and hepatic function.

Miscellaneous Antiseizure Drugs

- Give PO.
- Give with food to increase absorption.

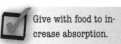 Give with food to increase absorption.

- Liquid form should not be given with other liquid drugs as precipitate can develop in stomach.
- Do not give within 14 days of MAOI.
- Assess CBC, electrolytes, liver, and kidney tests.
- Monitor I & O.
- Elderly may become confused and agitated.
- Therapeutic blood level is 4.0 to 12.0 mcg/mL.

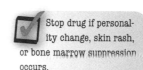

Liquid form should not be given with other liquid drugs as precipitate can develop in stomach.

Adjunct Antiseizure Drugs

- Give PO.
- Can give with food
- Assess CBC.
- Stop drug if personality change, skin rash, or bone marrow suppression occurs.
- Taper drug slowly.

Stop drug if personality change, skin rash, or bone marrow suppression occurs.

REFERENCES

1. Aschenbrenner D, Clevland L, Venable S. *Drug Therapy in Nursing.* Philadelphia, PA: Lippincott, Williams & Wilkins; 2006:278.

2. Youngkin E, Sawin K, Kissinger J, Israel D. *Pharmacotherapeutics: a Primary Care Clinical Guide.* Upper Saddle River, NJ: Pearson/Prentice Hall; 2005:629.

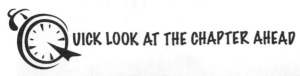

The central nervous system (CNS) stimulants are a small class of drugs that enhance the activity of the neurons in the CNS. They can cause seizure activity if given in therapeutic doses.[1] Their use is currently limited to the treatment of narcolepsy and attention deficit/hyperactivity disorder.

19

Central Nervous System Stimulants

TERM
☐ **dextroamphetamine (Dexedrine)**

Table 19-1 Central Nervous System

Prototype Drug	Related Drugs	Drug Classification
dextroamphetamine (Dexedrine)	amphetamine sulfate (Adderall) dexmethylphenidate (Focalin) methylphenidate (Ritalin, Concerta) Concerta) modafinil (Provigil) pemoline (Cylert)	Centrally acting stimulants

CENTRAL NERVOUS SYSTEM STIMULANTS CLIENT TEACHING

- Do not participate in activities requiring concentration until drug response is known.
- Do not breast-feed.
- Drug must be stopped gradually.
- For children, measure height and weight and report weight loss to physician.
- Insomnia and agitation need to be reported to physician.
- Physical and psychological dependence can develop.

 Do not participate in activities requiring concentration until drug response is known.

 Do not breast-feed.

 Drug must be stopped gradually.

 For children, measure height and weight and report weight loss to physician.

 Physical and psychological dependence can develop.

ACTION

- Excite the cortex and reticular activating system through liberating catecholamines from presynaptic neurons, which, in turn, cause an elevated stimulation of postsynaptic neurons.

USE

- Narcolepsy and attention deficit/hyperactivity disorder

ADVERSE EFFECTS AND SIDE EFFECTS

- *Pregnancy category C, except for pemoline (Cylert), which is category B*
- *CNS:* Restlessness, nervousness, headache, dizziness, insomnia
- *CV:* Tachycardia, palpitations, hypertension, angina, arrhythmias
- *Derm:* Rash
- *EENT:* Increased intraocular pressure, blurred vision, accommodation difficulties
- *GI:* Weight loss, anorexia, nausea, dry mouth, diarrhea, constipation, hepatic failure with pemoline (Cylert)
- *GU:* Impotence
- *Other:* Sweating, dystonia of extremities, head and neck

INTERACTIONS

- Concurrent use with guanethidine (Ismelin) decreases antihypertensive properties of guanethidine (Ismelin).
- Concurrent use with MAOIs can cause hypertensive crisis.
- Phenytoin (Dilantin) and tricyclic antidepressants increase effects of CNS stimulants.
- Sodium bicarbonate and acetazolamide (Dimox) slow down elimination.
- Ascorbic acid and ammonium chloride speed up elimination.
- Barbiturates and CNS stimulants antagonize each other.
- Concurrent use with furazolidone (Furoxone) increases effects of CNS stimulants on blood pressure.

CONTRAINDICATIONS

- Hypersensitivity
- Pregnancy

- Lactation
- Agitation
- Glaucoma
- Fatigue
- Heart disease
- Hypertension
- Seizure disorder

NURSING IMPLICATIONS

- Give PO.
- Sustained release tablet must be swallowed whole.
- Prevent insomnia by giving at least 6 hours before client goes to sleep.
- Monitor CBC, EKG, and weight.
- For children, stop or reduce drug dose to assess behavior and need to continue drug therapy.
- Assess blood pressure.

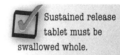

Sustained release tablet must be swallowed whole.

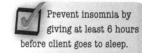

Prevent insomnia by giving at least 6 hours before client goes to sleep.

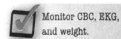

Monitor CBC, EKG, and weight.

REFERENCE

1. Lehne R. *Pharmacology for Nursing Care.* Philadelphia, PA: WB Saunders; 2007:387.

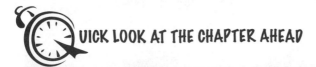

Anesthetics are a group of drugs that result in differing amounts of loss of sensation in the body. They are organized into two groups: general anesthetics and local anesthetics. The first general anesthetic, nitrous oxide (laughing gas), is still in use today. General anesthetics are able to produce amnesia, analgesia, and unconsciousness by creating widespread depression in the CNS.[1] The general anesthetics are given parenterally or by inhalation.

Local anesthetics are able to block sensation in a specific area of the body. Lidocaine (Xylocaine), is currently the most widely used local anesthetic. These drugs are potent nerve blockers and could cause toxicity problems if they were absorbed systemically. There are five types of local anesthetics: **topical, infiltration, nerve block, epidural,** and **spinal.**

20
Anesthetics

TERMS
☐ **thiopental (Pentothal)**
☐ **halothane (Fluothane)**
☐ **lidocaine (Xylocaine)**

Table 20-1 Anesthetics

Prototype Drug	Related Drugs	Drug Classification
thiopental (Pentothal)	droperidol (Inaspine) etomidate (Amidate) ketamine (Ketalar) methohexital (Brevital) midazolam (Versed) propofol (Diprivan)	Parenteral general anesthetics
halothane (Fluothane)	enflurane (Ethrane) isoflurane (Forane) nitrous oxide	Inhalation general anesthetics
lidocaine (Xylocaine)	benzocaine (Dermoplast) bupivacaine (Marcaine) chloroprocaine (Nesacaine) dibucaine (Nupercainal) levobupivacaine (Chirocaine) pramoxine (Prax) procaine (Novocaine) ropivacaine (Naropin)	Local anesthetics

ANESTHETICS CLIENT TEACHING

General Anesthetics

- The nurse should perform standard preoperative teaching, alleviate anxiety, and answer client's questions.
- Consciousness is lost quickly.

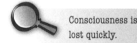
Consciousness is lost quickly.

Local Anesthetics

- The nurse performs standard preoperative teaching, alleviates anxiety, and answers client's questions.
- Report confusion, pain in injection site, faintness, and/or heart palpitations.
- As drug takes effect, the senses will be lost in the following order: temperature, pain, touch, position sense, and muscle tone. As drug wears off, senses return in reverse order.
- As drug wears off, pain will be felt.

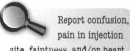
Report confusion, pain in injection site, faintness, and/or heart palpitations.

ACTION

General Anesthetics

- The exact action is not known. These agents are able to reduce the activity of the cerebral cortex and the reticular activating system.

Local Anesthetics

- Interfere with the initiation and conduction of impulses in nerve fibers by preventing the movement of calcium, potassium, and sodium through the fibers

 ## USE

General Anesthetics

- Given so that surgical procedures can be performed

Local Anesthetics

- Given so diagnostic, dental, and surgical procedures can be performed
- Also used to treat pain. Lidocaine (Xylocaine) is used to treat ventricular arrhythmias.

 ## ADVERSE EFFECTS AND SIDE EFFECTS

General Anesthetics

- *Pregnancy category C, except propofol (Diprivan), enflurane (Ethrane), and metholhexital (Brevital), which are category B, and midazolam (Versed), which is category D*
- *CNS:* Headache, extended somnolence, delirium
- *CV:* Hypotension, arrhythmias, shock, decreased cardiac output
- *F & E:* Acidosis

- *GI:* Hiccups, nausea, vomiting
- *GU:* Kidney damage
- *Resp:* Bronchospasm, laryngospasm, apnea, cough
- *Other:* Malignant hyperthermia

Local Anesthetics

- *Pregnancy category C, except for levobupivacaine (Chirocaine), lidocaine (Xylocaine), and ropivacaine (Naropin), which are category B*
- *CNS:* Tremors, dizziness, headache, restlessness, anxiety
- *CV:* Arrhythmias, hyper or hypotension, peripheral vasodilation, cardiac arrest
- *EENT:* Blurred vision
- *GI:* Nausea, vomiting
- *Resp:* Respiratory arrest

INTERACTIONS

General Anesthetics

- Concurrent use of midazolam (Versed) with thiopental (Pentothal), propofol (Diprivan), narcotics, inhaled anesthetics, or CNS depressants causes elevated toxicity of midazolam (Versed).
- Concurrent use with phenothiazines causes hypotension.
- Use with probenecid (Benemid) extends anesthesia effects.
- Valerian and kava-kava extend sedation.

Local Anesthetics

- Use with succinylcholine (Anectine) extends neuromuscular blockade.
- Concurrent use with quinidine, beta blockers, and cimetadine (Tagament) extends effects.
- Concurrent use with barbiturates decreases effects.
- Concurrent use with antihypertensives and MAOIs causes low blood pressure.

℞ CONTRAINDICATIONS

General Anesthetics

- Hypersensitivity
- Nonexistence of adequate veins
- Status asthmaticus
- Pregnancy
- Lactation
- Cautious use in cardiac disease, shock, hypotension, increased intracranial pressure, myasthenia gravis

Local Anesthetics

- Hypersensitivity
- Shock
- Heart block
- Pregnancy
- Lactation
- Cautious use in CHF, respiratory depression, renal and kidney disease, shock, elderly, and familial history of malignant hyperthermia

℞ NURSING IMPLICATIONS

General Anesthetics

- Give IV and by inhalation.
- IV solutions must be prepared just before administration and given immediately.
- Assess vital signs before, during, and after administration.
- Provide emotional support preoperatively.
- Administer preoperative medications on time.
- Monitor for nausea and vomiting, and institute appropriate measures to prevent aspiration.

 Give IV and by inhalation.

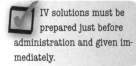 IV solutions must be prepared just before administration and given immediately.

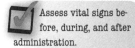 Assess vital signs before, during, and after administration.

- Assess postoperative pain and administer analgesics.
- Assess skin.

Local Anesthetics

- Give topically and IV.
- Topical preparation must be kept out of eyes.
- No topical administration to injured skin
- Lidocaine (Xylocaine) solution containing preservatives cannot be given for spinal or epidural block.
- Assess vital signs before, during, and after administration.
- Emergency equipment must be available during administration.
- Assess skin.

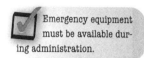

Emergency equipment must be available during administration.

REFERENCE

1. Karch A. *Focus on Nursing Pharmacology.* Philadelphia, PA: Lippincott, Williams & Wilkins; 2008:434.

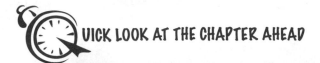

QUICK LOOK AT THE CHAPTER AHEAD

The anxiolytics and sedative-hypnotics are drugs that have depressant effects on the central nervous system (CNS). They currently rank among the most prescribed drugs in the world.[1] The hypnotics cause sleep to occur, while the anxiolytics and sedatives induce relaxation. The effects of these drugs are controlled by their dosages. Small doses of hypnotics can cause sedation, while high doses of the anxiolytics and sedatives can cause sleep. The barbiturates were previously used as anxiolytics, sedatives, and hypnotics but have been mostly replaced by the benzodiazepines, which are considered to be safer.[1] Both groups of drugs have been discussed previously in Chapter 18, and the reader should refer to that chapter for information on them. A third group of miscellaneous drugs that also effect sleep, sedation, and anxiety will be mentioned.

21

Anxiolytics and Sedative-Hypnotics

TERMS
☐ **phenobarbital (Luminal)**
☐ **diazepam (Valium)**

Table 21-1 Anxiolytics and Sedative-Hypnotics

Prototype Drug	Related Drugs	Drug Classification
phenobarbital (Luminal)	amobarbital (Amytal Sodium) butabarbital (Butisol) mephobarbital (Mebaral) pentobarbital (Nembutal) secobarbital (Seconal)	Barbiturates
diazepam (Valium)	alprazolam (Xanax) chlordiazepoxide (Librium) clonazepam (Klonopin) clorazepate (Tranxene) estazolam (ProSom) flurazepam (Dalmane) halazepam (Paxipam) lorazepam (Ativan) oxazepam (Serax) quazepam (Doral) temazepam (Restoril) triazolam (Halcion)	Benzodiazepines
There is no prototype for this classification	buspirone (BuSpar) chloral hydrate (Aquachloral) dexmedetomidine (Precedex) eszopiclone (Lunesta) ethchlorvynol (Placidyl) glutethimide (Doriglute) paraldehyde (Paral) ramelteon (Rozerem) zaleplon (Sonata) zolpidem (Ambien)	Miscellaneous drugs

ANXIOLYTICS AND SEDATIVE-HYPNOTICS CLIENT TEACHING

Barbiturates

• See client teaching on page 129 in Chapter 18.

Benzodiazepines

- See client teaching on page 129 in Chapter 18.

For All Miscellaneous Drugs

Do not abruptly stop drug.

- Do not breast-feed.
- Do not abruptly stop drug.
- No alcohol while taking drug
- Do not perform activities that require concentration until drug effects are known.
- Report any unusual effects to physician.
- Take exactly as directed.

No alcohol while taking drug

Do not perform activities that require concentration until drug effects are known.

 ACTION

Barbiturates

- See "Action" on page 130 in Chapter 18.

Benzodiazepines

- See "Action" on page 130 in Chapter 18.

Miscellaneous Drugs

Buspirone (BuSpar)

- Action is unknown.

Chloral hydrate (Aquachloral)

- Action is unknown.

Ethchlorvynol (Placidyl)

- Action is unknown.

Glutethimide (Doriglute)

- Same action as Barbiturates. See "Action" on page 130.

Paraldehyde (Paral)

+ Same action as Barbiturates. See "Action" on page 130.

Zaleplon (Sonata)

+ Same action as Benzodiazepines. See "Action" on page 130.

Zolpidem (Ambien)

+ Same action as Benzodiazepines. See "Action" on page 130.

USE

Barbiturates

+ See "Use" on page 131.

Benzodiazepines

+ See "Use" on page 131.

Miscellaneous Drugs

Buspirone (BuSpar)

+ Anxiety

Chloral hydrate (Aquachloral)

+ Preoperative sedation and sleep

Dexmedetomidine (Precedex)

+ Sedation in mechanically ventilated and newly intubated patients

Eszopiclone (Lunesta)

+ Insomnia

Ethchlorvynol (Placidyl)

+ To treat short intervals (no longer than a week) of insomnia

Glutethimide (Doriglute)

+ Preoperative sedation, during first stage of labor and for short intervals of insomnia

Paraldehyde (Paral)

- Sedation in delirium tremens and seizures from drug intoxication, tetanus, status epilepticus, and eclampsia

Ramelteon (Rozerem)

- Insomnia in patients who have difficulty falling asleep

Zaleplon (Sonata)

- Brief interval of insomnia

Zolpidem (Ambien)

- Brief interval of insomnia

ADVERSE EFFECTS AND SIDE EFFECTS

Barbiturates

- *Pregnancy category D, except for butabarbital (Butisol), which is category C*
- See "Adverse Effects and Side Effects" on pages 132–133.

Benzodiazepines

- *Pregnancy category D, except for clonazepam (Klonopin) and ox- azepam (Serax), which are category C; and estazolam (Prosom), flurazepam (Dalmane), quazepam (Doral), temazepam (Restoril), and triazolam (Halcion), which are category X*
- See "Adverse Effects and Side Effects" on page 133.

Miscellaneous Drugs

- *Pregnancy category C, except for buspirone (BuSpar) and zolpidem (Ambien), which are category B*

Buspirone (BuSpar)

- *CNS:* Headache, dizziness, drowsiness
- *GI:* Nausea

Chloral Hydrate (Aquachloral)

- *GI:* Diarrhea, nausea, vomiting

Dexmedetomidine (Precedex)

- *CV:* Hypotension
- *GI:* Nausea

Eszopiclone (Lunesta)

- *CNS:* Headache, sleepiness
- *CV:* Tachycardia
- *Other:* Unpleasant taste

Ethchlorvynol (Placidyl)

- *CNS:* Facial numbness, dizziness, headache, tremors
- *Derm:* Itchy rash
- *EENT:* Blurred vision
- *GI:* Aftertaste

Glutethimide (Doriglute)

- *CNS:* Vertigo, headache, agitation
- *EENT:* Blurred vision
- *GI:* Dry mouth, hiccups, "hangover"
- *Hematologic:* Blood disorders
- *Other:* Allergic reaction

Paraldehyde (Paral)

- *Derm:* Rash
- *GI:* Irritated oral and rectal mucous membranes

Ramelteon (Rozerem)

- *CNS:* Headache, dizziness
- *GI:* Nausea, diarrhea

Zaleplon (Sonata)

- *CNS:* Headache

Zolpidem (Ambien)

- *CNS:* Dizziness, headache, lethargy, anxiety; elderly can experience falls and confusion

- *EENT:* Diplopia
- *GI:* Stomach upset
- *Other:* Muscle ache

 ## INTERACTIONS

Barbiturates

- See "Interactions" on page 135.

Benzodiazepines

- See "Interactions" on page 135.

Miscellaneous Drugs

Buspirone (BuSpar)

- Elevates haloperidol (Haldol) levels with concurrent administration
- Use with trazodone (Desyrel) and MAOIs increases blood pressure and liver enzymes.
- The following will elevate levels of drug: grapefruit juice, ketoconazole (Nizoral), and erythromycin.
- Use with digoxin (Lanoxin) can elevate levels of digoxin.

Chloral Hydrate (Aquachloral)

- Additive CNS depression with other CNS depressants
- Concurrent use with warfarin (Coumadin) elevates anticoagulant effect.
- Alcohol can cause increased heart rate.

Dexmedetomidine (Precedex)

- Numerous interactions. Consult with physician before taking any other drug.

Eszopiclone (Lunesta)

- Numerous interactions. Consult with physician before taking any other drug.

Ethchlorvynol (Placidyl)

- Additive CNS depression with other CNS depressants
- Concurrent use with warfarin (Coumadin) decreases anticoagulant effect.

Glutethimide (Doriglute)

- Additive CNS depression with other CNS depressants
- Concurrent use with warfarin (Coumadin) decreases anticoagulant effect.
- Additional anticholinergic effects with tricyclic antidepressants

Paraldehyde (Paral)

- Additive CNS depression with other CNS depressants

Ramelteon (Rozerem)

- Grapefruit increases ramelteon (Rozerem) level.
- Rifampin (Rifadin) decreases ramelteon (Rozerem) level.

Zaleplon (Sonata)

- Additive CNS depressant effects with CNS depressants, melatonin, valerian
- Elevated blood levels of zaleplon with cimetadine (Tagmet)
- Elevated metabolism of zaleplon with rifampin (Rifadin)

Zolpidem (Ambien)

- Additive CNS depression with CNS depressants.

CONTRAINDICATIONS

Barbiturates

- See Contraindications on pages 136–137.

Benzodiazepines

- See Contraindications on page 137.

Miscellaneous Drugs

Buspirone (BuSpar)

* Pregnancy
* Lactation
* Use with alcohol
* Cautious use in liver and kidney disease

Chloral Hydrate (Aquachloral)

* Pregnancy
* Lactation
* Heart, kidney, or liver disease
* Hypersensitivity
* Oral route in clients with ulcer; known irritation of stomach or esophagus

Dexmedetomidine (Precedex)

* Labor and delivery
* Hypersensitivity

Eszopiclone (Lunesta)

* Alcohol
* Hypersensitivity
* Children less than 18 years of age

Ethchlorvynol (Placidyl)

* Pregnancy
* Lactation
* Children
* Severe pain
* Porphyria

Glutethimide (Doriglute)

* Pregnancy
* Lactation
* Children under 12 years of age
* Severe pain
* Kidney and liver disease

Paraldehyde (Paral)

- Pregnancy
- Lactation
- Respiratory and liver disease
- Ulcers or inflammation of GI tract
- Use with disulfiram

Ramelteon (Rozerem)

- Lactation
- Alcohol
- CNS depressants
- Hypersensitivity
- Liver disorders

Zaleplon (Sonata)

- Allergy to this drug
- Zolpidem (Ambien)
- Lactation

NURSING IMPLICATIONS

Barbiturates

- See "Nursing Implications" on pages 138–139.

Benzodiazepines

- See "Nursing Implications" on page 139.

Miscellaneous Drugs

Buspirone (BuSpar)

- Give PO.
- Effects on anxiety take at least a week or longer to be established.
- Assess apical pulse, blood pressure, dizziness, and nausea.

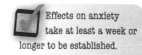
Effects on anxiety take at least a week or longer to be established.

Chloral hydrate (Aquacloral)

- Give PO and PR.
- Mix liquid form with fruit juice, water, or ginger ale.
- Suppository can be given with water-based lubricant
- Abruptly stopping drug can cause seizures and delirium.
- Allergic reactions can be seen 10 days after drug is started.
- Physical dependence can develop.

 Mix liquid form with fruit juice, water, or ginger ale.

 Suppository can be given with water-based lubricant

 Abruptly stopping drug can cause seizures and delirium.

 Allergic reactions can be seen 10 days after drug is started.

Dexmedetomidine (Precedex)

- Give IV.
- Assess cardiovascular status continuously.
- Use pump for administration.
- Assess for hypertension while loading dose is administered.

Eszopiclone (Lunesta)

- Give PO.
- Take just before bedtime.
- Client must be able to have 8 hours of sleep.
- Client needs assistance with ambulation after taking drug.
- Assess insomnia.

 Take just before bedtime.

 Client needs assistance with ambulation after taking drug.

Ethchlorvynol (Placidyl)

- Give PO.
- Milk or food slows absorption.
- Cannot be stopped quickly.
- Elderly may need reduced dose.
- Assess for hallucinations and confusion, as these signal a need for smaller dose or eliminating drug.

 Milk or food slows absorption.

 Elderly may need reduced dose.

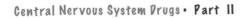 Assess for hallucinations and confusion, as these signal a need for smaller dose or eliminating drug.

Glutethimide (Doriglute)

- Give PO.
- Cannot be stopped quickly
- Client must get at least 4 hours of nighttime sleep to prevent daytime drowsiness.

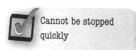

Cannot be stopped quickly

Paraldehyde (Paral)

- Give PO and PR.
- Has unpleasant taste and odor
- Mix with juice or milk to disguise taste and odor.
- If drug smells like vinegar, it must be thrown out.
- Do not use if open for more than 24 hours.
- Use glass or rubber to prepare drug as plastic will cause drug to convert into a toxic substance.
- Client's breath will have odor.

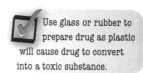

Has unpleasant taste and odor

Use glass or rubber to prepare drug as plastic will cause drug to convert into a toxic substance.

Ramelteon (Rozerem)

- Give PO.
- Do not administer after a high-fat meal.
- Administer within 30 minutes of bedtime.
- Assess insomnia.

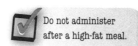

Do not administer after a high-fat meal.

Zaleplon (Sonata)

- Give PO.
- Absorption slowed by big or high-fat meal
- Can be taken within 4 hours of arising as no residual effects are seen.

Absorption slowed by big or high-fat meal

Zolpidem (Ambien)

- Give PO.
- Assess for depression and respiratory function.

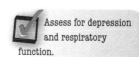

Assess for depression and respiratory function.

- Elderly will need lower dose.
- Food slows absorption.

REFERENCE

1. Aschenbrenner S, Cleveland L, Venable S. *Drug Therapy in Nursing*. Philadelphia, PA: Lippincott, Williams & Wilkins; 2006:229.

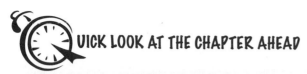

The antipsychotic drugs are used to treat diseases that interfere with thought processes. They are also called neuroleptic agents due to their neurological side effects and at one time were referred to as major tranquilizers. This group of drugs is divided into two other categories: the **typical and atypical antipsychotics**. The typical antipsychotics have been used for the past 50 years and were considered to be the principal drug treatment for schizophrenia. The atypical antipsychotics are newer drugs and have a low incidence of extrapyramidal effects when compared to the older drugs. A third drug that will be discussed in this chapter is lithium (Eskalith), which is a mood stabilizer, and is used to treat the mood swings in bipolar disorder.

22

Antipsychotics

TERMS
- [ ] **chlorpromazine (Thorazine)**
- [ ] **clozapine (Clozaril)**
- [ ] **lithium (Eskalith)**

Table 22-1 Antipsychotics

Prototype Drug	Related Drugs	Drug Classification
chlorpromazine (Thorazine)	fluphenazine (Prolixin) haloperidol (Haldol) loxapine (Loxitane) mesoridazine (Serentil) molindone (Moban) perphenazine (Trilafon) pimozide (Orap) prochlorperazine (Compazine) thioridazine (Mellaril) thiothixene (Navane) trifluoperazine (Stelazine) triflupromazine (Vesprin)	Typical antipsychotics
clozapine (Clozaril)	olanzapine (Zyprexa) quetiapine (Seroquel) risperidone (Risperdal) ziprasidone (Geodan)	Atypical antipsychotics
lithium (Eskalith)		Mood stabilizer

℞ ANTIPSYCHOTICS CLIENT TEACHING

Typical Antipsychotics

- Do not get liquid drug on your skin. If that happens, flush skin with lots of water.
- Take drug exactly as ordered.
- Report symptoms of tremors, restlessness, or facial muscle spasms to physician.
- Move slowly after taking drug to avoid orthostatic hypotension.
- No activities requiring concentration until drug reaction is known
- Report sexual problems to physician.
- Stay out of sun and use sunscreen if you have to be outdoors.

Do not get liquid drug on your skin. If that happens, flush skin with lots of water.

Report symptoms of tremors, restlessness, or facial muscle spasms to physician.

Move slowly after taking drug to avoid orthostatic hypotension.

- Report fever or sore throat to physician.
- No OTC drugs until checking with physician
- Do not drink alcohol.
- Urine may discolor to pink to reddish-brown.
- Do not stop taking drug until speaking with physician.

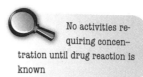

No activities requiring concentration until drug reaction is known

Do not drink alcohol.

Urine may discolor to pink to reddish-brown.

Atypical Antipsychotics

- Must have weekly blood work done to check WBC.
- Report fever or sore throat to physician.
- No activities requiring concentration until reaction to drug is known
- Move slowly after receiving drug to avoid orthostatic hypotension.
- No OTC drugs until checking with physician
- Do not breast-feed.
- Drug should be taken as ordered.

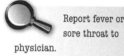

Report fever or sore throat to physician.

Mood Stabilizer

- No activities requiring concentration until reaction to drug is known
- Do not decrease or increase salt intake.
- Increase fluids to 2 to 3 L/day when beginning therapy and 1 L/day when therapy is continuing.
- Do not get pregnant.
- Do not breast-feed.
- Report fever or diarrhea to physician.
- Do not take any foods, liquids, or drugs that are high or low in sodium.

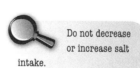

Do not decrease or increase salt intake.

Increase fluids to 2 to 3 L/day when beginning therapy and 1 L/day when therapy is continuing.

ACTION

Typical Antipsychotics

- Block a number of receptors for norepinephrine, histamine, acetylcholine, and dopamine inside and outside the CNS. It is believed that the therapeutic actions are caused by the blocking of the dopamine receptor sites.

Atypical Antipsychotics

- Block serotonin and dopamine receptor sites in the CNS

Mood Stabilizer

- Mechanism for altering the manic state is not understood, but drug does two things in the body: changes the movement of sodium in and out of muscle and nerve cells, and interferes with liberation of dopamine and norepinephrine from the neurons and increases their levels.

 ## USE

Typical Antipsychotics

- Schizophrenia and other psychotic disorders
- Attention deficit disorder in children
- Preoperative medication for agitation and anxiety
- Intractable hiccups
- Tetanus

Atypical Antipsychotics

- Schizophrenia

Mood Stabilizer

- Manic phase of bipolar disorder

ADVERSE EFFECTS AND SIDE EFFECTS

Typical Antipsychotics

- *Pregnancy category C*
- *CNS:* Extrapyramidal effects (tardive dyskinesia; dystonia; pseudoparkinsonism; akathisia), neuroleptic malignant syndrome, drowsiness, sedation, tremor, weakness, lightheadedness
- *CV:* Pulmonary edema, orthostatic hypotension, syncope, congestive heart failure, cardiac arrhythmias
- *Derm:* Rash, pruritis, photosensitivity
- *EENT:* Blurred vision, glaucoma, photophobia
- *Endocrine:* Irregular menses, galactorrhea, decreased libido, damaged temperature regulation
- *GI:* Constipation, dry mouth, liver disease, paralytic ileus
- *GU:* Urinary retention and hesitancy, priapism, impaired ejaculation
- *Hematologic:* Agranulocytosis, leukopenia
- *Resp:* Bronchospasm, dyspnea, laryngospasm
- *Other:* Pink to reddish-brown tinge to urine, weight gain

Atypical Antipsychotics

- *Pregnancy category C, except for clozapine (Clozaril), which is category B*
- *CNS:* Sedation, seizures, headache, insomnia
- *CV:* Tachycardia, EKG changes, orthostatic hypotension
- *GI:* Constipation, dry mouth, nausea
- *GU:* Urinary retention
- *Hematologic:* Agranulocytosis

Mood Stabilizer

- *Pregnancy category D*
- *CNS:* Fatigue, lethargy, headache, memory loss of recent events
- *CV:* EKG changes, hypotension, cardiac arrhythmias, edema
- *Derm:* Rash, pruritis, alopecia
- *Endocrine:* Diabetes insipidus, hyponatremia, hypothyroidism
- *EENT:* Tinnitus, blurred vision

- *GI:* Dry mouth, metal taste, anorexia, nausea, vomiting, abdominal pain
- *GU:* Incontinence of urine, oliguria, polyuria, elevated excretion of uric acid, albuminuria
- *Hematologic:* Leukocytosis
- *Other:* Weight gain

 ## INTERACTIONS

Typical Antipsychotics

- Additive CNS depressant effects if taken with alcohol or other known CNS depressant drug
- Concurrent use with the following increase effects of typical antipsychotics: lithium (Eskalith), meperidine (Demerol), haloperidol (Haldol), pimozide (Orap), propanol (Inderal), and barbiturates.
- Decreases action of antiseizure drugs.
- Concurrent use with TCAs causes low blood pressure and increases anticholinergic effects.
- Concurrent use with antidiarrheals and antacids slows absorption of atypical antipsychotics.
- Concurrent use with kava-kava elevates possibility of dystonia.

Atypical Antipsychotics

- Additive CNS depressant effects if taken with known CNS depressants
- Elevated levels of digoxin (Lanoxin) and warfarin (Coumadin) if taken with atypical antipsychotics
- Increased hypotension if taken with antihypertensives
- Increased anticholinergic effects if taken with anticholinergics

Mood Stabilizer

- Caffeine decreases lithium (Eskalith) levels.
- Nonsteroidal anti-inflammatory drugs (NSAIDs) increase lithium (Eskalith) levels.
- Elevated action of TCAs if given with them

- Concurrent use with haloperidol (Haldol), carbamazepine (Tegretol), and phenothiazines cause extrapyramidal effects and tardive dyskinesia.
- Concurrent use with methyloda (Aldomet) causes lithium (Eskalith) toxicity.

 ## CONTRAINDICATIONS

Typical Antipsychotics

- Hypersensitivity
- Parkinson's disease
- Coma
- Bone marrow depression
- Alcohol withdrawal
- Lactation
- Pregnancy
- Reye's syndrome
- Children under 6 months of age

Atypical Antipsychotics

- Lactation
- Pregnancy
- In client taking any bone marrow suppression drug or benzodiazepine
- Cautious use with antihypertensives, anticholinergics, or drugs affecting the CNS

Mood Stabilizer

- Lactation
- Pregnancy
- Clients receiving diuretics
- Clients with dehydration or low sodium
- Brain damage
- Kidney or heart disease
- Children under 12 years of age

NURSING IMPLICATIONS

Typical Antipsychotics

- Give PO, PR, IM, and IV.
- Routine oral dosing done at bedtime
- Liquid form can be mixed in fruit juice.
- Contact dermatitis caused by liquid form
- Sustained-release capsule must be swallowed whole.
- Client should lie down for 30 minutes after parenteral dose to prevent orthostatic hypotension.
- Assess CBC.
- Cannot be stopped abruptly
- Assess for signs of extrapyramidal effects and tardive dyskinesia and report promptly.
- Monitor for seizures.
- Monitor for anticholinergic effects and assist client in dealing with them. For example, offer ice chips, hard candy, and mouth care for dry mouth; encourage voiding for urinary retention.
- Sedative effects seen in early treatment
- Client and family need to be educated about psychotic disease.
- Compliance with drug can be a problem.

Routine oral dosing done at bedtime

Sustained-release capsule must be swallowed whole.

Client should lie down for 30 minutes after parenteral dose to prevent orthostatic hypotension.

Assess for signs of extrapyramidal effects and tardive dyskinesia and report promptly.

Compliance with drug can be a problem.

Atypical Antipsychotics

- Give PO.
- Do not stop abruptly.
- Monitor WBC.
- Assess for seizures, low blood pressure, rapid heart rate.

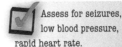
Assess for seizures, low blood pressure, rapid heart rate.

- Monitor temperature daily as elevation can occur during initial weeks of receiving drug.

Mood Stabilizer

- Give PO.
- Give with food.
- May take up to 2 weeks to see results of drug

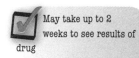

May take up to 2 weeks to see results of drug

- Monitor drug level.
- Assess for symptoms of toxicity as toxic levels are close to therapeutic levels.

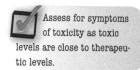

Assess for symptoms of toxicity as toxic levels are close to therapeutic levels.

- Assess weight daily.
- All symptoms of side effects must be reported to physician immediately.
- Assess thyroid tests.

QUICK LOOK AT THE CHAPTER AHEAD

An English doctor named James Parkinson was the first person to relate the symptoms of Parkinson's disease in 1817. This disease was at first called, "shaking palsy," and it took until 1960 before the reason for the signs and symptoms could be explained.[1] Parkinson's disease is a progressive, chronic, neurologic illness that affects the neurons in the substantia nigra area of the brain where dopamine is produced. This in turn causes an imbalance of the neurotransmitters, dopamine, and acetylcholine. The four classic symptoms of the disease are tremor, rigidity, bradykinesia (slow movement), and postural instability.[2] The main treatment for Parkinson's disease at this time is drug therapy. There currently is no cure for this disease.

There is a combination drug called Stalevo currently available. It is composed of carbidopa, levodopa, and entacapone, and is given in tablet form.[3]

23

Anti-Parkinson's Disease Drugs

TERMS
☐ biperiden (Akineton)
☐ levodopa (Dopar)
☐ tolcapone (Tasmar)

Table 23-1 Anti-Parkinson's Disease Drugs

Prototype Drug	Related Drugs	Drug Classification
biperiden (Akineton)	benztropine (Cogentin) diphenhydramine (Benadryl) procyclidine (Kemadrin) trihexyphenidyl (Artane)	Anticholinergics
levodopa (Dopar)	amantadine (Symmetrel) bromocriptine (Parlodel) carbidopa-levodopa (Sinemet) pergolide (Permax) pramipexole (Mirapex) ropinirole (Requip) selegiline (Eldepryl	Dopaminergics
tolcapone (Tasmar)	entacapone (Comtan)	Catechol-o-methyl transferase (COMT) inhibitor

ANTI-PARKINSON'S DRUGS CLIENT TEACHING

Anticholinergics

- Do not breast-feed.
- Suck on hard candy and perform frequent mouth care if you experience dry mouth.
- No activities requiring concentration until effects of drug are known
- Drug dose may be increased as you develop tolerance to the drug over time.
- Urinate before taking the drug if urinary retention is a problem.

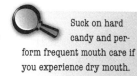

Suck on hard candy and perform frequent mouth care if you experience dry mouth.

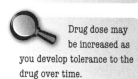

Drug dose may be increased as you develop tolerance to the drug over time.

COMT Inhibitors

- No hazardous activities until drug response is known
- No alcohol or sedative drugs
- Change positions slowly.
- Drug must not be stopped abruptly.

- Do not breast-feed.
- Notify physician of: fainting, hallucinations, severe diarrhea, increased loss of muscle control, or yellow eyes or skin.

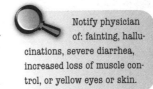

Notify physician of: fainting, hallucinations, severe diarrhea, increased loss of muscle control, or yellow eyes or skin.

Dopaminergics

- Do not breast-feed.
- Drug benefits may not be seen for weeks or months.
- Avoid foods high in protein and pyridoxine (Vitamin B_6).
- Check with physician before taking any OTC drugs.
- Urine and perspiration may turn dark in color.
- Drug must not be stopped abruptly.
- Change positions slowly.

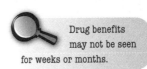

Drug benefits may not be seen for weeks or months.

Avoid foods high in protein and pyridoxine (Vitamin B_6).

ACTION

Anticholinergics

- Inhibit the action of acetylcholine in the CNS, which assists in keeping the ratio of acetylcholine to dopamine in proportion

Dopaminergics

- Elevate the level of dopamine in the substantia nigra, as well as excite the dopamine receptors located there

COMT INHIBITORS

- Inhibits enzyme COMT, which metabolizes levodopa. This leads to increased stimulation of dopamine in the brain.

USE

Anticholinergics

- Given to treat all types of Parkinson's disease in clients with minor symptoms who are unable to take dopaminergics or given with other anti-Parkinson's drugs
- Also, given to clients experiencing symptoms of Parkinson's disease from the use of antipsychotic drugs

Dopaminergics

- Given to treat idiopathic Parkinson's disease in clients with working dopamine receptors

COMT Inhibitors

- Adjunct to levodopa/carbidopa

 ## ADVERSE EFFECTS AND SIDE EFFECTS

Anticholinergics

- *Pregnancy category C*
- *CNS:* Muscle weakness, dizziness, drowsiness, agitation, hallucinations, delusions, confusion, depression
- *CV:* Increased heart rate, postural hypotension
- *EENT:* Photophobia, blurred vision
- *GI:* Constipation, nausea, vomiting, dry mouth

Dopaminergics

- *Pregnancy category C, except for pergolide (Permax) which is category B*
- *CNS:* Bradykinetic episodes (on-off phenomena), abnormal movements, bruxism, ballismus, fatigue, headache, confusion, agitation, insomnia, psychosis with hallucinations, delusions, and depression

- *CV:* Elevated heart rate, orthostatic hypotension, hypertension, edema
- *Derm:* Hair loss, rash, flushing, increased perspiration
- *EENT:* Blurred vision, diplopia, blepharospasm
- *GI:* Liver toxicity, dry mouth, nausea, vomiting, anorexia, flatulence, diarrhea, or constipation
- *GU:* Urinary incontinence or retention, priapism, postmenopausal bleeding, dark urine
- *Resp:* Abnormal breathing patterns, rhinorrhea
- *Other:* Dark urine or perspiration, weight loss or gain

COMT Inhibitors

- *Pregnancy category C*
- *CNS:* Dizziness, dyskinesia, daytime sleepiness, dystonia, hallucinations
- *CV:* Orthostatic hypotension
- *GI:* Nausea, diarrhea, liver failure

 INTERACTIONS

Anticholinergics

- Concurrent use with CNS depressants will increase sedation.
- Concurrent use with opiates, tricyclic antidepressants, quinidine (Quinidex Extentabs), phenothiazines, haloperidol (Haldol) elevates risk of anticholinergic side effects.

Dopaminergics

- Concurrent use with hydantoins, phenothiazines, and TCAs will cause the effects of the dopaminergics to be lessened.
- Concurrent use with pyridoxine (Vitamin B_6) decreases levels of the dopaminergics.
- If given with MAOIs, there is risk of hypertensive crisis.
- Kava-kava increases signs of parkinsonism.
- Food interferes with absorption.

COMT Inhibitors

- Concurrent use with levodopa elevates levodopa levels.
- Concurrent use with CNS depressants causes additive sedation.
- Do not give with nonselective MAOIs due to inhibition of catecholamine metabolism.

CONTRAINDICATIONS

Anticholinergics

- Genitourinary or GI obstruction
- Myasthenia gravis
- Narrow-angle glaucoma
- Lactation
- Pregnancy
- Cautious use in cardiac arrhythmias, liver disease, and hypo- or hypertension
- Allergy

Dopaminergics

- Allergy
- History of melanoma
- Closed-angle glaucoma
- History of psychosis
- Pregnancy
- Lactation
- Children under 2 years of age
- Cautious use in respiratory disease, cardiac disease, diabetes mellitus, peptic ulcer disease

COMT Inhibitors

- Pregnancy
- Known hypersensitivity

NURSING IMPLICATIONS

Anticholinergics

- Give PO, IM, IV.
- Can give with food
- IM should be injected slowly into large muscle mass.
- IV should be infused slowly: 2.0 mg/min.
- Assess for euphoria, postural hypotension, and abnormal coordination after IV administration.
- Assess swallowing.
- Give frequent mouth care for mouth dryness.
- Hot temperatures require decreased dosing.
- Assess I & O.

 Can give with food

 IM should be injected slowly into large muscle mass.

 IV should be infused slowly: 2.0 mg/min.

Dopaminergics

- Give PO.
- Can give with food except for foods high in protein and pyridoxine (Vitamin B_6)
- Tablets can be crushed.
- Assess for any untoward reactions and report immediately as dose is dependent on client's response to drug.
- Assess bowel function.
- Assess I & O.
- Monitor the following lab tests: hepatic and renal function, CBC, serum K, and glucose.

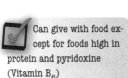 Can give with food except for foods high in protein and pyridoxine (Vitamin B_6)

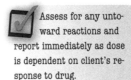 Assess for any untoward reactions and report immediately as dose is dependent on client's response to drug.

COMT Inhibitors

- Give PO.
- Nausea very common at initial stages of therapy.

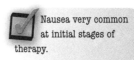 Nausea very common at initial stages of therapy.

- Assess liver function studies.
- Assess International Normalized Ratio and Prothrombin Time when drug given with warfarin (Coumadin).
- Assess for signs of liver failure (yellow skin and eyes, dark urine).

REFERENCES

1. Lilley L, Harrington S, Snyder J. *Pharmacology and the Nursing Process.* Philadelphia, PA: Mosby; 2007:210.

2. Lilley L, Harrington S, Snyder J. *Pharmacology and the Nursing Process.* Philadelphia, PA: Mosby; 2007:211.

3. Karch A. *Focus on Nursing Pharmacology.* Philadelphia, PA: Lippincott , Williams & Wilkins; 2008:393.

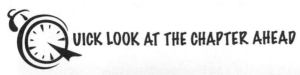

The skeletal muscle relaxants are a group of drugs that bring relief to the muscle spasm and spasticity that often occur in trauma or disease of the neuromuscular system. These drugs offer pain relief and are frequently used along with physical therapy and rest in the treatment of muscle spasms. Many of the skeletal muscle relaxants act directly on the spinal cord and brain, and dantrolene (Dantrium) works on muscle fibers.

24

Skeletal Muscle Relaxants

TERMS
- ☐ **baclofen (Lioresal)**
- ☐ **dantrolene (Dantrium)**

Table 24-1 Skeletal Muscle Relaxants

Prototype Drug	Related Drugs	Drug Classification
baclofen (Lioresal)	carisoprodol (Soma) chlorphenesin (Malate) chlorzoxazone (Paraflex) cyclobenzaprine (Flexeril) metaxalone (Skelaxin) methocarbamol (Robaxin) orphenadrine (Banflex) tizanidine (Zanaflex)	Centrally acting
dantrolene (Dantrium)	botulinum toxin type A (Botox)	Peripherally-acting

SKELETAL MUSCLE RELAXANTS CLIENT TEACHING

Centrally Acting

- Do not breast-feed.
- No activities requiring concentration until drug reaction is known
- No OTC drugs unless approved by physician
- Do not stop taking drug as hallucinations and psychotic behavior may develop.
- No alcohol as this will cause additional CNS depression
- Report any adverse effects to physician as these are usually dose related and can be eliminated if dose of drug is decreased.

No activities requiring concentration until drug reaction is known

Do not stop taking drug as hallucinations and psychotic behavior may develop.

Report any adverse effects to physician as these are usually dose related and can be eliminated if dose of drug is decreased.

Peripherally Acting

- Do not breast-feed.
- No activities requiring concentration until drug reaction is known
- No alcohol or OTC drugs

No alcohol or OTC drugs

- Signs of liver toxicity such as jaundice, dark-colored urine, abdominal pain, or clay-colored stools must be reported to physician immediately. Liver toxicity typically happens within 3–12 months of taking drug.
- Injection of botulinum toxin type A (Botox) lasts 3–4 months and needs to be repeated.

ACTION

Centrally Acting

- It is not understood how these drugs work. However, it is believed that these drugs depress the CNS and interfere with elevated muscle contraction and tone through the prevention of nerve impulses.

Peripherally Acting

- Prohibits contraction of muscle fiber by preventing calcium from leaving muscle tubules.
- Botulinum toxin type A (Botox) prevents release of acetylcholine.

USE

Centrally Acting

- Given as an adjunct to treat pain and muscle spasms of spinal cord injuries and musculoskeletal disorders

Peripherally Acting

- Treats muscle spasms that are found in such disorders as multiple sclerosis, cerebral palsy, spinal cord injury, and cerebrovascular accident
- Also used to treat malignant hyperthermia
- Cervical dystonia
- Improve frown wrinkles
- Strabismus
- Severe hyperhidrosis

ADVERSE EFFECTS AND SIDE EFFECTS

Centrally Acting

- *Pregnancy category C, except for cyclobenzaprine (Flexeril), which is category B*
- *CNS:* Sleeplessness, headache, confusion, fatigue, weakness, dizziness, drowsiness
- *CV:* Hypotension, cardiac arrhythmias
- *EENT:* Strabismus, blurred vision, double vision, miosis, mydriasis, tinnitus
- *GI:* Jaundice, nausea, vomiting, constipation
- *GU:* Urinary frequency and urgency, bed-wetting; discolorization of urine to orange to purple-red with chlorzoxazone (Paraflex)
- *Resp:* Nasal congestion

Peripherally Acting

- *Pregnancy category C*
- *CNS:* Muscle weakness, sleeplessness, seizures, drowsiness, fatigue, dizziness, headache, confusion, speech disturbances
- *CV:* Irregular blood pressure, fast heart beat
- *EENT:* Photophobia, double vision, blurred vision
- *GI:* Hepatitis, liver disease, nausea, vomiting, diarrhea, anorexia, taste alterations, dysphagia, GI bleeding
- *GU:* Urinary retention and frequency, bed-wetting, nocturia, crystalline urine with burning and pain on urination
- *Other:* Hypersensitivity, injection site reactions for botulinum toxin type A (Botox)

INTERACTIONS

Centrally Acting

- Concurrent use with CNS depressants will increase CNS depression.
- Elevated glucose levels with baclofen (Lioresal) requiring increased doses of insulin and sulfonylureas

Peripherally Acting

- Concurrent use with CNS depressants will increase CNS depression.
- Concurrent IV use with calcium channel blockers elevates risk of cardiovascular collapse.
- Elevated risk of liver toxicity if given concurrently in women under 35 who are taking estrogen
- Neuromuscular blockade is potentiated if given with aminoglycosides and neuromuscular blocking agents.

CONTRAINDICATIONS

Centrally Acting

- Children under 12 years of age
- Pregnancy
- Lactation
- Cautious use in kidney and liver disease, elderly, seizure disorder, diabetes mellitus
- Allergy

Peripherally Acting

- Children under 5 years of age
- Allergy
- Liver disease
- Pregnancy
- Lactation
- Muscle spasticity from rheumatic disorders
- Muscle spasms needed to maintain body function or balance
- Cautious use in women under 35 years of age, and in heart and respiratory disease
- Hypersensitivity

NURSING IMPLICATIONS

Centrally Acting

- Give PO.
- Can give with milk or food

- Intrathecal administration for baclofen (Lioresal)
- For intrathecal administration of baclofen (Lioresal), can only dilute with sterile, preservative free normal saline injection.
- Elderly need close observation as they are sensitive to these drugs.

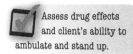

Elderly need close observation as they are sensitive to these drugs.

- If allergic reaction occurs, stop drug immediately.
- Assess drug effects and client's ability to ambulate and stand up.

Assess drug effects and client's ability to ambulate and stand up.

- Monitor lab work: liver function tests, blood glucose, blood pressure.

Peripherally Acting

- Give PO and IV; botulinum toxin type A (Botox) is given IM, IO, and SC.
- Capsule can be opened and drug mixed with any liquid if client is unable to swallow capsule. This should be refrigerated and only stored for a few days as there are no preservatives.
- IV form should be mixed with sterile water (20 mg of drug to 60 mL of sterile water) and used within 6 hours of mixing.
- IV form should be given via quick direct injection.
- Assess IV site and surrounding skin as IV form can be very irritating to tissues.

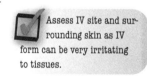

Assess IV site and surrounding skin as IV form can be very irritating to tissues.

- Assess the following during IV administration: EKG, VS, central venous pressure (CVP), and serum K.
- Effects of drug may take a week or more to be seen.

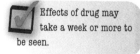

Effects of drug may take a week or more to be seen.

- Drug may be stopped after 45 days of treatment with no change in symptoms as liver toxicity may develop.
- Assess client's ability to walk and stand up.

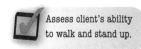

Assess client's ability to walk and stand up.

- Adverse effects usually last for the first 2 weeks of treatment and then dissipate.

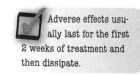

Adverse effects usually last for the first 2 weeks of treatment and then dissipate.

- Continually assess respiratory, cardiac, and GI functions.
- Monitor lab work: liver and kidney function tests, CBC.
- Injections of botulinum toxin type A (Botox) should be spaced at least 3 months apart and should be assessed for effectiveness at 1–2 weeks.

There are many types of migraine headache, but severe pain is something they all have in common. Arterial dilation is believed to be the cause of migraines. The Ergot Derivatives were the first group of drugs that were used to treat migraine headaches, and the second group, the Triptans, were developed in the 1990s.[1] The Triptans have proven to be very effective with less side effects than the Ergots.

25

Antimigraine Drugs

TERMS
- ☐ ergotamine (Ergomar)
- ☐ sumatriptan (Imitrex)

181

Table 25-1 Antimigraine Drugs

Prototype Drug	Related Drugs	Drug Classification
ergotamine (Ergomar)	dihydroergotamine (Migranal)	Ergot derivatives
sumatriptan (Imitrex)	almotriptan (Axert) eletriptan (Relpax) frovatriptan (Frova) naratriptan (Amerge) rizatriptan (Maxalt) zolmitriptan (Zomig)	Triptans

 ## ANTIMIGRAINE DRUGS CLIENT TEACHING

Ergot Derivatives

- Do not breast-feed.
- Take drug as soon as migraine headache begins.
- Must talk with physician before increasing dose
- The following must be reported to physician: nausea, vomiting, irregular heartbeat, muscle pain or weakness in extremities, and cold fingers.
- Extremities must be kept warm.
- After taking drug, lie down in dark, quiet room for 2–3 hours.

Take drug as soon as migraine headache begins.

After taking drug, lie down in dark, quiet room for 2–3 hours.

Triptans

- Do not breast-feed.
- Must learn how to use autoinjector for SC dose.
- Do not take within 24 hours of an Ergot Derivative or any other Triptan.
- Contact physician if experiencing angina or hypersensitivity.
- Do not take any new prescription or OTC drug until checking with physician.

Do not take within 24 hours of an Ergot Derivative or any other Triptan.

Contact physician if experiencing angina or hypersensitivity.

ACTION

Ergot Derivatives

* Act directly on the cranial and peripheral smooth muscles and has depressant effect on central vasomotor centers

Triptans

* Vasoconstrict the cranial carotid arteries

 ## USE

Ergot Derivatives

* Prevent/stop migraine and other vascular headaches

Triptans

* Treatment of migraine headaches

 ## ADVERSE EFFECTS AND SIDE EFFECTS

Ergot Derivatives

* *Pregnancy category X*
* *CNS:* Drowsiness, confusion
* *CV:* Intermittent claudication, irregular pulse
* *Derm:* Cold skin
* *GI:* Nausea, vomiting
* *Other:* Muscle weakness

Triptans

* *Pregnancy category C*
* *CNS:* Dizziness, vertigo, numbness, tingling
* *CV:* angina, coronary artery spasm, myocardial infarction

- *GI:* Diarrhea, nausea, vomiting
- *Other:* Muscle aching

INTERACTIONS

Ergot Derivatives

- Increased risk of gangrene and peripheral ischemia if taken with beta blockers

Triptans

- Increased risk of vasoconstriction if taken within 2 weeks of an MAOI
- Increased vasoactivity if combined with an Ergot Derivative
- Increased toxicity if taken with St. John's Wort

CONTRAINDICATIONS

Ergot Derivatives

- Pregnancy
- Sepsis
- Hypersensitivity
- Liver or kidney disease
- Severe pruritis
- History of cardiac problems
- Hypertension
- Malnutrition

Triptans

- Pregnancy
- Use in children
- Hypersensitivity
- Coronary artery disease

NURSING IMPLICATIONS

Ergot Derivatives

- Give SL.
- Tablet cannot be crushed.
- No smoking, eating, or drinking while tablet is in place
- Nausea and vomiting are very common and may require an antiemetic.
- Clients on high doses for long periods need assessment for increased headaches.
- If client has peripheral vascular disease, assess for peripheral ischemia.

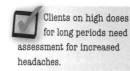
Nausea and vomiting are very common and may require an antiemetic.

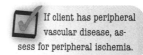
Clients on high doses for long periods need assessment for increased headaches.

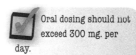
If client has peripheral vascular disease, assess for peripheral ischemia.

Triptans

- Give PO, SC, and intranasal.
- Inform client there will be pain and redness at the injection site, which will resolve in 1 hour.
- Oral dosing should not exceed 300 mg. per day.
- A second tablet can be taken 2 hours after the first tablet if symptoms aren't alleviated.
- Assess and report chest pain.
- Expect pain relief within 10 minutes of SC injection.

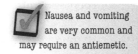
Oral dosing should not exceed 300 mg. per day.

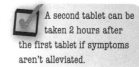
A second tablet can be taken 2 hours after the first tablet if symptoms aren't alleviated.

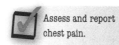
Assess and report chest pain.

REFERENCE

1. Karch A. *Focus on Nursing Pharmacology.* Philadelphia, PA: Lippincott, Williams & Wilkins; 2008:426.

PART II · QUESTIONS

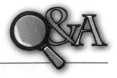

1. Morphine is contraindicated in all of the following EXCEPT:
   a. Increased intracranial pressure.
   b. Respiratory depression.
   c. Hyperthyroidism.
   d. Prostatic hypertrophy.

2. The nurse should assess for which of the following side effects in a client receiving an opioid agonist-antagonist?
   a. Constipation
   b. Hyperventilation
   c. Tinnitus
   d. Tremors

3. The antidote for an overdose of acetaminophen (Tylenol) is:
   a. None at this time.
   b. Acetylcysteine (Mucomyst).
   c. Protamine sulfate.
   d. Amyl nitrite.

4. A client who has been taking a selective serotonin reuptake inhibitor (SSRI) for a week calls you, the office nurse, and reports that his symptoms of depression are not improved. Your best response to the client is:
   a. "Your symptoms should be better by now."
   b. "You need a different drug."
   c. "It may take 4 weeks for your symptoms to improve."
   d. "Double the dose of your medication each day."

5. Which of the following is NOT a tricyclic antidepressant?
   a. Imipramine (Tofranil)
   b. Sertraline (Zoloft)
   c. Amitriptyline (Elavil)
   d. Doxepin (Sinequan)

6. The nurse knows which of the following about the MAOIs?
   a. Baseline EKG must be done before starting drug.
   b. Entire dose must be taken at bedtime.
   c. Weigh client weekly when taking these drugs.
   d. Taper drug slowly when discontinuing.

7. The drug of choice for treating tonic-clonic seizures in adults is:
   a. Phenobarbital (Luminal).
   b. Diazepam (Valium).
   c. Phenytoin (Dilantin).
   d. Carbamazepine (Tegretol).

8. Which of the following should the nurse teach the client no matter what antiseizure drug he is receiving?
   a. Take with food.
   b. Do not drink alcohol.
   c. Your urine will change color.
   d. Stay out of the sun.

9. The succinimides are given to treat which of the following seizures?
   a. Absence seizures
   b. Tonic-clonic seizures
   c. Partial seizures
   d. Atonic seizures

10. The nurse should teach the client all of the following about CNS stimulants EXCEPT:
    a. Weekly weight must be measured.
    b. Take the drug just before bedtime.
    c. Do not abruptly stop taking the drug.
    d. Physical and psychological dependence on this drug can develop.

11. If a local anesthetic is given to a client who is taking a MAOI, what problem can occur?
    a. Excess sedation
    b. Low blood pressure
    c. Elevated pulse
    d. Manic behavior

12. The nurse would instruct the client to take buspirone (BuSpar) with all of the following fluids EXCEPT:
    a. Milk.
    b. Orange juice.
    c. Apple juice.
    d. Grapefruit juice.

13. The nurse should assess an elderly client taking a barbiturate for which of the following side effects?
    a. Hypertension
    b. Dyspnea
    c. Agitation
    d. Tachycardia

14. The herb, kava-kava, should not be taken with a benzodiazepine because there will be
    a. Increased CNS depressant effects.
    b. Decreased level of the benzodiazepine.
    c. Increased seizure activity.
    d. Decreased absorption of the benzodiazepine.

15. The atypical antipsychotics act by:
    a. Changing the movement of sodium in and out of nerve cells.
    b. Liberating norepinephrine from the neurons.
    c. Blocking dopamine and serotonin receptors.
    d. Blocking histamine and acetylcholine receptors.

16. The nurse should teach which of the following to the client who is taking lithium (Eskalith)?
    a. Stay out of the sun.
    b. Your urine will turn reddish-brown.
    c. Do not get the liquid form of the drug on your skin.
    d. Increase your fluid intake.

17. Extrapyramidal effects occur more often in which of the following medications?
    a. Clozapine (Clozaril)
    b. Haloperidol (Haldol)
    c. Risperidone (Risperdal)
    d. Lithium (Eskalith)

18. Which of the following can occur if levodopa (Dopar) is taken with a MAOI?
    a. Hypertensive crisis
    b. Increased signs of Parkinsonism
    c. Decreased absorption of levodopa (Dopar)
    d. Decreased blood level of levodopa (Dopar)

19. An anticholinergic drug to treat Parkinson's disease would be contraindicated in the client with:
    a. History of melanoma.
    b. History of psychosis.
    c. Myasthenia gravis.
    d. Closed-angle glaucoma.

20. A client who has been taking dantrolene (Dantrium) for 4 days reports that he/she has no improvement in his/her muscle spasms. The best response for the nurse to give him/her about this is
    a. "You should have seen an improvement already."
    b. "Increase your dose by an additional tablet each day."
    c. "Wait for another week to see if improvement occurs."
    d. "You need a new drug to treat your muscle spasms."

21. Which of the following should the nurse teach the client about the Triptans?
    a. The tablet needs to be placed under the tongue.
    b. Nausea and vomiting are very common while taking this drug.
    c. The client must keep the extremities warm while taking this drug.
    d. The client cannot take more than 300 mg of this drug per day.

PART II • ANSWERS

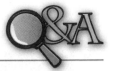

1. **The correct answer is c.** Morphine is contraindicated in hypothyroidism along with the other options listed.

2. **The correct answer is a.** A client receiving an opioid agonist-antagonist can experience the following GI symptoms: dry mouth, nausea, vomiting, constipation, and altered taste.

3. **The correct answer is b.** Acetylcysteine (Mucomyst), a mucolytic used in the treatment of chronic pulmonary conditions, is the antidote for acetaminophen (Tylenol) poisoning.

4. **The correct answer is c.** Antidepressants in general can take up to 4 weeks to relieve symptoms of depression.

5. **The correct answer is b.** Sertraline (Zoloft) is an SSRI.

6. **The correct answer is d.** MAOIs must be tapered slowly when they are discontinued to avoid adverse effects.

7. **The correct answer is c.** Phenytoin (Dilantin) is the drug of choice for treating tonic-clonic seizures in adults.

8. **The correct answer is b.** Alcohol has CNS depressant effects that would increase the already existing CNS depressant effectives of the antiseizure drug the client is taking.

9. **The correct answer is a.** The succinimides specifically treat absence seizures.

10. **The correct answer is b.** CNS Stimulants should be taken at least 6 hours before the client goes to sleep to prevent insomnia.

11. **The correct answer is b.** Concurrent use of MAOIs and antihypertensive drugs with local anesthetics can cause hypotension.

12. **The correct answer is d.** If grapefruit juice is taken with buspirone (BuSpar), the serum level of buspirone (BuSpar) will become elevated.

13. **The correct answer is c.** The elderly can experience confusion and agitation when taking a barbiturate.

14. **The correct answer is a.** Concurrent use of kava-kava or valerian with a benzodiazepine will increase CNS depressant effects.

15. **The correct answer is c.** The atypical antipsychotics act by blocking both dopamine and serotonin receptor sites in the CNS.

16. **The correct answer is d.** A client beginning therapy of lithium (Eskalith) should increase fluid intake to 2 to 3 L/day, and the client on continuing therapy should have 1 L of fluid per day.

17. **The correct answer is b.** Extrapyramidal effects occur most often with the typical Antipsychotics, and haloperidol (Haldol) belongs to that group.

18. **The correct answer is a.** Concurrent use of levodopa (Dopar) with a MAOI increases the risk of hypertensive crisis, and the two drugs should not be taken concurrently.

19. **The correct answer is c.** Anticholinergics are contraindicated in clients with myasthenia gravis

20. **The correct answer is c.** The effects of dantrolene (Dantrium) can take at least a week or longer to be seen.

21. **The correct answer is d.** The client should not take more than 300 mg of a Triptan per day. The other answers are all client teaching that should be done for the Ergot derivatives.

III

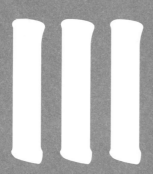

Autonomic Nervous System Drugs

Nancy Elaine Clarkson, MEd, RN, BC

The cholinergic drugs have the same effect in the body as the neurotransmitter, acetylcholine (ACh). Thus, they stimulate sites in the parasympathetic nervous system (PSNS). They are also called parasympathomimetics because their action is identical to that of the PSNS. This group of drugs has the ability to act either indirectly or directly on receptor sites. Due to the fact that they work on sites all over the body, the effects of these drugs are quite extensive as are their adverse effects.

26

Cholinergic Drugs

TERMS
- ☐ bethanechol (Urecholine)
- ☐ neostigmine (Prostigmine)
- ☐ donepezil (Aricept)

Table 26-1 Cholinergic Drugs

Prototype Drug	Related Drugs	Drug Classification
bethanechol (Urecholine)	carbachol (Miostat) cevimeline (Evoxac) pilocarpine (Pilocar)	Direct-acting cholinergic
neostigmine (Prostigmine)	ambenonium (Mytelase) edrophonium (Tensilon) physostigmine (Antilirium) pyridostigmine (Mestinon)	Indirect-acting cholinergics
donepezil (Aricept)	galantamine (Reminyl) rivastigmine (Exelon) tacrine (Cognex)	Indirect-acting cholin- ergics for Alzheimer's disease

CHOLINERGIC DRUGS CLIENT TEACHING

Direct-Acting Cholinergics

- Do not breast-feed.
- No activities that require concentration until response to drug is known
- Change position slowly.
- Be aware that blurred vision may occur.
- To prevent fainting, do not stand for long periods of time.
- For eye preparations, do not insert soft contact lenses until 15 minutes after instilling drug to prevent staining lenses.

No activities that require concentration until response to drug is known

Be aware that blurred vision may occur.

For eye preparations, do not insert soft contact lenses until 15 minutes after instilling drug to prevent staining lenses.

Indirect-Acting Cholinergics (Including Those for Alzheimer's Disease)

- Do not breast-feed.
- Frequent changes in dosing may occur.
- Drug may need to be taken during the night.

Frequent changes in dosing may occur.

- Keep a written record of drug response for physician.
- Avoid standing for long periods to prevent fainting.
- Signs of GI bleeding (eg, pain, bloody stools, coffee-ground emesis) need to be reported to physician immediately.

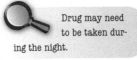

Drug may need to be taken during the night.

 ## ACTION

Direct-Acting Cholinergics

- Attach to the ACh receptor sites and directly stimulate them

Indirect-Acting Cholinergics

- Prevent ACh from being destroyed by acetylcholinesterase (AChE), thus enabling more ACh to be able to have direct effect on the receptor. The direct action of ACh on its receptor causes stimulation.

Indirect-Acting Cholinergics for Alzheimer's Disease

- Cross the blood brain barrier and keep level of ACh high in the cerebral cortex by blocking AChE

 ## USE

Direct-Acting Cholinergics

- Bethanechol (Urecholine) is used to treat nonobstructive urinary retention and neurogenic bladder in adults and children under 8 years of age.
- Carbachol (Miostat) and pilocarpine (Pilocar) are used as eye medications to treat miosis and glaucoma.
- Cevimeline (Evoxac) is used to treat dry mouth in Sjögren's Syndrome.

Indirect-Acting Cholinergics

- Used to diagnose and treat myasthenia gravis and to reverse action of nondepolarizing neuromuscular blocking drugs
- Four drugs are specifically used in the treatment of mild to moderate Alzheimer's disease.

ADVERSE AND SIDE EFFECTS

Direct-Acting Cholinergics

- *Pregnancy category C*
- *CNS:* Headache
- *CV:* Heart block, dizziness, hypotension
- *EENT:* Tearing, miosis, blurred vision
- *GI:* Diarrhea, nausea, vomiting, salivation, spontaneous defecation
- *GU:* Spontaneous urination
- *Resp:* Dyspnea, asthma attack
- *Other*: Hypothermia, increased perspiration

Indirect-Acting Cholinergics

- *Pregnancy category C*
- *CNS:* Drowsiness, headache, dizziness
- *CV:* Cardiac arrest, hypotension, heart block, bradycardia
- *EENT:* Blurred vision, tearing, miosis
- *GI:* Spontaneous defecation, diarrhea, nausea, vomiting, abdominal cramps, salivation
- *GU:* Urinary urgency
- *Resp:* Dyspnea, cough, increased bronchial secretions
- *Other:* Increased perspiration, flushing, fasciculations, weakness, fatigue, paralysis, muscle cramps

Indirect-Acting Cholinergics for Alzheimer's Disease

- See "Adverse Effects and Side Effects" for Indirect-Acting Cholinergics.

INTERACTIONS

Direct-Acting Cholinergics

- Concurrent use with AChE inhibitors increases cholinergic effects.
- The following oppose the effects of bethanechol (Urecholine): atropine, epinephrine, quinidine, procainamide (Pronestyl).

Indirect-Acting Cholinergics

- Concurrent use with nonsteroidal anti-inflammatory drugs (NSAIDs) can elevate risk of GI bleeding.
- Atropine, quinidine, and procainamide (Pronestyl) block the effects of these drugs.

Indirect-Acting Cholinergics for Alzheimer's Disease

- See "Interactions" for Indirect-Acting Cholinergics.
- Tacrine (Cognex) increases blood levels of theophylline.
- The following speed up elimination of donepezil (Aricept): phenytoin (Dilantin), rifampin (Rifadin), carbamazepine (Tegretol), dexamethasone (Decadron).

 CONTRAINDICATIONS

Direct-Acting Cholinergics

- Parkinsonism
- Seizure disorder
- Myocardial infarction
- Coronary artery disease
- Hyper- or hypotension
- Bradycardia
- Chronic obstructive pulmonary disease
- Asthma
- Hyperthyroidism
- Recent urinary or GI surgery

- Pregnancy
- Lactation
- Children less than 8 years of age

Indirect-Acting Cholinergics

- Pregnancy
- Lactation
- Allergy
- Hypotension
- Bradycardia
- Urinary or intestinal obstruction

Indirect-Acting Cholinergics for Alzheimer's Disease

- See "Contraindications" for Indirect-Acting Cholinergics.

NURSING IMPLICATIONS

Direct Acting Cholinergics

- Give PO, SC, and ophthalmically.
- Decrease nausea and vomiting by giving oral dose on empty stomach.
- Atropine is the antidote.
- Do not administer IM or IV.
- Monitor I & O.
- Assess pulse and blood pressure during and after SC administration.
- Assess pulmonary status.
- Employ safety measures such as assisting client with walking.

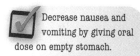
Decrease nausea and vomiting by giving oral dose on empty stomach.

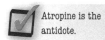
Atropine is the antidote.

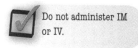
Do not administer IM or IV.

Indirect-Acting Cholinergics (Including Those for Alzheimer's Disease)

- Give PO, SC, IM, and IV.
- The amount of medication in oral doses is greater than parenteral doses due to poor oral absorption.

- Can give with milk or food
- Give IV dose undiluted.
- Client should urinate within 1 hour after first dose when given for urinary retention.
- Assess pulmonary status.
- Assess vital signs when dose is adjusted for treatment of myasthenia gravis.
- Cholinergic crisis (overdose) typically occurs 1 hour after administration.

 Can give with milk or food

 Client should urinate within 1 hour after first dose when given for urinary retention.

 Assess pulmonary status.

 Cholinergic crisis (overdose) typically occurs 1 hour after administration.

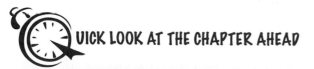

The anticholinergic drugs interfere or block the effects of acetylcholine (ACh) in the parasympathetic nervous system (PSNS). They are also called parasympatholytics or cholinergic blockers. They have actually been used therapeutically for many years,[1] although they are not used very often today.[2] They are derived from natural, synthetic, and semisynthetic sources.

27

Anticholinergic Drugs

TERM
☐ atropine

201

Table 27-1 Anticholinergic Drugs

Prototype Drug	Related Drugs	Drug Classification
atropine	dicyclomine (Bentyl) flavoxate (Urispas) glycopyrrolate (Robinul) homatropine (Isopto Homatropine) hyoscyamine (Anaspaz) ipratropium (Atrovent) methscopolamine (Pamine) propantheline (Pro-Banthine) scopolamine (Transderm Scop) trospium (Sanctura)	Anticholinergics

 ## ANTICHOLINERGIC DRUGS CLIENT TEACHING

- Dry mouth can be helped by chewing gum, sucking on hard candy, sipping fluids, rinsing mouth, or performing oral hygiene.
- No activities requiring concentration until drug effects are known
- Wear sunglasses.
- Urinate before taking drug.
- Increase intake of fluid and fiber to prevent constipation.
- Do not breast-feed.
- Stop eye drops if conjunctivitis, eye pain, dizziness, or heart palpitations occur.

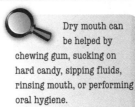
Dry mouth can be helped by chewing gum, sucking on hard candy, sipping fluids, rinsing mouth, or performing oral hygiene.

Wear sunglasses.

Urinate before-taking drug.

Increase intake of fluid and fiber to prevent constipation.

 ## ACTION

These drugs vie with ACh to attach to the muscarinic receptors in the PSNS. After they affix themselves to these receptors, nerve transmission is interrupted. While they can bind to receptors all over the body, they usually attach to receptors in the exocrine glands and in cardiac and smooth muscle.

 ## USE

- Decrease GI and pulmonary secretions
- Pupil dilation
- Bradycardia
- Antidote for cholinergic crisis (overdose) and neuromuscular blockers
- Irritable bowel
- Pylorospasm
- Ureteral colic
- Bladder relaxation
- Obstetric amnesia
- Motion sickness
- Cycloplegia
- Amanita mushroom poisoning
- Chronic obstructive pulmonary disease (COPD)

 ## ADVERSE EFFECTS AND SIDE EFFECTS

- *Pregnancy category C, except for dicyclomine (Bentyl), glycopyrrolate (Robinul), and ipratropium (Atrovent), which are category B*
- *CNS:* Hallucinations, confusion, depression, headache, dizziness, irritability, seizures, fatigue, drowsiness
- *CV:* Atrial or ventricular fibrillation, ventricular tachycardia, heart palpitations, hyper- or hypotension, bradycardia
- *Derm:* Rash; urticaria; flushed, dry skin
- *EENT:* Increased intraocular pressure, blurred vision, mydriasis, photophobia, cyclopegia
- *GI:* Paralytic ileus, dry mouth, dysphagia, nausea, vomiting, constipation
- *GU:* Impotence, dysuria, urinary retention and hesitancy

INTERACTIONS

- Additive anticholinergic effects with monoamine oxidase inhibitors, anti-Parkinson's drugs, antihistamines, tricyclic antidepressants, quinidine, and procainamide (Pronestyl)
- Concurrent use with phenothiazines decreases their effectiveness and elevates risk of paralytic ileus.
- Concurrent use with levodopa (Dopar) decreases its effects.

 CONTRAINDICATIONS

- Allergy
- Glaucoma
- Peptic ulcer
- Paralytic ileus
- Abdominal obstruction
- Ulcerative colitis
- Enlarged prostate
- Obstruction of bladder
- Tachycardia
- Cardiac arrhythmias
- Liver or kidney disease
- Myasthenia gravis
- Pregnancy
- Lactation
- Cautious use in hypertension and brain trauma

 NURSING IMPLICATIONS

- Give PO, SC, IM, IV, and ophthalmically.
- Monitor I & O.
- Have client void before giving atropine.
- Assess vital signs.
- Parenteral administration can cause postural hypotension.

 Give PO, SC, IM, IV, and ophthalmically.

 Have client void before giving atropine.

- Assess effects of drug in infants and children. Death has occurred from systemic effects from eye drops.
- Elderly are sensitive to CNS effects of drug.
- Assess for "atropine fever" in elderly, infants, and children.

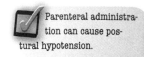

Parenteral administration can cause postural hypotension.

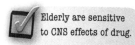

Elderly are sensitive to CNS effects of drug.

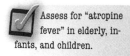

Assess for "atropine fever" in elderly, infants, and children.

REFERENCES

1. Lilley L, Harrington S, Snyder J, Aucker R. *Pharmacology and the Nursing Process.* St. Louis, MO: Mosby; 2007:306.

2. Karch A. *Focus on Nursing Pharmacology.* Philadelphia, PA: Lippincott, Williams & Wilkins; 2008:524.

QUICK LOOK AT THE CHAPTER AHEAD

The adrenergic drugs are able to imitate the effects of the sympathetic nervous system. They are also called sympathomimetic drugs and have a wide spectrum of use. These drugs are able to stimulate various adrenergic receptor sites. The drugs that stimulate both alpha and beta sites are called **nonselective adrenergic agonists,** while the ones that stimulate alpha sites are called alpha adrenergic agonists, and the ones that stimulate beta sites are called beta adrenergic agonists. The reader should note that the majority of beta adrenergic agonists are used in the treatment of respiratory disorders, and these are covered in Part IV: Respiratory System Drugs.

28

Adrenergic Drugs

TERMS
☐ epinephrine (Adrenalin)
☐ phenylephrine
  (Neo-Synephrine)
☐ isoproterenol (Isuprel)

Table 28-1 Adrenergic Drugs

Prototype Drug	Related Drugs	Drug Classification
epinephrine (Adrenalin)	dobutamine (Dobutrex) dopamine (Intropin) ephedrine (Efedron) mephentermine (Wyamine) metaraminol (Aramine) norepinephrine (Levophed)	Nonselective adrenergic agonists
phenylephrine (Neo-Synephrine)	clonidine (Catapres) methoxamine (Vasoxyl) midodrine (ProAmatine)	Alpha adrenergic agonists
isoproterenol (Isuprel)	ritodrine (Yutopar)	Beta adrenergic agonists

ADRENERGIC DRUGS CLIENT TEACHING

Nonselective Adrenergic Agonists

- Do not breast-feed.
- Nasal formulation can burn.
- Ophthalmic preparation should be given at bedtime and may burn.
- Report drug tolerance to physician.
- If allergic reaction to ophthalmic formulation occurs, stop drug and report to physician.

Nasal formulation can burn.

Alpha Adrenergic Agonists

- Ophthalmic preparation may burn and may stain contact lenses.
- Contact physician if no improvement in 5 days.
- Wear sunglasses for pupil dilation.
- Do not breast-feed.
- Report systemic effects to physician.

Ophthalmic preparation may burn and may stain contact lenses.

Contact physician if no improvement in 5 days.

Beta Adrenergic Agonists

- Do not breast-feed.
- Sputum and saliva may turn pink.
- Drug should be taken exactly as ordered.
- Refer to Part IV: Respiratory System Drugs.

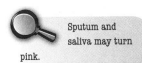

Sputum and saliva may turn pink.

 # ACTION

Nonselective Adrenergic Agonists

- Work on both alpha and beta receptor sites throughout the body. Through stimulation of these sites, the following occurs: pupil and bronchial dilation, increased perspiration, strengthening of cardiac contraction, elevated heart rate, breakdown of glucose, elevation of systolic blood pressure, decreased intraocular pressure, and increased respirations.

Alpha Adrenergic Agonists

- Stimulate alpha receptors but main action is in the vascular system where vasoconstriction is produced.

Beta Adrenergic Agonists

- Act on $beta_1$ and $beta_2$ receptors. Results of $beta_1$ stimulation are elevated heart rate and contractility and $beta_2$ stimulation is vasodilation.
- Refer to Part IV: Respiratory System Drugs.

 # USE

Nonselective Adrenergic Agonists

- Shock
- Congestive heart failure

- Hypotension
- Rhinitis
- Glaucoma
- Extension of effects of anesthesia
- Cardiac arrest

Alpha Adrenergic Agonists

- Shock
- Allergies and colds
- Glaucoma
- Allergic rhinitis
- Ear infection
- Supraventricular tachycardia
- Orthostatic hypotension

Beta Adrenergic Agonists

- Bronchospasm
- Shock
- Cardiac asystole
- Preterm labor
- Refer to Part IV: Respiratory System Drugs.

ADVERSE EFFECTS AND SIDE EFFECTS

Nonselective Adrenergic Agents

- *Pregnancy category C, except for mephentermine (Wyamine), metaraminol (Aramine), and norepinephrine (Levophed), which are category D*
- *CNS:* Headache, psychosis, nervousness, fear, tremors, dizziness, weakness, insomnia, Central Vascular Accident (CVA).
- *CV:* Palpitations, angina, arrhythmias, increased blood pressure
- *EENT:* Burning of eyes, tearing, iritis, burning of nose, rebound congestion, sneezing, nasal drying
- *F & E:* Increased lactic acid, metabolic acidosis
- *GI:* Nausea, vomiting

- *GU*: Urinary retention
- *Resp*: Pulmonary edema, dyspnea
- *Other*: Increased perspiration

Alpha Adrenergic Agonists

- *Pregnancy category C*
- *CNS*: Insomnia, dizziness, nervousness, anxiety, tremors
- *CV*: Increased blood pressure and heart rate, palpitations, arrhythmias
- *EENT*: Blurred vision, tearing, eye burning, rebound nasal congestion, nasal burning, sneezing
- *GI*: Anorexia, nausea, vomiting
- *GU*: Dysuria, decreased urine output
- *Other*: Increased perspiration

Beta Adrenergic Agonists

- *Pregnancy category C*
- *CNS*: Sleeplessness, anxiety, headache, tremors
- *CV*: Palpitations, increased heart rate, myocardial infarction, angina
- *Derm*: Rash
- *EENT*: Dilated pupils
- *GI*: Anorexia, nausea, vomiting
- *Resp*: Pulmonary edema, dyspnea, bronchospasm, coughing
- *Other*: Increased perspiration
- Refer to Part IV: Respiratory System Drugs.

 INTERACTIONS

Nonselective Adrenergic Agonists

- Additive effects with other adrenergic drugs
- Concurrent use with beta blockers causes increased blood pressure.
- Concurrent use with MAOIs and TCAs decrease effects of epinephrine (adrenalin).
- Use with general anesthetics causes elevated cardiac irritability.

Alpha Adrenergic Agonists

- Concurrent use with MAOIs can cause hypertensive crisis.
- Elevated blood pressure if used with oxytocics
- Concurrent use with TCAs has an additive effect.

Beta Adrenergic Agonists

- Additive effects with other adrenergic drugs
- Concurrent use with TCAs or oxytocics can cause high blood pressure.
- Irregular heart rhythms with concurrent use of general anesthetics.
- See Part IV: Respiratory System Drugs.

 ## CONTRAINDICATIONS

Nonselective Adrenergic Agonists

- Pregnancy
- Lactation
- Pheochromocytoma
- Cardiac arrhythmias
- General anesthetics
- Allergy
- Second stage of labor
- Hypovolemia

Alpha Adrenergic Agonists

- Pregnancy
- Lactation
- Allergy
- Narrow-angle glaucoma
- Hypertension
- Tachycardia
- Coronary artery disease

Beta Adrenergic Agonists

- Pregnancy
- Lactation
- Tachycardia
- Cardiogenic shock
- Allergy
- Pulmonary hypertension
- General anesthesia
- Refer to Part IV: Respiratory System Drugs.

 NURSING IMPLICATIONS

Nonselective Adrenergic Agonists

- Give PO, SC, IM, IV, ophthalmic, inhalation, and nasal instillation.
- For inhalation: do not administer with isoproterenol (Isuprel); client needs to be sitting upright; if symptoms not relieved in 20 minutes, report to physician.
- For ophthalmic use: if administered with miotic, give miotic first. Soft contacts should be taken out before drug administration and pressure applied to lacrimal duct to prevent systemic absorption.
- Tissue necrosis can occur from SC route so rotate sites.
- Incompatible with many IV drugs so check with pharmacy before giving.
- Assess vital signs and urine output during IV administration.
- Monitor I & O.

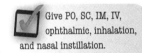
Give PO, SC, IM, IV, ophthalmic, inhalation, and nasal instillation.

For inhalation: do not administer with iso-proterenol (Isuprel); client needs to be sitting upright; if symptoms not relieved in 20 minutes, report to physician.

For ophthalmic use: if administered with miotic, give miotic first. Soft contacts should be taken out before drug administration and pressure applied to lacrimal duct to prevent systemic absorption.

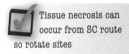
Tissue necrosis can occur from SC route so rotate sites

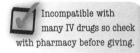
Incompatible with many IV drugs so check with pharmacy before giving.

Alpha Adrenergic Agonists

- Give PO, SC, IM, IV, nasal instillation, and ophthalmic.
- Nasal passageways should be open before nasal instillation.
- Apply pressure to lacrimal sac to prevent systemic absorption.
- Vital signs must be monitored during IV administration.
- Monitor IV administration closely to prevent overdose.

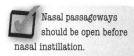

Nasal passageways should be open before nasal instillation.

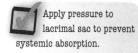

Apply pressure to lacrimal sac to prevent systemic absorption.

Beta Adrenergic Agonist

- Give PO, SC, IM, IV, and inhalation.
- Use IV pump for IV administration to keep drug administration at constant rate.
- IV solution formulation should be clear.
- Vital signs and EKG should be monitored continuously during IV administration.
- Stop if tolerance develops to prevent rebound bronchospasm.
- Refer to Part IV: Respiratory System Drugs.

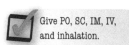

Give PO, SC, IM, IV, and inhalation.

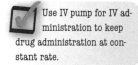

Use IV pump for IV administration to keep drug administration at constant rate.

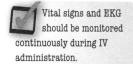

Vital signs and EKG should be monitored continuously during IV administration.

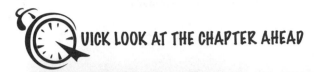

The adrenergic blocking agents attach to the adrenergic receptor sites and prevent stimulation of the SNS. They are also called sympatholytics. Alpha receptors are located on nerves, organs, muscles, and cells throughout the body. When these receptors are blocked, the following occur: pupil constriction, lowered blood pressure, vasodilation, and suppressed ejaculation. The beta receptors are located on the smooth muscles of the blood vessels and bronchioles and on the heart.

29

Adrenergic Blocking Agents

TERMS
☐ prazosin (Minipress)
☐ propranolol (Inderal)

Table 29-1 Adrenergic Blocking Agents

Prototype Drug	Related Drugs	Drug Classification

prazosin (Minipress)	doxazosin (Cardura)
	phenoxybenzamine
	  (Dibenzyline)
	phentolamine (Regitine)
	tamsulosin (Flomax)
	terazosin (Hytrin)
		Alpha adrenergic
		  blocking
		  agents

propranolol (Inderal)	acebutolol (Sectral) atenolol (Tenormin) betaxolol (Betoptic) bisoprolol (Zebeta) carteolol (Cartrol) esmolol (Brevibloc) metoprolol (Lopressor) nadolol (Corgard) penbutolol (Levatol) pindolol (Visken) sotalol (Betapace) timolol (Timoptic)	Beta-adrenergic blocking agents

ADRENERGIC BLOCKING AGENTS CLIENT TEACHING

Alpha Adrenergic Blocking Agents

- Do not breast-feed.
- Change position slowly.
- No activities that require concentration until drug effects are known
- Adverse effects tend to go away as dosing continues.
- Drug should be taken at same time daily.
- Learn how to take blood pressure and keep written record of what blood pressure was before each dose.
- No OTC drugs unless you check with physician
- Impotence needs to be reported immediately.

Change position slowly.

Drug should be taken at same time daily.

Learn how to take blood pressure and keep written record of what blood pressure was before each dose.

Beta Adrenergic Blocking Agents

- Do not breast-feed.
- No OTC drugs unless you check with physician
- No activities that require concentration until drug effects are known
- Do not stop drug abruptly.
- Change position slowly.
- Drug lowers intraocular pressure so all health care providers of the client need to be told.
- Low blood pressure may occur.
- Take drug exactly as prescribed.
- May suppress signs of low blood glucose

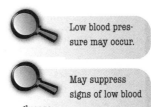

Low blood pressure may occur.

May suppress signs of low blood glucose

ACTION

Alpha Adrenergic Blocking Agents

- Prevent excitement of the SNS by competing with the neurotransmitter, norepinephrine at the adrenergic receptor site, or by occupation of the site without competition. Noncompetitive occupation is irreversible while the competitive occupation is reversible.

Beta Adrenergic Blocking Agents

- Prevent stimulation of adrenergic receptor sites from epinephrine and norepinephrine, which in turn blocks the action of the SNS

USE

Alpha Adrenergic Blocking Agents

- Hypertension
- Benign prostatic hypertrophy

- Hypertension associated with pheochromocytoma
- Vasoplastic diseases
- Frostbite
- Raynaud's disease
- Prevention of tissue necrosis accompanying extravasation from vasoconstrictive drugs

Beta Adrenergic Blocking Agents

- Myocardial infarction
- Cardiac arrhythmias
- Glaucoma
- Hypertension
- Angina
- Prophylaxis for migraine headache

ADVERSE EFFECTS AND SIDE EFFECTS

Alpha Adrenergic Blockng Agents

- *Pregnancy category C, except for doxazosin (Cardura) and tamsulosin (Flomax), which are category B*
- *CNS:* Drowsiness, sedation, headache, dizziness
- *CV:* Tachycardia, hypotension, palpitations, edema
- *Derm:* Rash, alopecia, itching
- *EENT:* Tinnitus, blurred vision
- *F & E:* Elevated BUN and serum uric acid
- *GI:* Nausea, vomiting, constipation, diarrhea, abdominal pain
- *GU:* Impotence, urinary incontinence and frequency
- *Other:* Increased perspiration, nosebleed

Beta Adrenergic Blocking Agents

- *Pregnancy category C, except for acebutolol (Sectral), pindolol (Visken), and sotalol (Betapace), which are category B, and atenolol (Tenormin), which is category D*
- *CNS:* Dizziness, fatigue, depression, sleeplessness, hallucinations, confusion, drowsiness

- *CV:* Heart block, congestive heart failure, bradycardia
- *Derm:* Itching, alopeicia, dry skin
- *EENT:* Tinnitus, hearing loss, conjunctivitis, dry eyes, visual changes
- *F & E:* Hyper- and hypoglycemia
- *GI:* Pancreatitis, nausea, vomiting, dry mouth
- *GU:* Impotence
- *Hematologic:* Agranulocytosis
- *Resp:* Bronchospasm, dyspnea
- *Other:* Fever, weight gain, muscle aches, sore throat

INTERACTIONS

Alpha Adrenergic Blocking Agents

- The following increase the effects of the alpha adrenergic blockers: epinephrine, antihypertensive drugs, nonsteroidal anti-inflammatory drugs, and central nervous system depressants.
- The following decrease the effects of the alpha adrenergic blockers: estrogens, birth control pills, and alpha adrenergic drugs.

Beta Adrenergic Blocking Agents

- The following increase the effects of the beta adrenergic blocking agents: phenytoin (Dilantin), digoxin (Lanoxin), other antihypertensives, furosemide (Lasix), cimetidine (Tagamet), IV verapamil (Calan), and quinidine.
- The following decrease the effects of the beta adrenergic blocking agents: atropine, antacids, and isoproterenol.

CONTRAINDICATIONS

Alpha Adrenergic Blocking Agents

- Pregnancy
- Lactation

- CVA
- Myocardial infarction
- Angina

Beta Adrenergic Blocking Agents

- Pregnancy
- Lactation
- Respiratory disorders that are associated with bronchoconstriction such as asthma
- Heart block
- Bradycardia

NURSING IMPLICATIONS

Alpha Adrenergic Blocking Agents

- Give PO, SC, IM, and IV.
- Give with food.
- First dose should be taken at hour of sleep to decrease chance of dizziness or postural hypotension.
- Assess blood pressure with each dose.
- May take 4 to 6 weeks before effects of drug are seen.
- Assess for "first-dose effect," which includes bradycardia, falling blood pressure, and fainting. Can occur 90 to 120 minutes after initial dose. Seen most often in clients with recent CVA, beta adrenergic drugs, and decreased plasma volume.

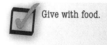

Give with food.

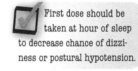

First dose should be taken at hour of sleep to decrease chance of dizziness or postural hypotension.

Beta Adrenergic Blocking Agents

- Give PO, IV, and ophthalmically.
- Blood pressure and apical pulse need to be taken before each dose.
- Long-acting forms must be swallowed whole.
- Cannot be stopped abruptly

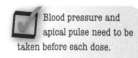

Blood pressure and apical pulse need to be taken before each dose.

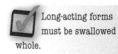

Long-acting forms must be swallowed whole.

- Cannot be given within 14 days of a monoamine oxidase inhibitor
- Can be given with or without food but must be given consistently the same way to decrease variations in absorption
- Monitor I & O.
- Daily weight
- Monitor the following lab tests: complete blood count, renal, and hepatic function.
- Do not give if client has any history of allergy, asthma, or chronic obstructive pulmonary disease, as bronchoconstriction can occur.
- Most adverse effects happen immediately after IV administration and when oral doses are given to the elderly and clients with renal disease.
- Salt intake may need restriction.
- Hypoglycemic effects seen in clients NPO for less than 12 hours.
- Assess extremities for impaired circulation.

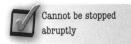
Cannot be stopped abruptly

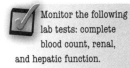
Monitor the following lab tests: complete blood count, renal, and hepatic function.

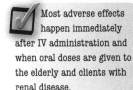
Most adverse effects happen immediately after IV administration and when oral doses are given to the elderly and clients with renal disease.

PART III • QUESTIONS

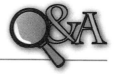

1. The antidote for a cholinergic overdose is:
   a. Atropine.
   b. Neostigmine (Prostigmin).
   c. Dopamine (Intropin).
   d. Propranolol (Inderal).

2. Which of the following drugs should not be taken with tacrine (Cognex)?
   a. Heparin
   b. Digoxin (Lanoxin)
   c. Theophylline (Theo-Dur)
   d. Ibuprofen (Advil)

3. The nurse instructs the client, who wears soft contact lenses, to do the following when administering pilocarpine (Pilocar) eye drops:
   a. The contacts need to be in your eyes before you take the pilocarpine (Pilocar) eye drops.
   b. You need to clean your contacts just before you put them in your eyes, and then take the pilocarpine (Pilocar) eye drops.
   c. Take the pilocarpine (Pilocar) eye drops and wait 15 minutes before inserting the contact lenses.
   d. Flush your eyes with sterile normal saline just before inserting the contact lenses and taking the pilocarpine (Pilocar) eye drops.

4. Which side effect could the nurse observe in a client taking atropine?
   a. Urinary frequency
   b. Peptic ulcer
   c. Pulmonary edema
   d. Increased intraocular pressure

5. Which receptors do the anticholinergics usually bind with? Receptors found in:
   a. Cerebral cortex.
   b. Cardiac muscle.
   c. Joints of the extremities.
   d. Peritoneum.

6. What happens if an anticholinergic is taken with levodopa (Dopar)?
   a. There is no effect.
   b. The effect of the levodopa (Dopar) is decreased.
   c. The effect of the anticholinergic is decreased.
   d. There are additive anticholinergic effects.

7. Which of the following statements about the nonselective adrenergic agonists is true?
   a. Stimulate alpha and beta receptors.
   b. Mostly used to treat respiratory disorders.
   c. Cause pupil constriction.
   d. All are pregnancy category C drugs.

8. The following is an alpha adrenergic agonist drug:
   a. Ritodrine (Yutopar).
   b. Dopamine (Intropin).
   c. Ephedrine (Efedron).
   d. Phenylephrine (Neo-Synephrine).

9. The nurse is aware of which of the following nursing implications of the nonselective adrenergic agonists?
   a. The client should be told to wear sunglasses.
   b. Rotate SC injection sites.
   c. Administer IV formulation on an IV pump.
   d. Sputum and saliva may turn pink.

10. All of the following statements about the adrenergic blocking agents are true EXCEPT . . . Adrenergic blocking agents:
    a. Are also called sympathomimetics.
    b. Stop stimulation of the sympathetic nervous system (SNS).
    c. Are used to treat hypertension.
    d. Should not be given to a client with asthma.

11. Alpha adrenergic blocking agents are used to treat the following disease:
    a. Glaucoma.
    b. Angina.
    c. Hypertension.
    d. Migraine headache.

12. A client with asthma has been ordered to receive a beta adrenergic blocking agent. What is the most appropriate action by the nurse?
    a. Give the medication.
    b. Decrease the dose of the medication.
    c. Call the physician.
    d. Give a bronchodilator with the beta blocker.

PART III · ANSWERS

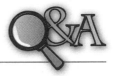

1. **The correct answer is a.** Atropine, which is an anticholinergic, is the antidote for a cholinergic overdose.

2. **The correct answer is c.** Theophylline (Theo-Dur) should not be taken with tacrine (Cognex) as tacrine (Cognex) increases the blood level of theophylline.

3. **The correct answer is c.** Pilocarpine (Pilocar) eye drops can stain soft contact lenses, so the contacts should be inserted 15 minutes after the eye drops have been taken.

4. **The correct answer is d.** Clients taking atropine can experience a number of eye problems along with increased intraocular pressure including: blurred vision, mydriasis, photophobia, and cyclopegia.

5. **The correct answer is b.** The anticholinergics typically bind with receptors found in cardiac and smooth muscle and in the exocrine glands.

6. **The correct answer is b.** If an anticholinergic is taken concurrently with levodopa (Dopar), the effect of the levodopa (Dopar) is decreased.

7. **The correct answer is a.** The nonselective adrenergic agonists act on both the alpha and beta receptors in the body.

8. **The correct answer is d.** Phenylephrine (Neo-Synephrine) is the prototype drug of the alpha adrenergic agonists.

9. **The correct answer is b.** Tissue necrosis can develop from SC injections, so sites must be rotated.

10. **The correct answer is a.** The adrenergic blocking agents are also called sympatholytics, because they prevent stimulation of the SNS.

11. **The correct answer is c.** The alpha adrenergic agents are used to treat hypertension, benign prostatic hypertrophy, vasoplastic diseases, frostbite, Raynaud's disease, and tissue necrosis that accompanies extravasation from vasoconstrictive drugs.

12. **The correct answer is c.** A client with asthma, allergies, or chronic obstructive pulmonary disease cannot receive a beta-blocker, because bronchoconstriction can occur. The physician must be consulted about this and change the client to another drug.

IV

Respiratory System Drugs

Marilyn J. Herbert-Ashton, MS, RN, BC

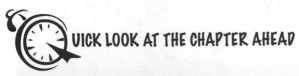

QUICK LOOK AT THE CHAPTER AHEAD

In 2002, the National Asthma Education and Prevention Program updated guidelines for diagnosing and managing asthma. Information on these guidelines can be found at http://www.nhlbi.nih.gov. Drugs are classified as long-term and quick relief medications with a stepwise approach to treatment.

Anticholinergic bronchodilators, antileukotriene agonists, synthetic glucocorticoids, and mast cell stabilizers are used for long-term control of asthma. Bronchodilators and xanthene derivatives are discussed in Chapter 31.

30
Antiasthmatic Drugs

TERMS
- ☐ ipratropium (Atrovent)
- ☐ zafirlukast (Accolate)
- ☐ budesonide (Pulmicort)
- ☐ cromolyn (Intal, Nasalcrom)

Table 30-1 Antiasthmatic Drugs

Prototype Drug	Related Drugs	Drug Classification
ipratropium (Atrovent)	iotropium bromide (Spiriva)	Anticholinergic bronchodilators and Beta$_2$ antagonist
	ipratropium/albuterol (Combivent)	Combination anticholinergic bronchodilator
zafirlukast (Accolate)	zileuton (Zyflo) montelukast (Singulair)	Antileukotriene antagonists
budesonide (Pulmicort)	beclomethasone (Beclovent, Vanceril flunisolide (AeroBid) fluticasone propionate (Flovent, Flonase) mometasone furoate (Elocon, Nasonex) triamcinolone acetonide (Azmacort, Nasacort)	Synthetic glucocorticoids
	salmeterol fluticasone (Advair Diskus)	Combination glucocorticoid and Beta$_2$ antagonist
cromolyn (Intal, Nasalcrom)	nedocromil (Tilade)	Mast cell stabilizers

ANTIASTHMATIC DRUGS CLIENT TEACHING

All Antiasthmatics

> Consult with health care provider before taking other OTC medications or herbal remedies.

- Follow directions and use medications as ordered.
- Consult with health care provider before taking other OTC medications or herbal remedies.
- Do not discontinue without consulting with health care provider.
- Do not double dose if a dose is missed.
- For inhaled agents, use a spacer if recommended by health care provider.
- Teach client how to use metered-dose inhaler. (See Chapter 31.)

Anticholinergic Bronchodilators

- Good mouth care, water, or hard candy helps to decrease dryness.
- If symptoms do not improve within 30 minutes after taking, contact health care provider.

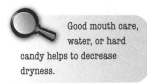

Good mouth care, water, or hard candy helps to decrease dryness.

- Keep a record of number of inhalations instead of floating canister in water to estimate how much drug is left in the canister.[1]
- Avoid getting drug into eyes.

Antileukotriene Antagonists

- Encourage follow-up with health care provider for periodic liver function enzyme testing.
- These drugs are used for prophylaxis and chronic asthma, but not acute asthma attacks.

These drugs are used for prophylaxis and chronic asthma, but not acute asthma attacks.

- Report symptoms of Churg-Strauss syndrome (generalized flu-like syndrome) to health care provider. Churg-Strauss syndrome is more apt to occur when weaning from systemic steroids. Occurs rarely but can be life-threatening.
- Take on an empty stomach.

Inhaled Synthetic Glucocorticoids

- Systemic glucocorticoids (see Chapter 51)
- To prevent fungal infections, rinse mouth after taking medication.
- Rinse mouthpiece in warm water after each use.

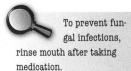

To prevent fungal infections, rinse mouth after taking medication.

- If using inhaled synthetic glucocorticoids and bronchodilator, use the bronchodilator first, and wait 5 minutes before using the glucocorticoid.

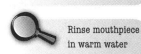

Rinse mouthpiece in warm water after each use.

- Inhaled synthetic glucocorticoids are not used to treat acute asthma attacks but should be continued if other agents are used. A systemic glucocorticoid may be ordered during an acute asthma attack.

- Contact health care provider if sore mouth or throat occurs.
- Allow 1 to 2 minutes between inhalations if a second inhalation is ordered.
- Use a spacer if recommended by health care provider.

Mast Cell Stabilizers

- Rinse mouth after taking medication to prevent dryness and throat irritation.
- If asthma symptoms do not improve in 4 weeks, worsen, or recur, contact health care provider.
- Intranasal use: inhale through nose during inhalation. Make sure nasal passages are clear before using.
- Opthalmic use: do not wear soft contact lenses.

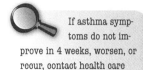

If asthma symptoms do not improve in 4 weeks, worsen, or recur, contact health care provider.

℞ ACTION

Anticholinergic Bronchodilators

- Antagonizes acetylcholine, which causes bronchodilation; action is slow and prolonged

Antileukotriene Antagonists

- Block leukotriene-mediated bronchoconstriction that decreases bronchial edema and inflammation seen in asthma

Synthetic Glucocorticoids

- Decrease inflammation and enhance beta-agonist activity[2]

Mast Cell Stabilizers

- May inhibit release of histamine and other mediators from mast cell.

USE

Anticholinergic Bronchodilators

- Prevention of bronchospasm in chronic obstructive pulmonary disease (COPD)
- Intranasal—allergic and nonallergic perennial rhinitis

Antileukotriene Antagonists

- Indicated to decrease the severity and frequency of asthma attacks, with improvement seen in about 1 week

Synthetic Glucocorticoids

- Treatment of chronic asthma
- Used intranasally for treatment of seasonal allergies. Rhinitis not responsive to other decongestants.

Mast Cell Stabilizers

- Prophylaxsis of asthma. These are not used to treat acute asthma attacks.
- Exercise-induced bronchospasm
- Perennial rhinitis

 ## ADVERSE EFFECTS AND SIDE EFFECTS

Anticholinergic Bronchodilator

- *Pregnancy category B, except for Tiotropium bromide (Spiriva), which is category C.*
- *CNS:* Headache, nervousness, blurred vision
- *EENT:* Sore throat, cough, dry mouth
- *GI:* GI irritation, nausea

Antileukotriene Antagonists

- *Pregnancy category B, although Zileuton (Zyflo) is a category C*
- *CNS:* Headaches, dizziness

- *GI:* nausea, vomiting, and diarrhea
- Increased incidence of infection over age 55
- Liver dysfunction (not seen with montelukast)
- Chrug-Strauss syndrome (seen with zafirlukast)

Synthetic Glucocorticoids

- *Pregnancy category C*
- *CNS:* Dizziness, headache
- *EENT:* Unpleasant taste, oral fungal infection, cough
- *GI:* GI distress

Mast Cell Stabilizers

- *Pregnancy category B*
- *CNS:* Dizziness, headache
- *GI:* Unpleasant taste
- *Resp:* Cough, bronchospasm, and throat irritation

INTERACTIONS

Anticholinergic Bronchodilators

- Additive anticholinergic effects with concurrent use of other anticholinergics

Antileukotriene Antagonists

Zileuton (Zyflo)
- Concurrent use with warfarin increases risk of bleeding.
- Concurrent use with theophylline decreases zafirukast and zileuton levels.

Zafirlukast (Accolate)
- Concurrent use with aspirin increases zafirukast levels.
- Concurrent use with erythromycin decreases zafirlukast levels.

Zileuton (Zyflo)
- Concurrent use with propranolol increases propranolol levels.

Montelukast (Singulair)

- Concurrent use with phenobarbital decreases montelukast levels.

Synthetic Glucocorticoids

- Few interactions as these drugs are given by inhalation

Mast Cell Stabilizers

- None significant

CONTRAINDICATIONS

Anticholinergic Bronchodilators

- Hypersensitivity to ipratropium, atropine, and derivatives
- Propellant used to make inhaled ipratropium has a cross-sensitivity to antigen causing peanut allergies. Inhaled ipratropium is contraindicated in clients with peanut allergies.[3]

Antileukotriene Antagonists

- Hypersensitivity
- Breast-feeding

Synthetic Glucocorticoids

- Hypersensitivity

Mast Cell Stabilizers

- Hypersensitivity
- Status asthmaticus

NURSING IMPLICATIONS

All Antiasthmatics

- Monitor vital signs throughout treatment.

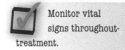
Monitor vital signs throughout-treatment.

- Assess lung sounds and respiratory function throughout treatment.

Anticholinergic Bronchodilators

- Administered by inhalation or intranasally
- Contact health care provider if severe bronchospasm present so that an alternative medication may be ordered.
- If administered with other inhalation medications, administer adrenergic bronchodilator first, followed by ipratropium, then corticosteroid, and wait 5 minutes between medications.

> If administered with other inhalation medications, administer adrenergic bronchodilator first, followed by ipratropium, then corticosteroid, and wait 5 minutes between medications.

Antileukotriene Antagonists

- Available orally
- Periodically monitor liver function studies.
- Monitor and report symptoms of Churg-Strauss syndrome especially if being weaned from systemic steroids.

> Monitor and report symptoms of Churg-Strauss syndrome especially if being weaned from systemic steroids.

Synthetic Glucocorticoids

- Monitor for adverse effects and report to health care provider.

Mast Cell Stabilizers

- Available by inhalation or intranasally, opthalmic use for allergy
- Do not administer during an acute asthma attack or status asthmaticus.
- If taking before exercise or exposure to allergy, take at least 10 to 15 minutes before exposure.

> Do not administer during an acute asthma attack or status asthmaticus

REFERENCES

1. McKenry L, Tessler E, Hogan M. *Mosby's Pharmacology in Nursing*, 22nd ed. St. Louis, MO: Elsevier Mosby; 2006:709.

2. Lilley L, Harrington S, Snyder S. *Pharmacology and the Nursing Process,* 5th ed. St. Louis, MO: Mosby; 2007:559.

3. Karch A. *Focus on Nursing Pharmacology.* Philadelphia, PA: Lippincott, Williams & Wilkins; 2008:910.

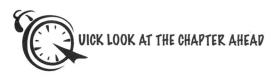

Bronchodilators dilate the bronchi and bronchioles and include two classes of drugs: the **beta-agonists** and **xanthine derivatives**. The beta-agonists are also called sympathomimetic bronchodilators. They are broken down into three classifications related to the specific receptors that they stimulate. Classifications include: nonselective alpha-beta-agonists that stimulate the alpha, $beta_1$, and $beta_2$ receptors; nonselective beta-agonists that stimulate $beta_1$ and $beta_2$ receptors; and selective $beta_2$-agonists that stimulate only $beta_2$ receptors.[1] The alpha-beta-agonist, epinephrine, is discussed in Chapter 28.

31

Bronchodilator Drugs

TERMS
- ☐ epinephrine (adrenalin, Primatene, Bronkaid)
- ☐ albuterol (Proventil, Ventolin, Volmax)
- ☐ theophylline (Theo-Dur, Slo-bid)

235

Table 31-1 Brochodilator Drugs

Prototype Drug	Related Drugs	Drug Classification
epinephrine (Adrenalin, Primatene, Bronkaid)	isoproterenol solution (Isuprel) isoetharine HCL (Bronkosol) metraproterenol (Alupent)	Beta-agonists (Sympathomimetics) or Alpha-beta-agonist (Epinephrine) Beta$_1$-Beta$_2$-agonist (isoproterenol, isoetharine HCL & metraproterenol) (Nonselective beta-agonists)
albuterol (Proventil, Ventolin, Volmax)	bitolterol (Tornalate) formoterol (Foradil) levalbuterol (Xopenex) pirbuterol (Maxair) salmeterol (Serevent) terbutaline (Brethaire, Bricanyl)	Beta$_2$-agonist
theophylline (Theo-Dur, Slo-bid)	aminophylline (Truphylline) dyphylline (Dilor, Lufyllin)	Xanthine derivatives

BRONCHODILATOR DRUGS CLIENT TEACHING

All Bronchodilators

- Check with health care provider before taking OTC medications and herbal remedies.
- Take exactly as prescribed and do not double up on missed doses.

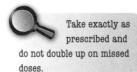

Take exactly as prescribed and do not double up on missed doses.

Beta-Agonists

- Report adverse effects such as feeling jittery, palpitations, chest pain, restlessness, insomnia, or other symptoms to health care provider.
- Take oral medication with meals to decrease GI upset.

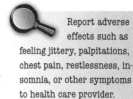

Report adverse effects such as feeling jittery, palpitations, chest pain, restlessness, insomnia, or other symptoms to health care provider.

Xanthines

- Avoid caffeine, as caffeine acts as a xanthine during therapy.
- Take with food if GI upset occurs.
- Do not crush or chew enteric-coated or sustained-release products.
- Report adverse effects such as palpitations, chest pain, nausea, vomiting, weakness, dizziness, or other symptoms to health care provider.
- Avoid tobacco use as nicotine increases the metabolism of xanthines.

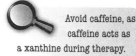

Avoid caffeine, as caffeine acts as a xanthine during therapy.

Metered-Dose Inhaler

- Instruct client on proper use of metered-dose inhaler (MDI). If taking a bronchodilator and steroid, take the bronchodilator first to open up the airways, followed by the steroid.
- Fast-acting bronchodilators, such as albuterol, should be taken before slower or longer acting bronchodilators, such as salmeterol.
- If taking a beta-agonist with an anticholinergic, take the beta-agonist before taking the anticholinergic, ipratropium.
- Canister contains measured doses of medication.

Instruct client on proper use of metered-dose inhaler (MDI). If taking a bronchodilator and steroid, take the bronchodilator first to open up the airways, followed by the steroid.

Proper Use of the Inhaler

- Shake the canister thoroughly before using.
- Exhale fully and place mouthpiece in mouth or about 1.5 inches away from mouth.
- Inhale slowly and deeply while pressing down the canister.
- Remove mouthpiece while holding breath for as long as possible, then exhale slowly with pursed lips.
- Rinsing mouth after use decreases dryness in mouth and prevents systemic absorption.
- Clean mouthpiece of MDI with warm water to remove secretions and dry.
- If a second dose is ordered, wait 1 to 2 minutes between doses.

- Keep a record of number of inhalations.
- Suggest a spacer, especially in children, as it helps to deliver the full dose and decreases the taste of medication.
- Avoid getting into eyes.

 ## ACTION

Nonselective Beta$_1$-Beta$_2$-Agonists

- Stimulate beta$_1$ receptors in the heart and beta$_2$ receptors in the heart and lung; relax bronchial smooth muscle and dilate trachea and bronchi by increasing levels of cyclic adenosine monophosphate (cAMP). Will see more cardiac adverse effects due to beta$_1$ receptor stimulation in the heart.

Selective Beta$_2$-Agonists

- Predominately stimulate the beta$_2$ receptors in the lungs and increase levels of cAMP, causing bronchodilation

Xanthine Derivatives

- Increase cAMP causing bronchodilation
- Also have diuretic and positive inotropic and chronotropic effects, and cause gastric acid secretion and CNS stimulation.
- Xanthine contains caffeine, so caffeine intake should be minimized while taking.

 ## USE

Beta-Agonists

- Bronchial asthma, bronchitis, bronchospasm, and other pulmonary disease

Alpha-Beta-Agonists

- Also used to treat hypotension and shock

Selective Beta$_2$-Agonists

- Also used to treat hyperkalemia

Bitolterol (Tornalate)

- Has a long onset of action and is used for prophylaxis of bronchospasm in clients over age 12

Formoterol (Foradil)

- Used for maintenance treatment of asthma and prophylaxis of bronchospasm in clients over age 5 with reversible obstructive airway disease
- Also used to prevent exercise-induced bronchospasm in clients over age 12

Isoproterenol (Isuprel)

- Also indicated for heart block, shock, and ventricular dysrhythmias.

Salmeterol (Serevent)

- Has a long-onset of action and is indicated for maintenance therapy of asthma, prevention of bronchospasm in selected clients over age 4 with reversible airway disease, and prevention of exercise-induced asthma

Terbutaline (Brethaire, Bricanyl)

- Also indicated to prevent premature labor in pregnant women

Xanthine Derivatives

- Prevention and treatment of bronchial asthma, bronchitis, and chronic obstructive pulmonary disease (COPD).

ADVERSE EFFECTS AND SIDE EFFECTS

Nonselective Beta$_1$-Beta$_2$-Agonists

- *Pregnancy category C*
- *CV:* Palpitations, tachycardia, hypertension, and cardiac arrest

- *CNS:* Anxiety, tremors, insomnia, dizziness, and headache
- *Endocrine:* Hyperglycemia
- *GI:* Nausea, vomiting

Selective Beta$_2$-Agonists

- *Pregnancy category C, except terbutaline (Brethaire, Bricanyl), which is category B*
- *CV:* Palpitations, hypertension
- *CNS:* Tremors, nervousness, restlessness, headache, and insomnia
- *Endocrine:* Hyperglycemia
- *GI:* Nausea, vomiting

Xanthine Derivatives

- *Pregnancy category C*
- *CV:* Tachycardia, dysrhythmias, and palpitations
- *CNS:* Anxiety, headache, insomnia, seizures, and tremors
- *GI:* Anorexia, nausea, vomiting, and cramps

INTERACTIONS

All Bronchodilators

- Concurrent use with sympathomimetics can increase cardiac and CNS stimulation.

Beta-Agonists

- Concurrent use with monoamino oxidase inhibitors (MAOIs) may cause hypertensive crisis.
- Concurrent use of beta-blockers may antagonize therapeutic effects.
- Increased risk of hypokalemia if taken with potassium-sparing diuretics
- Concurrent use with caffeine may increase stimulation effects.

Xanthine Derivatives

- Increased theophylline levels with concurrent use of: allopurinal, benzodiazepines cimetidine, erythromycin, oral contraceptives, influenza vaccine, interferon, beta-blockers, and corticosteroids
- Nicotine may increase metabolism and decrease effectiveness of xanthines.
- Concurrent use of ginseng or caffeine may increase stimulation effects.
- Concurrent use with St. John's wort may decrease effectiveness of xanthine derivatives.

CONTRAINDICATIONS

All Bronchodilators

- Hypersensitivity

Beta-Agonists and Xanthine Derivatives

- Tachydysrhythmias

NURSING IMPLICATIONS

All Bronchodilators

- Monitor vital signs.
- Assess lung sounds.
- Encourage fluids unless contraindicated.
- Careful monitoring of the elderly as they are more susceptible to adverse reactions

Assess lung sounds.

Encourage fluids unless contraindicated.

Beta-Agonists

- Available by inhalation
- Albuterol, metaproterenol, and terbutaline are also available orally.
- Isoproterenol (Isupril) is also available IV and SL.

- Terbutaline (Brethaire, Bricanyl) is also available SC.
- Oral medication can be given with food to decrease GI effects.
- Monitor cardiac status and report changes to health care provider.
- Salmeterol (Serevent): warning of small but significant increase in use of life-threatening asthma episodes. Study showed that African American clients had a greater risk of asthma-related deaths as compared to other groups.[2]

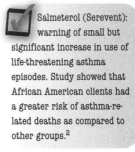

Xanthine Derivatives

- Available PO, parenterally, or rectally
- Give over 24 hours to maintain therapeutic levels.
- Monitor theophylline levels: therapeutic range 10.0 to 20.0 mcg/mL.
- Use an infusion pump and give slowly when administered IV.
- IV rate should not exceed 20.0 to 25.0 mg/minute.
- Wait 4 to 6 hours after IV therapy is discontinued before giving first dose orally.
- Monitor intake and output.
- Monitor for drug toxicity and notify health care provider if toxicity occurs.
- Oral drug can be given with food if GI effects occur.
- Clients with a cardiac history should be monitored for EKG changes or chest pain.

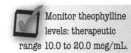

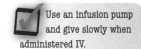

REFERENCES

1. Lilley L, Harrington S, Snyder J. *Pharmacology and the Nursing Process,* 5th ed. St. Louis, MO: Mosby; 2007:553.

2. Karch A. *Focus on Nursing Pharmacology.* Philadelphia, PA: Lippincott, Williams & Wilkins; 2008:908.

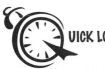

Antihistamines are also known as H_1 antagonists and directly compete with histamine for specific receptor sites. Antihistamines are categorized as **first generation,** which include the chemical classes of alkylamines, ethanolamines, ethylenediamines, phenothiazines, piperidines, and **second generation** or nonsedating agents. Sedation is a problem seen with first generation antihistamines. Diphenhydramine (Benadryl) is the prototype drug for the first generation antihistamines, and loratadine (Claritin) is the prototype drug for the second generation (nonsedating) antihistamines.

32

Antihistamine Drugs

TERMS
- ☐ diphenhydramine (Benadryl)
- ☐ loratadine (Claritin)

Table 32-1 Antihistamine Drugs

Prototype Drug	Related Drugs	Drug Classification
diphenhydramine (Benadryl)	clemastine (Tavist) dimenhydrinate (Dramamine) trimethobenzamide HCL (Arrestin, Benzacot, Tigan, others)	First generation antihistamines— Traditional antihistamines (Ethanolamines)
There is no prototype for this classification	brompheniramine (Dimetane) chlorpheniramine (Chlor-Trimeton) dexchlorpheniramine (Polaramine)	(Alkylamines)
There is no prototype for this classification	tripelennamine (Pyribenzamine)	(Ethylenediamines)
There is no prototype for this classification	buclizine (Bucladin-S) meclizine (Antivert) cyclizine (marezine) promethazine (Phenergan) trimeprazine (Temaril)	(Phenothiazines)
There is no prototype for this classification	azatadine (Optimine) cyproheptadine (Periactin) hydroxyzine (Atarax, Vistaril, others)	(Piperidines)
loratadine (Claritin)	azelastine (Astelin) cetirizine (Zyrtec) desloratadine (Clarinex) fexofenadine (Allegra)	Second generation antihistamines— Nonsedating antihistamines

ANTIHISTAMINES DRUGS CLIENT TEACHING

- Avoid driving or operating heavy machinery.
- Avoid alcohol and taking other CNS depressants.
- If possible, take at bedtime to avoid daytime sedation.
- Inform health care provider and dentist if taking antihistamines.

Avoid driving or operating heavy machinery.

Avoid alcohol and taking other CNS depressants.

- Take with food to decrease GI upset.
- Encourage fluids and hard candy to minimize anticholinergic effects of dry mouth.
- Consult with health care provider before taking other OTC or herbal preparations.
- Wear sunscreen and protective clothing to prevent photosensitivity.
- As many of these drugs are available OTC, take as directed.

 ## ACTION

All Antihistamines

- H_1 blockers block the effects of histamine by competing for H_1 receptor sites.
- Second-generation, nonsedating antihistamines do not cross the blood brain barrier, which reduces or prevents sedation.
- Second-generation antihistamines have a longer duration of action and fewer anticholinergic effects than first-generation antihistamines.

 ## USE

All Antihistamines

- Rhinitis, allergies, colds, nausea, adjunctive therapy of anaphylaxis, motion sickness, vertigo, Parkinson's disease, and as a sleep aid (first generation antihistamines)

 ## ADVERSE EFFECTS AND SIDE EFFECTS

All Antihistamines

- *Anticholinergic effects:* First generation antihistamines: dry mouth, dilated pupils, urinary retention, tachycardia, and constipation; second generation antihistamines have minimal effects

- *CNS:* Sedation in first generation antihistamines, although this is rarely seen with second generation antihistamines; paradoxical excitation
- *Derm:* Photosensitivity
- *EENT:* Blurred vision
- *GI:* Dry mouth, GI upset, diarrhea, or constipation
- *GU:* Urinary retention

First Generation Antihistamines and Second Generation Antihistamines

- *Pregnancy category B, although azelastine (Astelin), brompheniramine (Dimetane), cyclizine (Marezine), promethazine (Phenergan), and hydroxyzine (Atarax, buclizine (Bucladin-S), triamethobenzamide HCL (Arresten, Benzacot, Tigan), Vistaril, and others are category C. Those in unclassified pregnancy category include tripelennamine (Pyribenzamine) and trimeprazine (Temaril).*

 INTERACTIONS

All Antihistamines

- Concurrent use with alcohol, other CNS depressants, antidepressants, kava-kava, valerian, and chamomile may cause additive CNS depression.
- Concurrent use with MAOIs can intensify antihistamine effects.
- Concurrent use of erythromycin or ketoconazole with loratadine and fexofenadine increases concentrations of loratadine and fexofenadine.

 CONTRAINDICATIONS

All Antihistamines

- Hypersensitivity
- Lactation

- Clients with lower respiratory tract disease
- Acute asthma attacks
- Cautious use with bladder neck obstruction, narrow angle glaucoma, and stenosing peptic ulcer

 NURSING IMPLICATIONS

All Antihistamines

- Give PO; some antihistamines may also be given SC, IM, IV, PR, or topically.
- Azelastine (Astelin) is available as a nasal and opthalmic agent.
- Monitor vital signs.
- Assess lung sounds, secretions, and allergy symptoms.
- Unless contraindicated, encourage fluid intake.

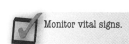
Monitor vital signs.

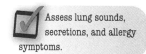
Assess lung sounds, secretions, and allergy symptoms.

- If client undergoing allergy testing, discontinue antihistamine use for at least 4 days before testing, as antihistamines may decrease skin response to allergy test.
- When antihistamines are used as a sleep aid, ie, diphenhydramine (Benadryl), they should be given at least 20 minutes before bedtime.
- Antihistamines used for motion sickness should be given at least 30 minutes before exposure to situations that may cause motion sickness.

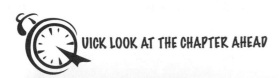

Decongestants are used to decrease nasal congestion caused by stimulation of the alpha$_1$-adrenergic receptors on nasal blood vessels, which causes vasoconstriction, in turn shrinking mucous membranes and relieving congestion.[1] Decongestants are available orally and topically. Oral decongestants have a delayed onset with prolonged and less potent effects, while topical decongestants produce rapid and potent effects. Topical steroid decongestants are discussed in Chapter 30.

33

Decongestant Drugs

TERM

☐ ephedrine (Pretz-D)

Table 33-1 Decongestant Drugs

Prototype Drug	Related Drugs	Drug Classification
ephedrine (Pretz-D)	naphazoline (Privine) oxymetazoline (Afrin, Dristan) phenylephrine (NeoSynephrine, Coricidin, others) pseudo-ephedrine hydrochloride (Sudafed, Dorcol, Decofed) tetrahydrozoline (Tyzine) xylometazoline (Otrivin)	Decongestants (Sympathomimetics)

Sympathomimetics are discussed in more detail in Chapter 28.

DECONGESTANT DRUGS CLIENT TEACHING

- Avoid concurrent use of OTCs and herbal remedies without consulting health care provider.
- Avoid caffeine while taking decongestants.
- May cause cardiac or CNS stimulation, such as palpitations, restlessness, or insomnia. Report symptoms to health care provider.
- Take exactly as directed.
- Topical decongestants (sympathomimetics) should not be taken for more than 3 to 5 days to avoid rebound congestion.
- Contact health care provider if symptoms persist for more than a week or if a rash occurs.
- Encourage fluids unless contraindicated.
- Avoid taking near bedtime to prevent insomnia.

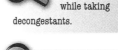

Avoid caffeine while taking decongestants.

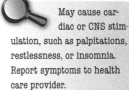

May cause cardiac or CNS stimulation, such as palpitations, restlessness, or insomnia. Report symptoms to health care provider.

ACTION

- Causes vasoconstriction through stimulation of the alpha$_1$-adrenergic receptors on the nasal blood vessels causing shrinkage of the nasal membranes

USE

- Congestion seen with acute or chronic rhinitis, sinusitis, and colds

ADVERSE EFFECTS AND SIDE EFFECTS

- *Pregnancy category C*
- *CV:* Hypertension, palpitations, and tachycardia, dyspnea (seen more frequently with oral agents)
- *CNS:* Stimulation, headache, nervousness, restlessness, and dizziness (seen more frequently with oral agents)
- *GI:* Nausea & vomiting
- *Other:* Rebound congestion with topical agents, fever

INTERACTIONS

- Concurrent use with other sympathomimetics can increase toxicity.
- Concurrent use with MAOIs can cause hypertensive crisis.

CONTRAINDICATIONS

- Hypersensitivity
- Hypertension (oral use)
- Coronary artery disease (oral use)

NURSING IMPLICATIONS

- Many decongestants are OTC agents.
- Monitor vital signs and assess lung sounds and congestion periodically throughout therapy.
- Monitor for hypertension, palpitations, or tachycardia and report symptoms to health care provider.

> Monitor vital signs and assess lung sounds and congestion periodically throughout therapy.

REFERENCE

1. Lehne RA. *Pharmacology for Nursing Care,* 6th ed. Philadelphia, PA: Saunders/Elsevier; 2007:885.

QUICK LOOK AT THE CHAPTER AHEAD

Coughing serves a protective purpose in removing secretions and foreign substances from the respiratory tract. The cough center is located in the medulla and is triggered when the cough reflex receptors found in the bronchi, alveoli, and pleura are stimulated and in turn, stretched.[1] There are situations when coughing is not beneficial, for example, after certain surgeries (eg, a tonsillectomy) when coughing may be harmful or for a dry nonproductive cough, as in bronchitis.

The two categories of antitussives are opioid and nonopioid antitussives. The nonopioid antitussives are less effective than the opioid antitussives. Dextromethorpan (Vicks 44, Robitussin DM) is the most popular antitussive of both categories.

If used properly, the opioid antitussives should not lead to dependency. They are rarely used as sole agents.

Prescription antitussives are usually indicated when OTC preparations have not been effective.

34

Antitussive Drugs

TERMS
- ☐ **dextromethorphan (Vicks Formula 44, Robitussin DM)**
- ☐ **diphenhydramine (Benylin, Benadryl)**
- ☐ **codeine (Dimetane-DC, Tussar SF)**

Table 34-1 Antitussive Drugs

Prototype Drug	Related Drugs	Drug Classification
dextromethorphan (Vicks Formula 44, Robitussin DM)		Nonopioid antitussive
	benzonatate (Tessalon)	Nonopioid antitussive (locally acting)
diphenhydramine (Benylin, Benadryl)	There are no related drugs at this time	Antitussive, antihistamine
codeine (Dimetane-DC, Tussar SF)	hydrocodone (Hycodan)	Opioid antitussive

 ## ANTITUSSIVE DRUGS CLIENT TEACHING

- Avoid concurrent use of OTCs and herbal remedies without consulting with physician.
- Use an antitussive for a dry, nonproductive cough.
- Avoid driving or operating heavy machinery while taking antitussives as they may cause drowsiness.
- Encourage fluid intake unless contraindicated.
- Avoid drinking fluids for at least 30 minutes after taking an antitussive.
- Contact health care provider if cough persists for more than a week, or if a rash, fever, or persistent headache occurs.

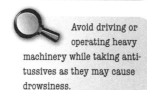

Use an antitussive for a dry, nonproductive cough.

Avoid driving or operating heavy machinery while taking antitussives as they may cause drowsiness.

 ## ACTION

Nonopioid Antitussives

- Suppress the cough reflex through direct action to the cough center.[1] They do not cause addiction nor CNS depression like the opioid antitussives. They are available OTC.

Nonopioid Antitussives (Locally Acting)

* Anesthetize or numb the stretch receptors and keep the cough reflex from being stimulated in the medulla.[1] Available only by prescription.

Antitussive, Antihistamines

* Antagonize histamine effects at H receptor sites, CNS depressant and anticholinergic effects, and suppress cough. Available OTC.

Opioid Antitussives

* Narcotic analgesics available by prescription only. Suppress the cough reflex through direct action to the medullary cough center, with analgesic effects.[2]

 ## USE

All Antitussives

* Symptomatic relief for nonproductive coughs or in situations (eg, surgical) when coughing may be harmful

 ## ADVERSE EFFECTS AND SIDE EFFECTS

Nonopioid Antitussives

* *Pregnancy category UK*
* *CNS:* Dizziness, drowsiness
* *GI:* Nausea

Nonopioid Antitussives (Locally Acting)

* *Pregnancy category C*
* *CNS:* Dizziness, headache, and sedation

- *Derm:* Pruitus
- *EENT:* Nasal congestion
- *GI:* Constipation, nausea

Antitussive, Antihistamines

- *Pregnancy category B*
- *CNS:* Drowsiness, anticholinergic effects, headache, and dizziness
- *GI:* Dry mouth, anorexia, constipation, and diarrhea
- *Derm:* photosensitivity

Opioid Antitussives

- *Pregnancy category C*
- *CV:* Hypertension
- *CNS:* Confusion, sedation, and headache
- *GI:* Constipation, nausea, and vomiting
- *GU:* Urinary retention
- *Resp:* Respiratory depression

INTERACTIONS

Nonopioid Antitussives

- Concurrent use with MAOIs may cause serotonin syndrome.
- Additive CNS depression with alcohol, antihistamines, anti-depressants, sedative/hypnotics, and opioids

Nonopioid Antitussives (Locally Acting)

- Additive CNS depression with alcohol, antihistamines, sedative/hypnotics, and opioids

Antitussive, Antihistamines

- Additive CNS depression with alcohol, antihistamines, sedative/hypnotics, and opioids

- Additive anticholinergic effects with tricyclic antidepressants, disopyramide, or quinidine
- MAOIs intensify and prolong anticholinergic effects of antihistamines.

Opioid Antitussives

- Additive CNS depression with alcohol, antihistamines, anti-depressants, MAOIs, and sedative/hypnotics

 # CONTRAINDICATIONS

All Antitussives

- Hypersensitivity
- Should not be used for chronic productive coughs

Nonopioid Antitussives

- Clients taking MAOIs or selective serotonin reuptake inhibitors
- May contain alcohol and should be avoided by recovering alcoholics

Nonopioid Antitussives (Locally Acting)

- Cross hypersensitivity to benzonatate or related compounds (tetracaine)[2]

Antitussive, Antihistamines

- Acute asthma attacks
- Lactation
- Liquid products may contain alcohol and should be avoided by recovering alcoholics.

Opioid Antitussives

- Clients with severe respiratory disorders or respiratory depression
- Seizure disorders
- Increased intracranial pressure

NURSING IMPLICATIONS

All Antitussives

- All antitussives are administered orally.
- Assess cough, lung sounds, and type and amount of sputum.

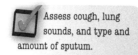

Assess cough, lung sounds, and type and amount of sputum.

Nonopioid Antitussives

- Do not give fluids immediately after administering to prevent dilution of drug.
- Shake oral suspensions before giving.

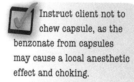

Do not give fluids immediately after administering to prevent dilution of drug.

Nonopioid Antitussives (Locally Acting)

- Instruct client not to chew capsule, as the benzonate from capsules may cause a local anesthetic effect and choking.

Instruct client not to chew capsule, as the benzonate from capsules may cause a local anesthetic effect and choking.

Antitussive, Antihistamine

- See "Nursing Implications" for all antitussives.

Opioid Antitussives

- Assess for constipation.
- Antidote: naloxone (Narcan).
- Prolonged use can lead to physical or psychological dependence.

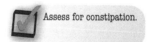

Assess for constipation.

REFERENCES

1. Lilley LL, Harrington S, Snyder J. *Pharmacology and the Nursing Process,* 5th ed. St. Louis, MO: Mosby; 2007:544.

2. Karch A. *Lippincott's Nursing Drug Guide.* Philadelphia, PA: Lippincott, Williams & Wilkins; 2007:318.

3. Karch A. *Lippincott's Nursing Drug Guide.* Philadelphia, PA: Lippincott, Williams & Wilkins; 2007:169.

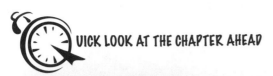

Expectorants stimulate the flow of respiratory tract secretions, which makes the cough more effective. Mucolytics work directly on mucus to make it more watery, which makes the cough more productive.

Efficacy of expectorants is questionable, but they are popular over-the-counter (OTC) drugs that are found in cold and cough preparations. Guaifenesin (Robitussin) is a widely used and popular expectorant. Expectorants can be given as a single agent or in combination with other drugs.

35
Expectorant Drugs

TERMS
☐ guaifenesin (Robitussin, others)
☐ acetylcysteine (Mucomyst)

Table 35-1 Expectorant Drugs

Prototype Drug	Related Drugs	Drug Classification
guaifenesin (Robitussin, others)	There are no related drugs at this time	Expectorants
acetylcysteine (Mucomyst)		Mucolytics (Antidote: acetaminophen [Tylenol]) (cystic fibrosis drug)
	dornase alfa (Pulmozyme)	

EXPECTORANT DRUGS CLIENT TEACHING

- Avoid concurrent use of OTCs and herbal remedies without consulting with physician.
- Dispose of tissues and secretions properly.
- Cough effectively by sitting up, taking several slow deep breaths before coughing.
- Encourage fluid intake to help liquefy secretions, unless contraindicated.
- Report fever, cough, headache, or other symptoms lasting longer than 1 week to health care provider.

Encourage fluid intake to help liquefy secretions, unless contraindicated.

Guaifenesin (Robitussin)

- Liquid product may contain alcohol and sugar, and recovering alcoholics and diabetic clients should avoid use.

Liquid product may contain alcohol and sugar, and recovering alcoholics and diabetic clients should avoid use.

Acetylcysteine (Mucomyst)

- Has a characteristic rotten egg odor due to release of hydrogen sulfide
- Use good oral hygiene during therapy.

Use good oral hygiene during therapy.

ACTION

Expectorants

- Reduces viscosity of secretions by increasing respiratory tract fluid, which mobilizes and allows for expectoration of mucus.

- Also indirectly irritates the gastrointestinal (GI) tract, which can cause nausea and GI upset.

Mucolytics

- Decreases viscosity of pulmonary secretions. Splits links in the respiratory mucoprotein molecules into smaller, more soluble, and less viscous strands.[2]
- In acetaminophen (Tylenol) overdose, it alters hepatic metabolism to decrease liver injury.

 USE

All Expectorants

- Relief of coughs associated with viral upper respiratory tract infections

Mucolytics

- Adjunct treatment of thick tenacious mucus in cystic fibrosis and bronchiopulmonary disease
- Antidote for acetaminophen (Tylenol) toxicity
- Dornase alfa (Pulmozyine) used for management of cystic fibrosis

 ADVERSE EFFECTS AND SIDE EFFECTS

Expectorants

- *Pregnancy category C*
- *GI*: GI upset, nausea, and vomiting

Mucolytics

- *Pregnancy category B*
- *CNS:* Dizziness, drowsiness
- *GI:* Nausea, stomatitis, hepatoxicity, unpleasant odor (sulfur in drug may smell like rotten eggs)
- *Resp:* Bronchospasm, hemoptysis, rhinorrhea

Dornase Alfa (Pulmozyme)

• *Resp:* cough pharyngitis, wheezes
• *Other:* conjunctivitis, chest pain

INTERACTIONS

Expectorants (Guaifenesin [Robitussin])

• None significant

Mucolytics

• Acetylcysteine (Mucomyst) contains hydrogen sulfide and will discolor iron, copper, and harden rubber.

CONTRAINDICATIONS

All Expectorants and Mucolytics

• Hypersensitivity

Expectorants

• Some guaifenesin-containing products contain alcohol and should be avoided by recovering alcoholics.

Mucolytics

• Status asthmaticus and increased intracranial pressure
• Dornase alfa (Pulmozyme) hypersensitivity, chinese hamster ovary cell products

NURSING IMPLICATIONS

All Expectorants and Mucolytics

• Assess lung sounds and cough including: type, frequency, and characteristics.

Assess lung sounds and cough including: type, frequency, and characteristics.

Expectorants

- All expectorants are available orally.

Acetylcysteine (Mucomyst)

- Available by inhalation via nebulizer, instillation via endotracheal tube and orally
- Monitor vital signs.
- Encourage coughing after administering.
- Keep suction equipment at bedside.
- Suction if indicated after treatment (eg, debilitated or elderly clients).
- Maintain good oral hygiene.
- Percussion and postural drainage may assist client in eliminating secretions.
- Administer treatment at least 30 minutes to 1 hour before meals to prevent nausea.
- Use within 48 hours after opening and store in refrigerator.

> ✓ Keep suction equipment at bedside.

> ✓ Administer treatment at least 30 minutes to 1 hour before meals to prevent nausea.

Dornase alfa (Pulmozyme)

- Store in refrigerator and protect from light.
- Review use of nebulizer.

Antidotal Use of Acetylcysteine (Mucomyst)

- Give immediately, if 24 hours or less, since acetaminophen injestion.[1]
- Monitor liver function tests, electrolytes, blood urea nitrogen, acetaminophen levels, and cardiac function.
- Oral use: mix with colar or soft drinks tube use: can be given with water, and use within one hour.[1]

REFERENCES

1. Karch AM. *Lippincott's Nursing Drug Guide*. Philadelphia, PA: Lippincott, Williams & Wilkins; 2007:74.

2. Karch AM. *Lippincott's Nursing Drug Guide*. Philadelphia, PA: Lippincott, Williams & Wilkins; 2008:894.

PART IV · QUESTIONS

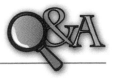

1. Which bronchodilator has selective beta$_2$-agonist effects?
   a. Albuterol (Proventil, Ventolin, Volmax)
   b. Epinephrine (Adrenalin)
   c. Isoproterenol (Isuprel)
   d. Theophylline (Theo-Dur, Slo-Bid)

2. Which of the following is a side effect of theophylline (Theo-Dur, Slo-Bid)?
   a. Increased appetite
   b. Increased intraocular pressure
   c. Hemolytic anemia
   d. Tachycardia

3. All of the following should be included in a teaching plan for a client taking theophylline (Theo-Dur, Slo-Bid) EXCEPT:
   a. Minimize caffeine intake.
   b. Take drug with food if GI upset occurs.
   c. Notify the health care provider if there is an increase in appetite.
   d. Do not crush or chew enteric coated or sustained-release form of drug.

4. Which of the following drugs is indicated for prophylaxsis of asthma and may take up to 4 weeks to be effective?
   a. Cromolyn (Intal, Nasalcrom)
   b. Beclomethasone (Beclovent, Vanceril)
   c. Ipratropium (Atrovent)
   d. Zafirlukast (Accolate)

5. Of the following, which antiasthmatic drug may cause oral fungal infections?
   a. Cromolyn (Nasalcrom)
   b. Beclomethasone dipropionate (Vanceril)
   c. Ipratropium bromide (Atrovent)
   d. Zafirlukast (Accolate)

6. Which of the following should the nurse include when teaching a client taking zafirlukast (Accolate)?
   a. Take with food.
   b. Double up on a dose if missed.
   c. Discontinue taking if symptom-free.
   d. Periodic liver function testing may be required.

7. Antihistamines used to treat motion sickness should be given at least how long before exposure to motion?
   a. 10 minutes
   b. 15 minutes
   c. 20 minutes
   d. 30 minutes

8. Which of the following adverse effects is more commonly seen in first generation antihistamines than in second generation antihistamines?
   a. Drowsiness
   b. GI upset
   c. Photosensitivity
   d. Weight gain

9. Which of the following should be included in teaching plan for a client taking decongestants?
   a. Take at bedtime.
   b. For best effects, use topical decongestants for at least 7 days.
   c. Limit fluid intake.
   d. Avoid caffeine during therapy.

10. Which of the following are adverse effects of decongestants?
    a. Bradycardia
    b. Hypotension
    c. Nervousness
    d. Neutropenia

11. Which antitussive is thought to work by anesthetizing or numbing the cough receptors?
    a. Benzonatate (Tessalon)
    b. Codeine (Dimetane-DC, Tussar SF)
    c. Dextromethorphan (Vicks Formula 44, Robitussin-DM)
    d. Diphenydramine (Benylin Cough Syrup)

12. Which of the following antitussives should be swallowed without chewing, as chewing may cause an anesthetic effect on the oral mucosa?
    a. Benzonatate (Tessalon)
    b. Codeine (Dimetane-DC, Tussar SF)
    c. Dextromethorphan (Vicks Formula 44, Robitussin-DM)
    d. Diphenydramine (Benylin Cough Syrup)

13. Which should be included in a teaching care plan for a client taking an antitussive?
    a. Restrict fluids.
    b. Encourage the client to drink water immediately after taking a cough syrup.
    c. Encourage the client to take an antitussive for a productive cough.
    d. Avoid drinking alcohol while taking an antitussive.

14. Which drug may cause a rotten egg odor due to its release of hydrogen sulfide?
    a. Acetylcysteine (Mucomyst)
    b. Acetaminophen (Tylenol)
    c. Codeine (Dimetane-DC, Tussar SF)
    d. Guaifenesin (Robitussin, others)

PART IV • ANSWERS

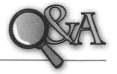

1. **The correct answer is a.** Albuterol (Proventil) is a selective beta$_2$-agonist. Epinephrine has nonselective alpha, beta$_1$, and beta$_2$ effects, isoproterenol (Isuprel) has nonselective beta$_1$ and beta$_2$ effects, and theophylline (Theo-Dur, Slo-Bid) is a xanthine derivative.

2. **The correct answer is d.** Tachycardia is a side effect of theophylline (Theo-Dur, Slo-Bid). Increased intraocular pressure and hemolytic anemia are not side effects of theophylline. Anorexia is also a side effect of theophylline.

3. **The correct answer is c.** Theophylline (Theo-dur, Slo-Bid) may cause a decrease in appetite. Caffeine intake should be minimized to reduce cardiac or CNS effects. The client can take with food if GI upset occurs. Enteric-coated or sustained release forms of the drug should not be crushed or chewed.

4. **The correct answer is a.** Cromolyn (Intal, Nasalcrom) is a mast cell stabilizer, used in prophylaxis of asthma, and may take up to 4 weeks to be effective.

5. **The correct answer is b.** Beclomethasone (Beclovent, Vanceril) is a synthetic glucocorticoid that may cause oral fungal infections. It is important that the nurse instruct the client to rinse mouth and mouthpiece after administration of drug to prevent oral fungal infections.

6. **The correct answer is d.** Periodic liver function testing may be required as zafirlukast (Accolate) may cause hepatic dysfunction. Zafirlukast should be taken on an empty stomach, doses should not be doubled up if missed, and clients should continue taking if symptom-free.

7. **The correct answer is d.** Antihistamines used to treat motion sickness should be given at least 30 minutes before exposure to motion.

8. **The correct answer is a.** Drowsiness is more commonly seen in first generation antihistamines. Second generation antihistamines do not cross the blood brain barrier, which reduces drowsiness. GI upset and photosensitivity are seen with both categories of antihistamines. Weight gain may be seen as an adverse effect of loratadine, a second generation antihistamine.

9. **The correct answer is d.** Caffeine can cause cardiac stimulation, which is also an adverse effect of decongestants (sympathomimetics). Decongestants can cause insomnia and should not be taken at bedtime. Topical decongestants can cause rebound hypertension with repeated use and should not be used for more than 3 to 5 days. Unless contraindicated, fluid intake should be encouraged.

10. **The correct answer is c.** Decongestants are sympathomimetics and can cause tachycardia, hypertension, and nervousness. Neutropenia is not an adverse effect of decongestants.

11. **The correct answer is a.** Benzonatate (Tessalon) is thought to work by anesthetizing or numbing the cough receptors. Codeine, Dextromethorphan (Vicks Formula 44, Robitussin-DM), Diphyenydramine (Benylin Cough Syrup) directly suppress the cough reflex through a direct action on the cough center.

12. **The correct answer is a.** Benzonatate (Tessalon) should not be chewed, as chewing may cause an anesthetic effect on the oral mucosa.

13. **The correct answer is d.** Clients should avoid drinking alcohol while taking an antitussive to prevent further CNS depression, such as drowsiness and sedation.

    Fluids should be encouraged unless contraindicated for the client. The client should not drink water immediately after taking a cough syrup but should wait to prevent diluting the antitussive agent and antitussives are indicated for a dry nonproductive cough.

14. **The correct answer is a.** Acetylcysteine (Mucomyst) is a mucolytic agent and may release hydrogen sulfide and cause a rotten egg odor. Acetylcysteine (Mucomyst) is also the antidote for acetaminophen (Tylenol) overdose.

V

Anti-Inflammatory and Antirheumatoid Drugs

Marilyn J. Herbert-Ashton, MS, RN, BC

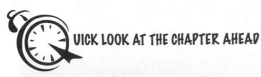

Nonsteroidal anti-inflammatory drugs (NSAIDs) have analgesic, antipyretic, anti-inflammatory, and anti-platelet effects. The NSAIDs are one of the most frequently prescribed groups of drugs, and include a variety of drugs.

Salicylic acid was the first drug in this class to be identified, and in 1899 aspirin became available and widely used. NSAIDs were developed because of aspirin's adverse effects including gastric irritation, bleeding, and renal impairment. NSAIDs are generally better tolerated and associated with less serious toxic effects, especially in clients with chronic diseases.[1]

36
Nonsteroidal Anti-Inflammatory Drugs (NSAIDs)

TERMS
☐ acetylsalicylic acid (aspirin, ASA, others)
☐ ibuprofen (Motrin, Advil, others)
☐ indomethacin (Indocin)
☐ celecoxib (Celebrex)

Table 36-1 Nonsteroidal Anti-Inflammatory Drugs (NSAIDs)

Prototype Drug	Related Drugs	Drug Classification
acetylsalicylic acid (aspirin, ASA, several product names)	choline magnesium (Tricosal) choline salicylate (Anthropan) balsalazide (Colazal) diflunisal (Dolobid) mesalamine (Pentasa, others) magnesium salicylate (Magan) olsalazine (Dipentum) salsalate (Disalcid, others) sodium salicylate (Dodd's Pills) sodium thiosalicylate (Rexolate)	Salicylates
ibuprofen (Motrin, Advil, others)	fenoprofen (Nalfon) flurbiprofen (Ansaid) ketropfen (Orudis) naproxen (Naprosyn, Aleve) oxaprozin (Daypro)	Propionic acids
indomethacin (Indocin)	diclofenac potassium (Cataflam) diclofenac sodium (Voltaren) etodolac (Lodine) ketorolac (Toradol) sulindac (Clinoril) tolmetin (Tolectin)	Acetic acids
celecoxib (Celebrex)	There are no related drugs at this time	Cyclooxygenase-2 enzyme inhibitors (COX-2 inhibitors)
There is no prototype for this classification	piroxicam (Feldene) meloxicam (Mobic)	Oxicams
There is no prototype for this classification	diflunisal (Dolobid) meclofenamate (Meclomen) mefenamic acid (Ponstel)	Fenamic acids
There is no prototype for this classification	nabumetone (Relafen)	Nonacidic NSAIDs (namphthylalkanone)

NONSTEROIDAL ANTI-INFLAMMATORY DRUGS CLIENT TEACHING CLOSER LOOKS

- NSAIDs generally cause gastrointestinal (GI) upset and can be taken with a full glass of fluid or food.
- Report signs of bleeding: nose, gums emesis, stool, urine, and petechiae; rash; ringing in ears; dizziness; difficulty breathing; or severe upset stomach.
- Avoid combined use of alcohol, aspirin, anticoagulants, thrombolytic agents, or other OTC or prescription-use NSAIDs to prevent increased risk of bleeding.
- Clients with aspirin sensitivity should avoid taking NSAIDs, as there may be a cross sensitivity.
- Inform health care provider of medication regime before surgery, treatment, or dental procedures.
- Do not crush or take enteric-coated tablets with dairy products or antacids.
- To prevent Reye's syndrome, avoid giving aspirin to children under age 18.
- Consult with health care provider before taking herbals as some may cause an increased risk of bleeding.

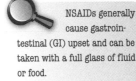

NSAIDs generally cause gastrointestinal (GI) upset and can be taken with a full glass of fluid or food.

Clients with aspirin sensitivity should avoid taking NSAIDs, as there may be a cross sensitivity.

ACTION

Aspirin and NSAIDs block the effects of prostaglandins by inhibiting the enzyme cyclooxygenase. Cyclooxygenase initiates the formation of prostaglandins from arachidonic acid. By blocking prostaglandins, undesirable effects such as pain and inflammation are relieved. NSAIDs act on the hypothalamus to inhibit prostaglandin E_2 to produce an antipyretic effect. NSAIDs, including aspirin, have antiplatelet effects, but vary in degree and mechanism. For example, aspirin has antiplatelet effects for the life span of the platelets, because it binds irreversibly with cyclooxygenase. This binding prevents synthesis of thromboxane A$_2$, while other NSAID antiplatelet effects last only while the drug is in the bloodstream, because they reversibly bind with cyclooxygenase.

The COX-2 inhibitors target COX-2 prostaglandins without interfering with COX-1 prostaglandins. There are fewer GI effects including bleeding, as well as less frequent administration with COX-2 inhibitors.

USE

Salicylates

- Mild to moderate pain, antipyretic, inflammatory disorders including rheumatoid arthritis and osteoarthritis, and prophylaxis of myocardial infarction, transischemic attacks, and other thromboembolic disorders
- Balsalazide (Colazal) used to treat mild to moderate acute ulcerative colitis
- Osalazine (Dipentum) and mesalamine (Pentasa, others) used to treat ulceratine colitus and inflammatory bowel desease
- Sodium thiosalicylate (Rexolate) used to treat acute gout, rheumatic fever, and muscular pain

Propionic Acid NSAIDs

Ibuprofen (Advil, Motrin)

- Mild to moderate pain, dysmenorrhea, and antipyretic inflammatory disorders including rheumatoid arthritis and osteoarthritis

Acetic Acid NSAIDs

Indomethacin (Indocin)

- Closure of patent ductus arteriosis (PDA), antirheumatic, and gout. Due to the potential for toxicity, indomethacin is not routinely used for analgesic and antipyretic effects, and is available only by prescription.

Ketorolac (Toradol)

- Little anti-inflammatory action, but is a potent analgesic similar to opioid analgesics. Used as a short-term (up to 5 days) analgesic that can be given orally, IV, IM, or ophthalmically and is the only NSAID that can be given via these routes.

COX-2 Inhibitors

Celecoxib (Celebrex)

- Rheumatoid arthritis and osteoarthritis

Oxicams

Piroxicam (Feldene)

- Rheumatoid arthritis and osteoarthritis

Meloxicam (Mobic)

- Osteoarthritis

Fenamic Acids

- Older agents and not used commonly

Meclofenamic Acid (Meclomen)

- Mild to moderate pain, rheumatoid arthritis, osteoarthritis, primary dysmenorrhea

Mefenamic Acid (Ponstel)

- Moderate pain and primary dysmenorrhea

Nonacidic NSAIDs (Naphthylalkanone)

- Relatively new NSAID

Nabumetone (Relafen)

- Rheumatoid arthritis and osteoarthritis

ADVERSE EFFECTS AND SIDE EFFECTS

Salicylates

- *Pregnancy category C, Aspirin category D, Mesalamine (Pentasa, others) category B.*

Aspirin

- Most common: Gastric distress, heartburn, nausea, GI bleeding, GI ulceration
- GI effects appear to be more common with aspirin use than with other NSAIDs
- Salicylism, which includes tinnitus, dizziness, headache, sweating, compensated respiratory alkalosis, and metabolic acidosis
- Increased bleeding time, anemia from blood loss, hypersensitivity, and Reye's syndrome
- Reye's syndrome is associated with the use of aspirin by children with influenza and chickenpox.

Propionic Acid NSAIDs

- *Pregnancy category B (category D in third trimester)*

Ibuprofen (Advil, Motrin)

- *CNS:* Headache, dizziness, and drowsiness; psychic effects
- *CV:* Edema, dysrhythmias
- *EENT:* Tinnitus, hearing loss, blurred vision
- *GI:* Bleeding, nausea, vomiting, abdominal discomfort, dyspepsia, and epigastric distress
- *GU:* Nephrotoxicity
- *Hematologic:* Prolonged bleeding times, blood dyscrasias
- *Other:* Hypersensitivity, hepatitis

Acetic Acid NSAIDs

- *Pregnancy category B drugs include indomethacin (Indocin), diclofenac potassium (Cataflam), diclofenac sodium (Voltaren), tolmetin (Tolectin); pregnancy category C drugs include etodolac (Lodine) and ketorolac (Toradol), but are category D in third trimester; and included in pregnancy category UK is sulindac (Clinoril), which is category D in third trimester.*

COX-2 Inhibitors

- *Pregnancy category C*
- *GI:* Produces few GI effects, but GI bleeding and epigastric discomfort, nausea, dyspepsia have occurred
- *Other:* Potential for increased cardiovascular events, hypertension, edema, dizziness, fatigue, and rash

Oxicams

- *Pregnancy category D*
- Potent drugs that tend to produce severe GI toxicities

Fenamic Acids

- *Pregnancy category B drugs include meclofenamic acid (Meclomen); pregnancy category C includes mefenamic acid (Ponstel) and diflunisal (Dolobid). These drugs are category D in third trimester.*

Nonacidic NSAIDs (Naphthylalkanone)

- *Pregnancy category C (category D in third trimester)*
- Produce less GI effects, but GI bleeding and abdominal pain, diarrhea, nausea, and dyspepsia can occur
- See ibuprofen for other adverse and side effects.

 INTERACTIONS

Salicylates and NSAIDs

- Concurrent use with alcohol, salicylates, and other NSAIDs may increase risk of GI bleeding.
- Concurrent use with anticoagulants and thrombolytics may increase risk of bleeding.

- Concurrent use with loop diuretics decreases diuretic effects.
- Concurrent use with beta-blockers decreases antihypertensive effect.
- Concurrent use with corticosteroids may increase ulcerogenic effects.
- Salicylates can increase serum alkaline phosphatase, alanine aminotransferease (ALT), and aspartate aminotransferease (AST).

CONTRAINDICATIONS

Salicylates and NSAIDs

- Hypersensitivity
- Cross sensitivity with salicylates and other NSAIDs
- Active GI bleeding and ulcer disease
- Use cautiously with clients with renal, hepatic, and cardiovascular disease.
- Pregnancy, especially in the third trimester, and lactation

Salicylates

- History of bleeding
- Vitamin K deficiency
- Children under age 12 or children with flu-like conditions

NSAIDs

- Asthma

NURSING IMPLICATIONS

- Monitor for gastric distress and bleeding.
- Monitor vital signs for hypertension (due to fluid retention) and dysrhythmias.
- Discard aspirin if it smells like vinegar (acetic acid).

 Monitor for gastric distress and bleeding.

 Monitor vital signs for hypertension (due to fluid retention) and dysrhythmias.

- Clients with a history of nasal polyps, asthma, and allergies are at increased risk to develop hypersensitivity reactions.
- Monitor renal and hepatic and blood studies.
- Monitor for therapeutic effects: reduction in pain, fever, and range of motion for clients with arthritis at least 1 to 2 hours after administering.
- For clients taking aspirin, teach them the signs of salicylism and to contact their health care provider if symptoms occur.
- The elderly are more prone to adverse effects, so lower doses may be indicated.

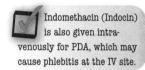

Indomethacin (Indocin) is also given intravenously for PDA, which may cause phlebitis at the IV site.

- Indomethacin (Indocin) is also given intravenously for PDA, which may cause phlebitis at the IV site.
- Ketolorlac (Toradol) is available PO, IV, or IM.

REFERENCE

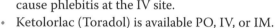

1. Lilley L, Harrington S, Snyder J. *Pharmacology and the Nursing Process,* 5th ed. St. Louis, MO: Mosby; 2007:677.

Although nonsteroidal anti-inflammatory drugs (NSAIDs) are used in treatment of rheumatoid arthritis, the antirheumatoid drugs have different effects. Antirheumatoid drugs, in addition to their anti-inflammatory and antiarthritic effects, also have immunomodulating effects, which prevent the movement of various cells into inflamed, damaged areas.[1] This halts the progression of the disease and reduces inflammatory symptoms.

Antirheumatoid drugs are also known as disease-modifying antirheumatoid drugs (DMARD). They have a slow onset of action and are generally given over long periods of time.

37

Antirheumatoid Drugs

TERMS
- ☐ hydroxychloroquine (Plaquenil)
- ☐ methotrexate (Rheumatrex)
- ☐ aurothioglucose (Solganal)

Table 37-1 Antirheumatoid Drugs

Prototype Drug	Related Drugs	Drug Classification
hydroxychloroquine (Plaquenil)		Disease modifying antirheumatics (DMARDs) Also an antimalarial
	anakinra (Kineret)	Also an interleukin-1 receptor antagonist
	infliximab (Remicade)	Also a monoclonal antibody and tumor necrosis factor (TNF) blocker
	adalimumab (Humira)	TNF blocker
methotrexate (Rheumatrex)	etanercept (Enbrel)	Also an antineoplastic, immunosuppressant, and TNF blocker
	lefunomide (Arava)	Also an antineoplastic and immuno-suppressant
	penicillamine (Cuprimine)	Also an aniturolithic and antidote (chelating agent)
aurothioglucose (Solganal)	auranofin (Ridaura) gold sodium thiomalate (Myochrysine)	Gold compounds

 ## Antirheumatoid Drugs Client Teaching

- Antirheumatoid drugs are generally given until remission, followed by maintenance doses indefinitely.
- Take antirheumatoids as prescribed and consult with health care provider before taking OTCs or herbal products.
- Use sunscreen and protective clothing to prevent photosensitivity reactions.
- Use a soft toothbrush to brush teeth.
- Avoid use of antirheumatoid agents during pregnancy and lactation.
- Periodic laboratory tests are indicated to monitor for side effects of antirheumatoids, including liver and renal function studies, CBC, and platelets.

> Periodic laboratory tests are indicated to monitor for side effects of antirheumatoids, including liver and renal function studies, CBC, and platelets.

- Report symptoms of upper respiratory infection, sore throat, fever, bleeding/bruising, dyspnea, wheezing, or cough to health care provider.
- Monitor for skin reactions such as rash, dermatitis, pruritus, stomatitis, and report to health care provider.

Report symptoms of upper respiratory infection, sore throat, fever, bleeding/bruising, dyspnea, wheezing, or cough to health care provider.

Hydroxychloroquine (Plaquenil)

- Baseline and periodic ophthalmic exams.

Baseline and periodic ophthalmic exams.

Penicillamine (Cuprimine)

- Taste acuity may be altered.

Taste acuity may be altered.

Methotrexate (Rheumatrex), Etanercept (Enbrel), Leflunomide (Arava), adalimumab (Humira), anakinra (Kineret)

- Avoid vaccinations with live vaccines during therapy.

Avoid vaccinations with live vaccines during therapy.

Leflunomide (Arava)

- May cause dizziness and clients should avoid activities requiring alertness (driving, operating heavy machinery) until reaction to drug is known

May cause dizziness and clients should avoid activities requiring alertness (driving, operating heavy machinery) until reaction to drug is known

ACTION

Disease-Modifying Antirheumatic Drugs

Hydroxychloroquine (Plaquenil)

- Antimalarial agent, with anti-inflammatory effects. The exact action is unknown. It may take up to 6 months to see therapeutic effects.

Anakinra (Kineret)

* Blocks activity of interleukin-1 (IL-1)

Infliximab (Remicade)

* Interferes with the effects of tumor necrosis factor (TNF).

Adaliumab (Humira)

* Interferes with the effects of TNF.

Anakinra (Kineret)

* Rheumatoid arthritis unresponsive to other DMARDs.

Infliximab (Remicade)

* Moderate to severe rheumatoid arthritis and Crohn's disease.

Adalimumab (Humira)

* Rheumatoid arthritis is unresponsive to other DMARDs in patients over age 18.

Methotrexate (Rheumatrex)

* An antineoplastic and immunosuppressant agent
* Therapeutic effects may be seen in 3 to 6 weeks.
* Interferes with folic acid metabolism and has immunosuppressant effects

Etanercept (Enbrel)

* Binds and neutralizes TNF.
* It may be used concurrently with methotrexate.

Leflunomide (Arava)

* Has antiproliferative, anti-inflammatory, and immunosuppresive effects

Penicillamine (Cuprimine)

* Also an antiurolithic and antidote for chelating agents
* Antirheumatic effects: exact mechanism of action is unknown.

Gold Compounds

* It may take 4 to 6 months to see therapeutic effects.

Auranofin (Ridaura)

- Anti-inflammatory, antirheumatic, and immunomodulating effects. Contains 29% active gold compound.

Aurothioglucose (Solganal) and Gold Sodium Thiomalate (Myochrysine)

- Anti-inflammatory, antirheumatic, and immunomodulating effects. Contains 50% active gold compound.

 USE

Disease-Modifying Antirheumatic Drugs

Hydroxychloroquine (Plaquenil)

- Severe rheumatoid arthritis

Anakinra (Kineret)

- Rheumatoid arthritis unresponsive to other DMARDs.

Infliximab (Remicade)

- Moderate to severe rheumatoid arthritis and Crohn's disease.

Adalimumab (Humira)

- Rheumatoid arthritis is unresponsive to other DMARDs in patients over age 18.

Methotrexate (Rheumatrex)

- Severe rheumatoid arthritis

Etanercept (Enbrel)

- Moderate to severe rheumatoid arthritis for patients who have responded inadequately to other disease-modifying antirheumatics

Leflunomide (Arava)

- Active rheumatoid arthritis

Penicillamine (Cuprimine)

- Rheumatoid arthritis that has not responded adequately to conventional therapy

Gold Compounds

- Rheumatoid arthritis and may prevent joint degeneration. It is most useful if given before joint degeneration occurs.

ADVERSE EFFECTS AND SIDE EFFECTS

Disease-Modifying Antirheumatic Drugs

Hydroxychloroquine (Plaquenil)

- *Pregnancy category C*
- *Derm:* Dermatitis, pruritus
- *EENT:* The most serious toxicity is retinopathy. May also see visual disturbances
- *GI:* Nausea, vomiting, diarrhea, abdominal cramping, and hepatotoxicity
- *Hematologic:* Agranulocytosis, aplastic anemia

Anakinra (Kineret)

- *Pregnancy category B*
- *CNS:* Headache, dizziness, seizures
- *Derm:* Injection site reaction
- *GI:* nausea, vomiting
- *Hematologic:* neutropenia
- *Other:* serious infections

Infliximab (Remicade)

- *Pregnancy category B*
- *CV:* Heart failure
- *CNS:* Headache, dizziness, seizures
- *Derm:* Rash, urticaria
- *GI:* nausea, vomiting, abdominal pain
- *Hematologic:* Anemia
- *Other:* Anaphylaxis

Adalimumab (Humira)

- *Pregnancy category B*
- *CNS:* Headache

- *Derm:* Injection site reaction
- *GI:* Abdominal pain, nausea
- *Other:* Serious infections, anaphylaxis

Methotrexate (Rheumatrex)

- *Pregnancy category X*
- *Derm:* Pruritus, allopecia, urticaria, and photosensitivity
- *EENT:* Blurred vision
- *GI:* Hepatoxicity, nausea, vomiting, and stomatitis
- *Hematologic:* Thrombocytopenia, leukopenia
- *GU:* Nephropathy
- *Resp:* Pulmonary fibrosis

Etanercept (Enbrel)

- *Pregnancy category B*
- Most common side effect is an injection site reaction that usually subsides in 3 to 5 days.
- *Resp:* Upper respiratory tract infection, cough, rhinitis, pharyngitis, and sinusitis

Leflunomide (Arava)

- *Pregnancy category X*
- *Derm:* Alopecia, rash
- *GI:* Diarrhea, elevated liver enzymes
- *Resp:* Respiratory tract infection

Penicillamine (Cuprimine)

- *Pregnancy category D*
- *Derm:* Dermatologic disorders, rash, and hypersensitivity
- *EENT:* Blurred vision
- *GI:* Altered taste, diarrhea, and hepatoxicity
- *GU:* Proteinuria
- *Hematologic:* Thrombocytopenia leukopenia, aplastic anemia

Gold Compounds

- *Pregnancy category C*
- *Derm:* Dermatitis, rash, pruritus, hypersensitivity reactions with Aurothioglucose (Solganal) and gold sodium thiomalate (Myochrysine)

- *GI:* Diarrhea, nausea, stomatitis, abdominal cramping, increased liver enzymes
- *GU:* Proteinuria, hematuria, tubular necrosis with Aurothioglucose (Solganal) and gold sodium thiomalate (Myochrysine)
- *Hematologic:* Thrombobycytopenia, agranulocytosis, leukopenia
- *Resp:* Interstitial pneumonitis, cough

 INTERACTIONS

Disease-Modifying Antirheumatic Drugs

- Concurrent use with other hepatotoxic drugs increases risk of hepatoxicity.

Hydroxychloroquine (Plaquenil)

- Hematologic toxicity is increased if taken with penicillamine.

Anakinra (Kineret)

- Do not give with live vaccines.
- Risk of severe infection increases if given with etanercept and Tumor Necrosis Factor (TNF) blocking agents.

Infliximab (Remicade)

- Do not give with live vaccines.

Adalimumab (Humira)

- Do not give with live vaccines.

Methotrexate (Rheumatrex)

- Avoid concurrent use with NSAIDs. NSAIDs increase toxicity of methotrextate.
- Concurrent use with echinacea decreases the effects of methotrexate.

Penicillamine (Cuprimine)

- Cross sensitivity with penicillin may exist.
- Avoid administering with iron or antacids, as iron and antacids decreases absorption of penicillamine.

Gold Compounds

- Increased risk of severe toxicity with concurrent use with anti-malarials, cytotoxic, immunosuppressive, or penicillamine.

CONTRAINDICATIONS

Disease-Modifying Antirheumatic Drugs

- Hypersensitivity
- Pregnancy and lactation
- Acute infection
- Cautious use with history of liver disease, alcoholism, or renal disease

Gold Compounds

- Hypersensitivity to gold
- Blood dyscrasias
- Severe diabetes millitus
- Impaired renal or hepatic function
- Congestive heart failure and hypertension
- Recent radiation therapy
- Pregnancy or lactation

NURSING IMPLICATIONS

For All Antirheumatoids

- Assess client periodically for pain, swelling, and range of motion.

Disease-Modifying Antirheumatic Drugs

Hydroxychloroquine (Plaquenil)

- Give PO.
- Monitor CBC and platelet counts for agranulocytosis and aplastic anemia.
- Avoid using in clients with psoriasis as it may precipitate an attack.

- Administer with food or milk to decrease gastrointestinal effects.
- Avoid alcohol while taking hydroxycholorquine.
- Children are more apt to develop toxic effects than adults.

Anakinra (Kineret)

- Available SC.
- Do not use if solution is cloudy, discolored, or if a particulate is present.
- Do not use a filter and protect from light.
- Neutrophil counts should be monitored throughout therapy.

Infliximab (Remicade)

- Available IV
- Give over 2 hours.
- Monitor CBC and vital signs.
- Do not give if patient has an active infection.
- Monitor for infection.
- Monitor for anaphylaxis.

Adalimumab (Humira)

- Available SC.
- Monitor for infection.

Methotrexate (Rheumatrex)

- Give PO for rheumatoid arthritis
- Monitor renal and liver function studies and CBC.
- Monitor for symptoms of pulmonary toxicity, which may begin with a nonproductive cough.
- Assess for bleeding, check stools for occult blood, and use soft toothbrush to brush teeth.

Etanercept (Enbrel)

- Needle cover contains latex: avoid handling if you have latex allergies.
- Administer SC in the upper arm, abdomen, or thigh.

Leflunomide (Arava)

- Give PO.
- Monitor liver function tests.

- Treatment of severe toxicity or overdose; in this case, cholestyramine or activated charcoal acts as an antidote
- Use of aspirin, low-dose corticosteroids, and NSAIDs may be used during leflunomide therapy.

Penicillamine (Cuprimine)

- Give PO.
- Monitor I & O and weight.
- Monitor CBC, platelets, urine for protein, and liver function tests.
- Monitor for allergic reaction; cross sensitivity with penicillin may exist.
- Administer at least 1 hour before meals or 2 hours after meals.
- Clients with impaired nutrition may need pyridoxine (Vitamin B_6) supplements.

Gold Compounds

Auranofin (Ridaura) Oral Use

- Give PO.
- Aurothioglucose (Solganal) and gold sodium thiomalate (Myochrysine) IM use
- Monitor CBC, platelets, urine for protein, hematuria, and liver enzymes.
- Monitor intake and output.
- Monitor respiratory status.
- Monitor for bleeding and rashes.

Aurothioglucose (Solganal) and Gold Sodium Thiomalate (Myochrysine)

- Given deep IM and IV.
- Keep client recumbent for 10 minutes after injection and monitor for a vasomotor response.

REFERENCE

1. Lilley LL, Harrington S, Snyder J. *Pharmacology and the Nursing Process,* 5th ed. St. Louis, MO: Mosby; 2007:684.

Gout is an inflammatory disorder that results in acute joint pain and is associated with impaired uric acid metabolism. This causes hyperuricemia, which can be a result of increased serum uric acid levels or impaired uric acid excretion. Uric acid is the end product of purine metabolism. Purines are found in certain foods such as organ meats; consequently, gout was once known as the "rich man's disease." When purines are metabolized, they are converted from hypoxanthine to xanthine and then to uric acid. When uric acid levels are elevated, this may cause the uric acid crystals to collect in the tissues and joints and cause pain.[1]

Nonsteroidal anti-inflammatory drugs (NSAIDs) and glucocorticoids may also be used to treat gout. The NSAIDs are discussed in Chapter 36 and glucocorticoids in Chapter 51.

38
Antigout Drugs

TERM
☐ allopurinal (Zyloprim)

Table 38-1 Antigout Drugs

Prototype Drug	Related Drugs	Drug Classification
allopurinal (Zyloprim)	There are no related drugs at this time	Xanthine oxidase inhibitor
There is no prototype for this classification	colchicine	Colchicum autumnale alkaloid
There is no prototype tor this classification	probenecid (Benemid) sulfinpyrazone (Anturane)	uricosuric (Pyrazolone)

ANTIGOUT DRUGS CLIENT TEACHING

- Take medication exactly as prescribed.
- If a dose is missed, remember to take as soon as remembered.
- Increase fluid intake to at least 2000 mL/day to prevent urate stone formation.
- Follow an alkaline diet if ordered to prevent urate stone formation.
- Follow health care provider's instructions regarding diet therapy and decreasing alcohol consumption.
- Promptly report sore throats, bruising, petechiae, bleeding, fatigue, diarrhea, abdominal pain, and rash to the health care provider.
- Do not take aspirin with probenecid (Benemid) or sulfinpyrazone (Anturane) as it decreases the effectiveness of probenecid and sulfinpyrazone.

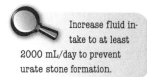

Increase fluid intake to at least 2000 mL/day to prevent urate stone formation.

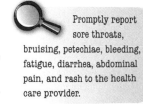

Promptly report sore throats, bruising, petechiae, bleeding, fatigue, diarrhea, abdominal pain, and rash to the health care provider.

Allopurinal (Zyloprim)

- May cause drowsiness and, thus, clients should not drive or operate heavy machinery until response to drug is known.

ACTION

Allopurinol (Zyloprim)

- Inhibits uric acid production and lowers serum uric acid levels.

Colchicine

- Not fully understood. Inhibits leukocyte migration.

Probenecid (Benemid) and Sulfinpyrazone (Anturane)

- Increases the excretion of uric acid in urine. Note: sulfinpyrazone is chemically similar to phenylbutazone.

USE

Allopurinol (Zyloprim)

- Used orally to treat chronic gout, and orally or IV to treat secondary hyperuricemia related to malignancies

Colchicine

- Used orally or IV to treat acute gout attacks and prophylactically for gout attacks

Probenecid (Benemid)

- Used orally in prophylaxis of gout attacks. Can worsen an acute gout attack and should not be given until the attack subsides. Also used to prolong effects of penicillin and related anti-infectives

Sulfinpyrazone (Anturane)

- Used orally to treat chronic gout. Also used to inhibit platelet aggregation

ADVERSE EFFECTS AND SIDE EFFECTS

Allopurinol (Zyloprim)

- *Pregnancy category C*
- *CNS:* Occasional drowsiness, headache
- *Derm:* Hypersensitivity, rash, fever, exfoliative dermatitis
- *GI:* Nausea, vomiting, diarrhea, and hepatitis
- *Hematologic:* Blood dyscrasias

Colchicine

- *Pregnancy category D*
- *GI:* Effects are most common and may cause nausea, vomiting, diarrhea, and abdominal pain
- *Hematologic:* Agranulcytosis thrombocytopenia
- *Renal:* Renal failure

Probenecid (Benemid)

- *Pregnancy category B*
- *CNS:* Headache
- *Derm:* Rash
- *Hematologic:* Aplastic anemia

Sulfinpyrazone (Anturane)

- *Pregnancy category C*
- *CNS:* Dizziness
- *Derm:* Rash
- *GI:* Effect most common and may include nausea, vomiting, abdominal pain, GI bleeding, and hepatic necrosis
- *Hematologic:* Rare agranulocytosis

INTERACTIONS

Allopurinol (Zyloprim)

- Increases action of oral anticoagulants, oral hypoglycemic agents, mercaptopurine, and azanthioprine
- The risk of rash increases if also taking ampicillin or amoxicillin.

Colchicine

- Avoid concurrent use of NSAIDs as they may cause additive GI effects.
- Concurrent use with bone marrow depressants, and radiation may cause increased bone marrow depression.

Probenecid (Benemid)

- Avoid aspirin use as aspirin decreases effects of probenecid.
- Increases blood levels of NSAIDs, allopurinol, penicillins, sulfon-amides, oral hypoglycemic agents. Note: there are multiple drug interactions.

Sulfinpyrazone (Anturane)

- Avoid aspirin use as aspirin decreases effects of sulfinpyrazone.
- Sulfinpyrazone increases the effects of warfarin and tolbutamide.

 ## CONTRAINDICATIONS

All Antigout Drugs

- Hypersensitivity

Probenecid (Benemid)

- Contraindicated in clients taking chronic high dose salicylate therapy

Sulfinpyrazone (Anturane)

- Peptic ulcer disease

NURSING IMPLICATIONS

Allopurinol (Zyloprim)

- Take with food to minimize GI irritation.
- Monitor CBC, uric acid levels, blood urea nitrogen, creatinine, aspartate aminotransferase, and liver function studies.
- Monitor I & O.
- Encourage a low purine diet (food high in purines: organ meats, turkey, venison, beer, codfish, anchovies, bacon).

Take with food to minimize GI irritation.

Monitor CBC, uric acid levels, blood urea nitrogen, creatinine, aspartate aminotransferase (AST), and liver function studies.

Monitor I & O.

Colchicine

- Administer on an empty stomach to promote absorption.
- Monitor I & O.
- Monitor for phlebitis with IV use.
- Monitor CBC, platelets.
- Monitor for toxicity symptoms (eg, nausea, vomiting, diarrhea, and abdominal pain).

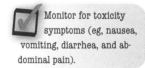
Monitor for toxicity symptoms (eg, nausea, vomiting, diarrhea, and abdominal pain).

Probenecid (Benemid)

- Give with food to decrease GI effects
- Monitor I & O.
- Monitor CBC, uric acid, liver, and renal function.
- Do not administer until acute attack subsides.
- Encourage fluid intake of at least 2000 mL daily.

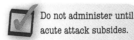
Do not administer until acute attack subsides.

Sulfinpyrazone (Anturane)

Give with food to decrease GI effects.

- Give with food to decrease GI effects.
- Encourage fluid intake of at least 2000 mL daily.

- Monitor intake and output.
- Avoid foods high in purines.
- Monitor CBC and uric acid levels.

REFERENCE

1. Lilley L, Harrington S, Snyder J. *Pharmacology and the Nursing Process*, 5th ed. St. Louis, MO: Mosby; 2007:684.

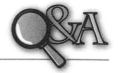

PART V · QUESTIONS

1. Of the following, which NSAID is also used to treat patent ductus arteriosis (PDA)?
   a. Ibuprofen (Advil, Motrin, others)
   b. Indomethacin (Indocin)
   c. Ketorolac (Toradol)
   d. Piroxicam (Feldene)

2. Which of the following NSAIDs has little anti-inflammatory action but is a potent analgesic similar to opioid analgesics?
   a. Ketorolac (Toradol)
   b. Naproxen (Naprosyn)
   c. Tolmetin (Tolectin)
   d. Sulindac (Clinoril)

3. Which drug inhibits COX-2 enzyme over COX-1?
   a. Ibuprofen (Advil, Motrin, others)
   b. Naproxen (Naprosyn, Aleve)
   c. Oxaprozin (Daypro)
   d. Celecoxib (Celebrex)

4. Client teaching concerning use of NSAIDs includes:
   a. Avoid giving acetaminophen to children under age 18.
   b. Take enteric-coated aspirin with an antacid to decrease GI side effects.
   c. Take NSAIDs on an empty stomach.
   d. Avoid combined use of NSAIDs with alcohol or aspirin.

5. Which of the following drugs is particularly beneficial in treating dysmenorrhea?
   a. Aspirin
   b. Acetaminophen (Tylenol)
   c. Ibuprofen (Advil, Motrin, others)
   d. Ketorolac (Toradol)

6. Signs and symptoms of Salicylism include all of the following EXCEPT:
   a. Headache.
   b. Hypothermia.
   c. Dizziness.
   d. Tinnitus.

7. Under which conditions are NSAIDs contraindicated?
   a. Diabetes Mellitus
   b. Hypothyroidism
   c. Hypotension
   d. Active GI bleeding

8. Which NSAID can be given parenterally, orally, and ophthalmically?
   a. Ketorolac (Toradol)
   b. Celecoxib (Celebrex)
   c. Meloxicam (Mobic)
   d. Naproxen (Naprosyn)

9. Which antirheumatoid drug is also used to treat malaria?
   a. Auranofin (Ridaura)
   b. Penicillamine (Cuprimine)
   c. Hydroxychloroquine (Plaquenil)
   d. Methotrexate (Rheumatrex)

10. Which antirheumatoid drug may alter taste acuity?
    a. Aurothioglucose (Solganal)
    b. Pencillamine (Cuprimine)
    c. Hydroxychloroquine (Plaquenil)
    d. Auranofin (Ridura)

11. Which antirheumatoid agent may cause dizziness, and clients should be instructed not to drive or operate heavy machinery until they know the response to this drug?
    a. Auranofin (Ridura)
    b. Pencillamine (Cuprimine)
    c. Leflunomide (Arava)
    d. Gold sodium thiomalate (Myochrysine)

12. Which statement is correct concerning antirheumatoid agents? Antirheumatoids:
    a. Are indicated for short-term use.
    b. Have immunomodulating effects.
    c. Are given at high doses during maintenance therapy.
    d. Have minor adverse effects.

13. Which antigout agent is also given to prolong the effects of penicillin?
    a. Allopurinol (Zyloprim)
    b. Colchicine
    c. Probenecid (Benemid)
    d. Sulfinpyrazone (Anturane)

14. Clients taking antigout medication should be instructed to:
    a. Increase fluid intake to at least 2000 mL per day.
    b. Drink alcoholic beverages to increase absorption of medication.
    c. Increase intake of turkey and organ meats.
    d. Continue to take medication even if diarrhea occurs.

PART V · ANSWERS

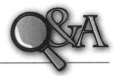

1. **The correct answer is b.** Indomethacin (Indocin) is used to treat PDA.

2. **The correct answer is a.** Ketorolac (Toradol) is a NSAID with little anti-inflammatory action but is a potent analgesic similar to opioid analgesics.

3. **The correct answer is d.** Celecoxib (Celebrex) is a COX-2 inhibitor that inhibits COX-2 enzyme over COX-1 enzyme.

4. **The correct answer is d.** Combining NSAIDs with alcohol or aspirin increases the risk of bleeding. Aspirin should be avoided in children under 18 to prevent Reye's syndrome. Enteric-coated aspirin should not be taken with an antacid as this will decrease the effectiveness and defeat the purpose of enteric-coated aspirin. NSAIDs should be taken with food to decrease GI side effects.

5. **The correct answer is c.** Ibuprofen (Advil, Motrin, others) is particularly beneficial in treating dysmenorrhea as it blocks the effect of prostaglandins. Ketorolac has little anti-inflammatory effect. Acetaminophen has little anti-inflammatory action, and aspirin is not as effective as ibuprofen in treating dysmenorrhea.

6. **The correct answer is b.** Hypothermia is not a symptom of salicylism. Headache, dizziness, and tinnitus are all classic signs of salicylism.

7. **The correct answer is d.** NSAIDs can cause bleeding and are therefore contraindicated in active GI bleeding.

8. **The correct answer is a.** Ketorolac (Toradol) is the only NSAID that can be given orally, IV, IM, or ophthalmically.

9. **The correct answer is c.** Hydroxychloroquine (Plaquenil) is also used to treat malaria.

10. **The correct answer is b.** Pencillamine (Cuprimine) may alter taste acuity.

11. **The correct answer is c.** Leflunomide (Arava) may cause dizziness, and clients should be instructed not to drive or operate heavy machinery until they know the response to the drug.

12. **The correct answer is b.** Antirheumatoids have immunomodulating effects, are not indicated for short-term use, are given at lower doses during maintenance therapy, and have some severe adverse effects including bone marrow suppression.

13. **The correct answer is c.** Probenecid (Benemid) prolongs the effects of penicillin.

14. **The correct answer is a.** Clients should increase their fluid intake to at least 2000 mL to help with excretion to prevent formation of uric acid stones. Alcohol, turkey, organ meats, and high purine foods exacerbate gout. Diarrhea is a sign of toxicity and the medication should be stopped.

VI

Cardiovascular Drugs

Marilyn J. Herbert-Ashton, MS, RN, BC

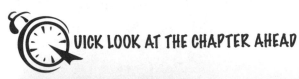

Cardiotonic-inotropic drugs, digitalis cardiac glycosides, and phosphodiesterase inhibitors, are used frequently to treat congestive heart failure (CHF). Recombinant Human type B natriuretic peptide is the newest class of medication used to treat heart failure. Cardiotonic-inotropic drugs also include adrenergic drugs.

Digitalis is derived from the foxglove plant and was initially used hundreds of years ago as an herbal remedy for fluid accumulation. It is one of the most commonly prescribed drugs in the world. Digoxin (Lanoxin, Lanoxicaps) is the most commonly prescribed digitalis glycoside.

39

Cardiotonic-Inotropic Drugs

TERMS
☐ digoxin (Lanoxin, Lanoxicaps)
☐ inamrinone lactate (Inocor)
☐ nesiritide (Natrecor)

Table 39-1 Cardiotonic-Inotropic Drugs

Prototype Drug	Related Drugs	Drug Classification
digoxin (Lanoxin, Lanoxicaps)	There are no related drugs at this time.	Digitalis cardiac glycoside
There is no prototype for this classification	digoxin immune FAB (Digibind)	Antidote-digoxin
inamrinone lactate (Inocor)	milrinone (Primacor)	Phosphodiesterase inhibitors (PDIs)
nesiritide (Natrecor)	There are no related drugs at this time.	Recombinant Human type B natriuretic peptide

CARDIOTONIC-INOTROPIC DRUGS CLIENT TEACHING

- Take radial pulse before taking medication.
- Contact health care provider if pulse is below 60 beats per minute or greater than 120 beats per minute in an adult, below 90 beats per minute in infants, and below 70 beats per minute in children through adolescence.
- Contact health care provider if experiencing visual changes, anorexia, nausea, vomiting, or if pulse is irregular.
- Take medication the same time daily and exactly as prescribed and do not abruptly stop taking.
- Avoid concurrent use of OTC drugs and herbal remedies without consulting health care provider.
- Carry or wear medical alert identification.
- Report signs and symptoms of digitalis toxicity immediately to health care provider.
- Weigh self daily.

Take radial pulse before taking medication.

Contact health care provider if pulse is below 60 beats per minute or greater than 120 beats per minute in an adult, below 90 beats per minute in infants, and below 70 beats per minute in children through adolescence.

Contact health care provider if experiencing visual changes, anorexia, nausea, vomiting, or if pulse is irregular.

- Notify health care provider if there is a weight gain of 1 to 2 pounds or more a day.
- If eating dairy products or taking antacids, take medication 2 hours before or after consuming.

ACTION

Cardiac Glycosides

Digoxin (Lanoxin, Lanoxicaps)

- Positive inotropic effect, which increases the force of myocardial contraction; negative chronotropic effect, which slows the heart rate; and negative dromotropic effect, which decreases conduction through the sinoatrial and atrioventricular (AV) nodes, with a prolonged refractory period through the AV node

Cardiac Glycosides Antidote

Digoxin Immune FAB (Digibind)

- Believed to work by binding to free digoxin or digitoxin, which blocks or reverses the drug effects and symptoms of toxicity
- It is an antibody produced in sheep.

Phosphodiesterase Inhibitors (PDIs)

Inamrinone Lactate (Inocor) and Milrinone (Primacor)

- Inhibit the enzyme phosphodiesterase, which produces a positive inotropic response and vasodilatation
- Inhibit phosphodiesterase, resulting in an increase in intracellular cyclic adenosine monophosphate

Recombinant Human Type-B Natriuretic Peptide

Nesiritide (Natrecor)

- Produced by recombinant DNA technology, and is identical to the hormone human type-B natriuretic peptide that has vasodilating effects on arteries and veins[1]

USE

Cardiac Glycosides

Digoxin (Lanoxin and Lanoxicaps)

- CHF, supraventricular dysrhythmias, atrial fibrillation and atrial flutter, and atrial tachycardia
- Also used to treat cardiogenic shock.

Digitalis Cardiac Glycosides Antidote

Digoxin Immune FAB (Digibind)

- For life-threatening overdosage of digitalis cardiac glycosides

Phosphodiesterase Inhibitors (PDIs)

Inamrinone Lactate (Inocor) and Milrinone (Primacor)

- Short-term management of CHF in clients unresponsive to digitalis cardiac glycosides, diuretics, and vasodilators

Recombinant Human Type-B Natriuretic Peptide

Nesiritide (Natrecor)

- Treatment of severe, life-threatening heart failure. It is not a first line drug to treat heart failure.[1]

 # ADVERSE EFFECTS AND SIDE EFFECTS

Cardiac Glycosides

- *Pregnancy category C*
- *CV:* Dysrhythmias, including bradycardia and tachycardia
- *CNS:* Fatigue, headache, confusion, convulsions
- *GI:* Anorexia, nausea, vomiting, and diarrhea
- *Visual:* Halo vision, colored vision (green or yellow)

Cardiac Glycosides Antidote

- *Pregnancy category C*
- *F & E:* Hypokalemia
- *CV:* Reactivation of CHF and arrhythmias

Phosphodiesterase Inhibitors (PDIs)

- *Pregnancy category C*

Inamrinone lactate (Inocor)

- *CV:* hypotension and arrhythmias
- *F & E:* Hypokalemia
- *GI:* Diarrhea, nausea, vomiting, and hepatoxocity with long-term use
- *Hematologic:* Thrombocytopenia

Milrinone Lactate (Primacor)

- *CV:* Hypotension, ventricular arrhythmias, angina pectoris, and chest pain
- *F & E:* Hypokalemia
- *Hematologic:* Thrombocytopenia

Recombinant Human Type-B Natriuretic Peptide

- *Pregnancy category C*
- *CV:* Hypotension, chest pain, or tightness; dysrhythmias, tachycardia
- *CNS:* Dizziness, headache, anxiety, weakness
- *GI:* Abdominal or stomach pain, vomiting

 ## INTERACTIONS

Cardiac Glycosides

- Thiazides, loop diuretics, laxative, corticosteroids, mezlocillin, piperacillin, tiracillin, and amphotericin B cause hypokalemia and increase risk of toxicity.

- Quinidine, cyclosporine, amiodarone, erythromycin, tetracycline, verapamil, diltazem, diclofenac, and propafenone lead to toxicity by increasing serum levels.
- Beta-adrenergic blockers, quinidine, and dispyramide may cause additive bradycardia.
- Antacids, antidiarrheals, cholestyramine, bleomycin, and colistipol decrease oral absorption, which reduces therapeutic effects.
- Concurrent use of hawthorn, ginseng, or licorice may increase toxicity.
- Eating large amounts of bran or concurrent use with psyllium may decrease absorption.
- Concurrent use with St. John's wort or psyllium reduces serum digoxin levels.
- Decreased serum levels may occur with thyroid hormones.

Cardiac Glycosides Antidote

- Inhibits therapeutic response to digoxin

Phosphodiesterase Inhibitors (PDIs)

- Phosphodiesterase inhibitors form precipitates when given in solution with furosemide (Lasix).[1]

Recombinant Human Type-B Natriuretic Peptide

- Hypotensive effects when given with diuretics & angiotensin converting enzyme inhibitors[1]

CONTRAINDICATIONS

Cardiac Glycosides

- AV block, hypersensitivity, uncontrolled ventricular arrhythmias

Cardiac Glycosides Antidote

- Cautious use in hypersensitivity to sheep proteins or products

Phosphodiesterase Inhibitors (PDIs)

- Hypersensitivity to bisulfites, Inamrinone lactate (Incor) or Milrinone (Primacor)
- Acute myocardial infarction, severe aortic or pulmonic valvular disease, ventricular dysrhythmias, and fluid volume deficit[2]

Recombinant Human Type-B Natriuretic Peptide

- Allergy to drug

 ## NURSING IMPLICATIONS

Cardiac Glycosides

- For rapid effects a larger loading or digitalizing dose may be given in divided doses over 12 to 24 hours.
- Monitor for digitalis toxicity.
- Monitor serum electrolytes.
- Give PO or IV.
- Differentiate Lanoxin from Lanoxicaps as dosage is different.
- Clients with hypokalemia, hypercalcemia, hypothyroidism, renal dysfunction, as well as the elderly are predisposed to digitalis toxicity.
- Assess apical pulse for one minute before administering. See "Client Teaching" on page 317 for pulse rates.
- Monitor EKG during loading dose.
- Monitor I & O, daily weights, and lung sounds.
- Monitor cardiac status.
- Monitor serum digoxin levels (0.5 to 2.0 ng/mL).
- May give with or without food. Note comments related to dairy products and antacids noted under "Client Teaching" on page 318.

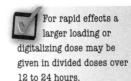
For rapid effects a larger loading or digitalizing dose may be given in divided doses over 12 to 24 hours.

Assess apical pulse for one minute before administering. See "Client Teaching" on page 317 for pulse rates.

Cardiac Glycosides Antidote

- Monitor vital signs and EKG throughout treatment.

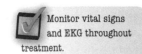
Monitor vital signs and EKG throughout treatment.

- Keep CPR equipment and crash cart nearby during administration.
- Monitor for re-emergence of CHF or arrhythmias.
- Monitor serum potassium levels.
- Serum digoxin levels are not valid for 5 to 7 days after administration.
- Administer a test dose for patients allergic to sheep or at high risk for allergy to digoxin immune FAB.
- Administer via IV infusion with a 0.22-μm filter; can be given direct IV push if cardiopulmonary arrest is imminent.

Phosphodiesterase Inhibitors (PDIs)

- Monitor EKG and vital signs, especially blood pressure.
- Monitor for hypotension, which is seen in toxicity.
- Discontinue use if excessive hypotension seen.
- Monitor I & O and daily weights.
- Monitor electrolytes and renal function and platelet counts.
- For IV administration, use an infusion pump.

Monitor for hypotension, which is seen in toxicity.

Inamrinone lactate (Inocor)

- Should be diluted with normal saline. Mixing with dextrose causes decomposition of drug.
- Monitor liver function.

Monitor liver function.

Recombinant Human Type-B Natriuretic Peptide

- Administer IV in a separate line.
- Hemodynamic monitoring of pulmonary artery pressure indicated to determine drug effectiveness[3]

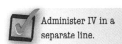

Administer IV in a separate line.

REFERENCES

1. Lilley L, Harrington S, Snyder J. *Pharmacology and the Nursing Process*, 5th ed. St. Louis, MO: Mosby; 2007:325.

2. Lilley L, Harrington S, Snyder J. *Pharmacology and the Nursing Process*, 5th ed. St. Louis, MO: Mosby; 2007:324.

3. Skidmore-Roth L. *Mosby's Nursing Drug Reference.* St. Louis, MO: Mosby Elsevier; 2007:717.

Antidysrhythmic drugs, also known antiarrhythmics, are indicated to prevent or treat dysrhythmias (arrhythmia). Dysrhythmias occur as a result of alterations in electrical impulses that regulate cardiac rhythm. It is important to note that antidysrhythmic drugs can also cause dysrhythmias or worsen existing ones. It is imperative that the nurse closely monitor clients during treatment.

The Vaughan Williams classification of antidysrhythmic drugs is a frequently used system based on the effect produced by a particular antidysrhythmic on the action potential. Four major groups of agents have been identified. Class I, also known as sodium channel blockers, is further broken down into Classes IA, IB, and IC, depending on their effects in phase 0, action potential duration, and effective refractory period. Class II drugs are beta-blockers that depress phase 4 depolarization. Class III potassium blockers prolong repolarization during phase 3. Class IV includes calcium channel blockers and depresses phase 4 depolarization and prolongs repolarization during phases 1 and 2.[1]

40

Antidysrhythmic Drugs

TERMS
☐ **bretylium (Bretylol)**
☐ **diltiazem (Cardizem)**
☐ **flecainide (Tambocor)**
☐ **lidocaine (Xylocaine)**
☐ **propranolol (Inderal)**
☐ **quinidine (Quinaglute)**

Table 40-1 Antidysrhythmic Drugs

Prototype Drug	Related Drugs	Drug Classification
There is no prototype for this classification	moricizine (Ethmozine)	Class I: Sodium channel blocker
quinidine (Quinaglute)	disopyramide (Norpace) procainamide (Pronestyl)	Class IA
lidocaine (Xylocaine)	mexiletine (Mexitil) tocainide (Tonocard)	Class IB
flecainide (Tambocor)	propafenone (Rythmol)	Class IC
propranolol (Inderal)	acebutolol (Sectral) esmolol (Brevibloc) sotalol (Betapace), also a Class III drug	Class II: Beta-blockers
bretylium (Bretylol)	amiodarone (Cordarone) dofetilide (Tikosyn) ibutilide (Corvert)	Class III: Potassium channel blockers
diltiazem (Cardizem)	verapamil (Calan)	Class IV: Calcium channel blockers
There is no prototype for this classification	adenosine (Adenocard)	Unclassified antidysrhythmic

ANTIDYSRHYTHMIC DRUGS CLIENT TEACHING

All Antidysrhythmics

- Take pulse and monitor rate and rhythm.
- Report any worsening of symptoms of dysrhythmia, chest pain, edema, shortness of breath, dizziness, or sudden weight gain.
- Carry medical identification.
- Contact health care provider before taking herbals or other OTC medications.
- Avoid caffeinated beverages as caffeine can cause an increase in arrhythmias.

Take pulse and monitor rate and rhythm.

Report any worsening of symptoms of dysrhythmia, chest pain, edema, shortness of breath, dizziness, or sudden weight gain.

Carry medical identification.

- Avoid driving or using heavy machinery if vision is blurred or you are dizzy.

Amiodarone (Cordarone)

- Wear sunscreen and protective clothing and avoid sun exposure.

Procainamide (Pronestyl)

- Notify health care provider if bleeding occurs or symptoms of lupus occur.

Disopyramide (Norpace) & dofetilide (Tikosyn)

- Change positions slowly and avoid alcohol.

Quinidine (Quinaglute)

- Report signs of bleeding, tinnitus, rash, and visual disturbances.

Quinidine (Quinaglute), disopyramide (Norpace), and procainamide (Pronestyl)

- Should have regular dental check-ups due to antimuscarinic effects of quinidine and side effects of dry mouth from disopyramide and procainamide

ACTION

Class I: Sodium Channel Blockers

Moricizine (Ethmozine)

- Exhibits characteristics of Class IA, IB, and IC. Blocks sodium channel in the myocardium, which prolongs PR interval and QRS duration, and suppresses prolonged automaticity

Class IA

Quinidine (Quinaglute)

- Decreases myocardial excitability, slows conduction velocity, and has anticholinergic effects

- Note: Procainadmide (Pronestyl) has weaker anticholinergic effects; disopyramide (Norpace) has stronger anticholinergic effects than quinidine.

Class IB

Lidocaine (Xylocaine)

- Blocks sodium channels and reduces automaticity in the ventricles and His-Purkinje system, accelerates repolarization, and has little or no effect on the EKG

Class IC

- Blocks sodium channels and decrease conduction velocity in the atria, ventricles, and His-Purkinje system

Class II: Beta-Blockers

- Block or reduce sympathetic nervous system stimulation to the heart and heart's conduction system, causing decreased heart rate, decreased myocardial contractility and automaticity, and delayed atrioventricular (AV) node conduction

Class III: Potassium Channel Blockers

- Prolong the refractory period by prolonging the action potential, which delays repolarization. The drugs in this class affect the heart differently and are not interchangeable.

Class IV: Calcium Channel Blockers

- Note: Calcium channel blockers are also discussed in Chapter 41.
- Block calcium channels in the heart and have a negative dromotropic effect (decrease conduction rate)

Unclassified Antidysrhythmics

Adenosine (Adenocard)

- Slows conduction time through the AV node and decreases automaticity in the sinoatrial (SA) node

USE

Class I: Sodium Channel Blockers

Moricizine (Ethmozine)

- Life-threatening ventricular dysrhythmias

Class IA

- Premature atrial contractions, atrial fibrillation, premature ventricular contractions, ventricular tachycardia, and Wolff-Parkinson-White syndrome
- Note: Quinidine (Quinaglute) is an unlabeled use is for malaria treatment.

Class IB

- Ventricular dysrhythmias
- Lidocaine (Xylocaine) is also used as a local anesthetic

Class IC

- Used when unresponsive to Class IB agents for supraventricular tachydysrhythmias

Class II: Beta-Blockers

Propranolol (Inderal)

- Note: Beta-blockers are also discussed in Chapter 28.
- Dysrhythmias caused by excessive sympathetic nerve activity, supraventricular dysrhythmias

Esmolol (Brevibloc)

- Short-term treatment of supraventricular tachycardia due to atrial fibrillation and atrial flutter

Acebutolol (Sectral)

- Ventricular dysrhythmias

Sotalol (Betapace)

- Usually used for life-threatening ventricular dysrhythmias, sustained ventricular tachycardia, and is similar to Class III antidysrhythmics

Class III: Potassium Channel Blockers

Amiodarone (Cordarone) and Bretylium (Bretylol)

- Life-threatening ventricular dysrhythmias unresponsive to Class IB and IC

Ibutilide (Corvert)

- Indicated for atrial dysrhythmias

Dafetilide (Tikosyn)

- Used to convert atrial fibrillation and atrial flutter to normal sinus rhythm; maintenance of normal sinus rhythm

Class IV: Calcium Channel Blockers

Diltiazem (Cardizem) and Verapamil (Calan)

- Paroxysmal supraventricular tachycardia (PSVT)
- Controls ventricular response to atrial fibrillation and atrial flutter

Unclassified Antidysrhythmics

Adenosine (Adenocard)

- Used to terminate PSVT, especially in clients who have failed to respond to verapamil

ADVERSE EFFECTS AND SIDE EFFECTS

Classes I, IA, IB, and IC

- *CV:* Dysrhythmias
- *CNS:* Dizziness, headache, confusion, and convulsions

- *GI:* Nausea, vomiting, and diarrhea
- *EENT:* Blurred vision

Specific Drug-Related Adverse and Side Effects

Moricizine (Ethmozine)

- *Pregnancy category B*
- *CNS:* Dizziness, headache, fatigue

Quinidine (Quinaglute)

- *Pregnancy category C*
- Cinchonism (tinnitus, hearing loss, blurred vision, GI upset)

Disopyramide (Norpace)

- *Pregnancy category C*
- *CV:* Cardiovascular depression, ventricular dysrhythmias, anti-cholinergic effects, and hypotension

Procainamide (Pronestyl)

- *Pregnancy category C*
- Systemic lupus erythematosus (SLE)

Class IB

Lidocaine (Xylocaine)

- *Pregnancy category C*
- *CNS:* Toxicity—drowsiness, convulsions, confusion, seizures
- *CV:* Hypotension, bradycardia

Mexiletine (Mexitil)

- *Pregnancy category C*
- Dizziness, tremor, nausea, vomiting

Tocainide (Tonocard)

- *Pregnancy category C*
- *Hematologic:* Angranulocytosis, thrombocytopenia, leukopenia
- *Resp:* Pulmonary edema, pulmonary fibrosis, pneumonia
- *Other:* Tremors, parasthesias, dizziness

Class IC

Flecainide (Tambocor) and Propafenone (Rythmol)

- *Pregnancy category C*
- Headaches, weakness, visual disturbances, constipation, dysrhythmias, chest pain, and irregular heartbeats

Class II: Beta-Blockers

Propranolol (Inderal) and Esmolol (Brevibloc)

- *Pregnancy category C, although acebutolol (Sectral) and sotalol (Betapace) are pregnancy category B agents*
- *CV:* Hypotension and bradycardia, may precipitate congestive heart failure (CHF)
- *CNS:* Fatigue, syncope

Class III: Potassium Channel Blockers

- *Pregnancy category C agents*
- Photosensitivity, corneal microdeposits (amiodarone, Cordarone)
- Pulmonary toxicity (amiodarone [Cordarone])
- Hepatitis and thyroid dysfunction (amiodarone [Cordarone])
- *GI:* Nausea and vomiting commonly seen with bretylium (Bretylol)
- Postural hypotension especially with bretylium (Bretylol)
- Dysrhythmias and toxicity especially with hypokalemia
- Ibutilide (Corvert) may cause torsades de pointes.
- Dofelitide (Tikosyn) may cause headache, fatigue, ventricular dysrhythmias, and lightheadedness.

Class IV: Calcium Channel Blockers

- *Pregnancy category C*
- *CV:* Hypotension, bradycardia, heart block, edema
- *Other:* Constipation

Unclassified Antidysrhythmics

Adenosine (Adenocard)

- *Pregnancy category C*
- Note: Adverse effects are short lived as the drug has an extremely short half life, and effects may last less than a minute.
- Frequently causes asystole for a few seconds

INTERACTIONS

Class I

- Digoxin and quinidine cause increased serum digoxin levels.
- Digoxin and Class IC agents increase serum digoxin levels.
- Digoxin and flecainide decrease urinary excretion of flecainide.
- Warfarin (Coumadin) and quinidine lead to hypothrombinemia.
- Nifedipine and quinidine decrease quinidine levels.
- Anticholinergic drugs increase anticholinergic effects.
- Neuromuscular blockers interact with quinidine, procainamide, and disopyramide, which leads to increased skeletal muscle relaxation.
- Cimetidine (Tagamet) and quinidine increase quinidine levels.
- Cimetidine and procainamide or moricizine increase levels of procainamide and moricizine.
- Anticonvulsants and quinidine or disopyramide increase the metabolism of both drugs.
- Toxicity may occur with concurrent administration of propranolol or cimetidine with lidocaine.

Class II

- Phenothiazines and antihypertensives interact with propranolol and acebutolol (sectrol) causing hypotension.
- Propanolol (Inderal) interacts with cimetidine, decreasing metabolism of propranolol.

Class III

- Concurrent use with digoxin leads to increased digoxin levels.
- Warfarin (Coumadin)—hypoprothrombinemia and increased clotting times
- Concurrent use with phenytoin (Dilantin) increases serum levels of phenytoin.
- Do not give dofetilide (Tikosyn) together with sotalol, disopyramide, quindine, amiodarone, or procainamide as it increases risk of life-threatening dysrhythmias.

Class IV

- Antidysrhythmics and antihypertensive agents increase the risk of hypotension and heart failure.
- Concurrent use with digoxin increases digoxin levels.
- Sulfonylureas, sulfonamide antibiotics, and aspirin increase adverse effects of Class IV drugs.

Unclassified Drugs

- Methylxanthines block receptors for adenosine.

CONTRAINDICATIONS

Class I

Moricizine (Ethmozine)

- Hypersensitivity, AV block, cardiogenic shock

Quinidine (Quinaglute)

- AV block, torsades de points, conduction defects, and hypersensitivity

Disopyramide (Norpace)

- See quinidine and procainamide.

Procainamide (Pronestyl)

- Hypersensitivity
- SLE
- Second, third, or complete heart block

Class IB

Lidocaine (Xylocaine)

- Hypersensitivity, SA or AV block, Stokes-Adams, or Wolff-Parkinson-White syndrome

Mexiletine (Mexitil)

- Hypersensitivity, second or third degree heart block, cardiogenic shock

Tocainide (Tonocard)

- Hypersensitivity, second or third degree heart block

Class IC

Flecainide (Tambocor) and Propafenone (Rythmol)

- Hypersensitivity, cardiogenic shock, AV block, non-life-threatening dysrhythmias

Class II: Beta-Blockers

- Hypersensitivity, asthma, bradycardia, cardiogenic shock, AV block

Class III: Potassium Channel Blockers

- Hypersensitivity
- Contraindicated in heart block

Class IV: Calcium Channel Blockers

- Hypersensitivity, acute myocardial infarction, cardiogenic shock heart block, severe hypotension, Wolff-Parkinson-White syndrome, pulmonary congestion

Unclassified Antidysrhythmics

Adenosine (Adenocard)

- Hypersensitivity, heart block, atrial fibrillation or flutter, ventricular tachycardia

NURSING IMPLICATIONS

Nursing Implications for All Antidysrhythmics

- Monitor vital signs before, during, and after treatment.
- Use a controller or pump for IV use.
- Monitor electrolytes, especially potassium.
- Monitor serum drug levels.
- Monitor EKG.
- Monitor weights and intake and output (I & O).
- Monitor for interactions; many antidysrhythmics interact with other antidysrhythmics.
- Implement safety measures.

Monitor vital signs before, during, and after treatment.

Monitor electrolytes, especially potassium.

Class I: Sodium Channel Blockers

Moricizine (Ethmozine)

- Give PO usually every 8 hours.
- Monitor I & O and weight.

Class IA

Quinidine (Quinaglute)

- Give PO, IM, or IV.
- May give with food to decrease GI upset
- Monitor for diarrhea and GI upset.

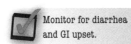
Monitor for diarrhea and GI upset.

Class IB

Lidocaine (Xylocaine)

- Give IV.
- Make sure vial states for "Cardiac Use"—noncardiac lidocaine contains epinephrine.
- Monitor neurological status and implement safety measures.

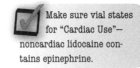
Make sure vial states for "Cardiac Use"—noncardiac lidocaine contains epinephrine.

Mexiletine (Mexitil) and Tocainide (Tonocard)

- Give PO.
- May give with food if GI upset occurs

Class IC

Flecainide (Tambocor) and Propafenone (Rythmol)

- Avoid concurrent use with other antidysrhythmic agents.
- Assess for symptoms of CHF.
- Give PO; may give with food if GI upset occurs

Class II: Beta-Blockers

- Propranolol (Inderal) is given PO or in life-threatening emergencies IV.
- Acebutolol (Sectral) and sotalol (Betapace) are given PO.
- Esmolol (Brevibloc) is given by IV infusion.
- Monitor for symptoms of CHF.
- May not see an increase in heart rate with exercise
- Withdraw gradually to prevent angina.
- If pulse is less than 60 beats per minute, withhold and notify health care provider.
- Take oral medication before meals.

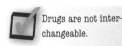
Propranolol (Inderal) is given PO or in life-threatening emergencies IV.

Class III: Potassium Channel Blockers

- Drugs are not interchangeable.

Amiodarone (Cordarone)

- Give PO or IV.
- Monitor hepatic and thyroid functions.

Drugs are not interchangeable.

Bretylium (Bretylol)

- Give IV or IM.
- Administer slowly to decrease adverse effects.
- Keep client in a supine position while receiving, until tolerance develops to minimize postural hypotension.

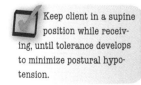
Keep client in a supine position while receiving, until tolerance develops to minimize postural hypotension.

dofetilide (Tikosyn)

- Given PO.
- Monitor EKG and creatine levels.

Ibutilide (Corvert)

- Give IV.

Class IV: Calcium Channel Blockers

Verapamil (Calan) and Diltazem (Cardizem)

- Give PO or IV; IV use is preferred for initial therapy.
- Monitor for CHF and hypotension.

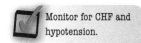

Monitor for CHF and hypotension.

Unclassified Antidysrhythmics

Adenosine (Adenocard)

- Give by IV bolus (6 mg) over 1 or 2 seconds. If first dose not effective, may give 12 mg in same manner after 1 to 2 minutes.
- Crash cart should be nearby when administering.
- Solution should be clear before administering.

Solution should be clear before administering.

REFERENCE

1. Lilley L, Harrington S, Snyder J. *Pharmacology and the Nursing Process,* 5th ed. St. Louis, MO: Mosby; 2007:338–339.

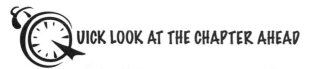
The nitrates, beta-blockers, and calcium channel blockers are the three main classes of drugs used to treat angina pectoris. The goal of treatment is to decrease pain, minimize frequency of attacks, prevent or delay myocardial infarction by reducing oxygen demand, and maintaining oxygen supply.[1]

The nitrates are the most frequently used antianginal drugs. Nitroglycerin has been used for treatment of angina since 1879.[1]

41

Antianginal Drugs

TERMS
- ☐ nifedipine (Procardia)
- ☐ nitroglycerin (Nitro-bid, Nitrostat, others)
- ☐ propranolol (Inderal)

Table 41-1 Antianginal Drugs

Prototype Drug	Related Drugs	Drug Classification
nitroglycerin (Nitro-bid, Nitrostat, others)	amyl nitrite isosorbide dinitrate (Isordil, Sorbitrate) isosorbide mononitrate (Imdur, ISMO)	Nitrates
propranolol (Inderal)	atenolol (Tenormin) metoprolol (Lopressor) nadolol (Corgard)	Beta-blockers
nifedipine (Procardia)	amlodipine (Norvasc) bepridil (Vascor) diltiazem (Cardizem) felodipine (Plendil) isradipine (Dynacirc) nicardipine (Cardene) nimodipine (Nimotop) nisoldipine (Sular) verapamil (Calan)	Calcium channel blockers

ANTIANGINAL DRUGS CLIENT TEACHING

Nitrates

- Change positions gradually to avoid orthostatic hypotension.
- Nitroglycerin can lose potency if exposed to light, moisture, or heat.
- Replace tablets 6 months after opening, as nitrates lose potency over time.
- Avoid alcohol, hot baths, saunas, and whirlpools, as they can cause vasodilatation and lead to hypotension and fainting.
- Teach side effects and adverse effects of nitrates, which include headaches (that can last up to 20 minutes), dizziness, facial flushing, increased heart rate, and lightheadedness.

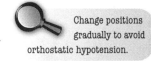

Change positions gradually to avoid orthostatic hypotension.

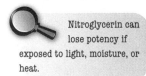

Nitroglycerin can lose potency if exposed to light, moisture, or heat.

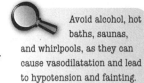

Avoid alcohol, hot baths, saunas, and whirlpools, as they can cause vasodilatation and lead to hypotension and fainting.

- Report to health care provider if dry mouth, severe headaches, or blurred vision occur.
- An analgesic can be given to treat headache.
- Discard cotton packing after opening bottle, as the packing may absorb the drug and lead to decreased potency.
- Encourage client to discontinue tobacco use, as tobacco causes vasoconstriction.
- Avoid OTC and herbal remedies without first consulting health care provider.
- Keep a journal documenting number and characteristics of anginal attacks, contributing factors and number of tablets taken, and adverse effects.

Sublingual Tablets

- If client has an acute anginal attack, teach client to lie down and take SL tablet as soon as possible; up to 3 nitroglycerin tablets every 5 minutes for 15 minutes may be taken; if no relief, emergency services should be notified for transport to the emergency room.
- Do not chew SL tablets. Place under tongue to dissolve. Do not swallow tablet.
- Tablet should burn slightly under the tongue, if not replace supply of tablets.[4]
- Do not eat food or smoke until tablet dissolves.

> If client has an acute anginal attack, teach client to lie down and take SL tablet as soon as possible; up to 3 nitroglycerin tablets every 5 minutes for 15 minutes may be taken; if no relief, emergency services should be notified for transport to the emergency room.

Buccal

- Place tablet between upper lip and gum to dissolve.

Chewable Tablets

- Chew thoroughly and hold in mouth 2 minutes before swallowing.

> Chew thoroughly and hold in mouth 2 minutes before swallowing.

Oral Sustained-Release Tablets or Capsules

- Take with a full glass of water on an empty stomach, swallowing whole medication.

Lingual Aerosol

- Do not shake when administering and hold can vertically and spray under the tongue. Do not swallow immediately.

Ointment

- Use applicator paper and follow directions for application (thin layer).
- Do not get ointment on hands as it can cause headache; wash hands after applying.
- Apply to a nonhairy site, remove old residue before applying, and rotate sites.

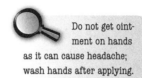

Do not get ointment on hands as it can cause headache; wash hands after applying.

Transdermal

- Avoid application to skin folds, irritated or hairy areas.
- Remove old application, remove old residue, apply at the same time daily, and rotate sites.
- Advise client that he or she can swim or bathe with patch on, and to apply a new patch after cleaning old residue if patch should fall off.

Advise client that he or she can swim or bathe with patch on, and to apply a new patch after cleaning old residue if patch should fall off.

Beta-Blockers

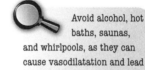

Avoid alcohol, hot baths, saunas, and whirlpools, as they can cause vasodilatation and lead to hypotension and fainting.

- Avoid alcohol, hot baths, saunas, and whirlpools, as they can cause vasodilatation and lead to hypotension and fainting.
- Do not abruptly discontinue as rebound hypertension can occur.
- Beta-blockers are indicated for long-term prevention of anginal attacks.
- Teach client to check pulse and notify health care provider if pulse rate is less than 60 beats per minute.
- Report edema, chest pain, palpitations, dyspnea, and fainting to health care provider.
- Change positions gradually to minimize orthostatic hypotension.

Calcium Channel Blockers

- Take pulse before taking.
- Report symptoms of edema, hypotension, headache, and dizziness to health care provider.
- Change positions gradually to minimize orthostatic hypotension.

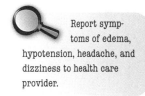

Report symptoms of edema, hypotension, headache, and dizziness to health care provider.

ACTION

Nitrates

- Decrease preload and afterload and reduce myocardial oxygen demand. Relax vascular smooth muscle, which decreases venous return and arterial blood pressure
- Nitroglycerin and amyl nitrite are rapid-acting agents, and isorbide dinitrate and isorbide mononitrate are long-acting agents.

Beta-Blockers

- Block the cardiac beta-adrenergic receptors to decrease heart rate, blood pressure, and contractility

Calcium Channel Blockers

- Decrease afterload and oxygen demand by dilating arterioles and decrease myocardial contractility; diltiazem (Cardizem) and verapamil (Calan) also decrease heart rate.

USE

- Nitrates, beta-blockers, and calcium channel blockers are indicated to treat stable and unstable angina; nitrates and calcium channel blockers are also indicated in treating variant angina[3]
- Beta-blockers and calcium channel blockers are also used in treatment of essential hypertension.

ADVERSE EFFECTS AND SIDE EFFECTS

Nitrates

- *Pregnancy category C*
- *CV:* Postural hypotension, tachycardia
- *CNS:* Headache, dizziness
- *Derm:* Contact dermatitis—ointment or transdermal nitroglycerine tolerance

Beta-Blockers

- *Pregnancy category C*
- *CV:* Hypotension, heart block, bradycardia, CHF, pulmonary edema
- *CNS:* unusual dreams, dizziness, depression, drowsiness, weakness
- *GU:* Decreased libido, impotence
- *Metabolic:* Altered glucose metabolism
- *Resp:* Wheezing, bronchospasm

Calcium Channel Blockers

- *Pregnancy category C*
- *CV:* Hypertension, bradycardia or tachycardia, palpitations, peripheral edema
- *CNS:* Headache, fatigue
- *Derm:* Flushing, rash, dermatitis
- *GI:* Constipation, nausea, vomiting

 ## INTERACTIONS

Nitrates

- Concurrent use with alcohol, antihypertensive agents, beta-blockers, calcium channel blockers, sildenafil (Viagra), tadalafil (Cialis), vardenafil (Levitra), or phenothiazines increases hypotensive effects of nitrates.[3]

Beta-Blockers

- Concurrent use with alcohol, antihypertensive agents, diuretics, calcium channel blockers, nitrates, and phenothiazine increases hypotensive effects of beta-blockers.
- Cimetidine increases beta-blocker effects.

Calcium Channel Blockers

- Concurrent use with alcohol, antihypertensive agents, or nitrates increases hypotensive effects of calcium channel blockers.
- Calcium channel blockers increase digoxin levels when taken with digoxin.
- Concurrent use with beta-blockers may cause bradycardia and AV block.
- Concurrent use with cimetidine increases blood levels of calcium channel blockers.

CONTRAINDICATIONS

Nitrates

- Hypersensitivity, severe anemia, severe hypotension, pericardial tamponade, or concurrent use with sildenafil (Viagra)

Beta-Blockers

- Heart block, bradycardia, pulmonary edema, hypersensitivity, cardiogenic shock, bronchospastic disease

Calcium Channel Blockers

- Cardiogenic shock, hypersensitivity, hypertension, second or third degree atrioventricular block

NURSING IMPLICATIONS

Nitrates

- Amyl nitrite is highly flammable and should be kept away from flames.

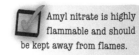

Amyl nitrate is highly flammable and should be kept away from flames.

- The dosages of the nitrates are not interchangeable.
- Monitor pulse and blood pressure.
- Store nitroglycerin and related drugs in their original containers and keep tightly closed.
- IV Nitroglycerin: Follow manufacturer's instructions and use glass bottles and tubing provided by manufacturer. Standard polyvinyl chloride tubing may absorb nitroglycerin; give as an infusion and use infusion pump. Do not mix nitroglycerin with other drugs.
- Headache may diminish when client develops drug tolerance.
- Remove transdermal patches before cardioversion or defibrillation to prevent burns.
- Wear gloves when preparing ointment to prevent headache. Use dose measuring applicators supplied by manufacturer. Avoid massaging or rubbing area.
- Rotate ointment and transdermal sites.
- Remove ointment or previous patch before applying new ointment or patch.
- Transdermal patch is usually worn 12 to 14 hours and then removed for 10 to 12 hours at night to prevent drug tolerance.
- Do not trim transdermal patch to alter dosage.

 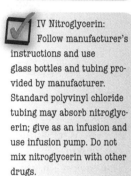

Monitor pulse and blood pressure.

IV Nitroglycerin: Follow manufacturer's instructions and use glass bottles and tubing provided by manufacturer. Standard polyvinyl chloride tubing may absorb nitroglycerin; give as an infusion and use infusion pump. Do not mix nitroglycerin with other drugs.

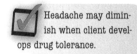

Headache may diminish when client develops drug tolerance.

Isosorbide Dinitrate (Isordil, Sorbitrate)

- Available PO, SL, in extended-release capsules, and in chewable tablet form

Isosorbide Monoitrate (Imdur, ISMO)

- Available PO, in immediate or sustained release forms

Beta-Blockers

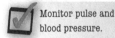

Monitor pulse and blood pressure.

- Monitor pulse and blood pressure.
- Assess frequency and characteristics of anginal attacks.
- Give PO for treatment of angina.

Calcium Channel Blockers

- Monitor pulse and blood pressure.
- Assess frequency and characteristics of anginal attacks.
- Calcium channel blockers given to treat angina are given PO, verapamil (Calan) and nicardipine (Cardene) is also available parenterally.
- Extended release tablets should not be chewed, opened, or broken.
- Encourage a high-fiber diet to prevent constipation.

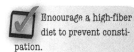
Encourage a high-fiber diet to prevent constipation.

REFERENCES

1. Lehne RA. *Pharmacology for Nursing Care,* 6th ed. Philadelphia, PA: Saunders Elsevier; 2007:574.

2. Lehne RA. *Pharmacology for Nursing Care,* 6th ed. Philadelphia, PA: Saunders Elsevier; 2007:572–573.

3. Lilley L, Harrington S, Snyder J. *Pharmacology and the Nursing Process,* 5th ed. St. Louis, MO: Mosby; 2007:356.

4. Lilley L, Harrington S, Snyder J. *Pharmacology and the Nursing Process,* 5th ed. St. Louis, MO: Mosby; 2007:755.

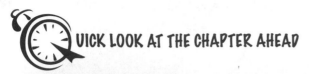

Hypertension is often known as the silent killer, as clients may be asymptomatic. There is an abnormal increase in blood pressure (BP) and without treatment, hypertension can lead to progressive deterioration of cardiac, renal, and ocular function, and cerebral vascular accident (CVA).

In clients diagnosed with hypertension, 90% of hypertensive cases are known as essential, idiopathic, or primary hypertension and the cause is not known. In 10% of the cases, the cause is known and is called secondary hypertension. It can be caused by pheochromocytoma, renal disease, eclampsia, or by other medications.[1] If the cause of secondary hypertension is cured, then the blood pressure generally returns to normal.

In 2003, the Joint National Committee on Prevention, Detection, Evaluation, and Treatment of High Blood Pressure, from the National Institutes of Health released its seventh report that provides a new guidelines for hypertension prevention and management.

The guideline states: "in individuals over age 50, systolic BP over 140 mmHg is a more important cardiovascular disease (CVD) risk factor than diastolic BP; the risks of CVD beginning at 115/75 mmHg, doubles with each increment of 20/10 mmHg; individuals who are normotensive at age 55 have a 90% lifetime risk for developing hypertension; a systolic BP of 120 to 139 mmHg or a diastolic BP of 80 to 89 mmHg should be considered as prehypertensive and requires lifestyle modifications; Thiazides should be used in treatment for most clients with uncomplicated hypertension, alone or in combination with other drugs from

42

Antihypertensive
Drugs

TERMS
☐ **captopril (Capoten)**
☐ **clonidine (Catapres)**
☐ **losartan (Cozaar)**
☐ **prazosin (Minipress)**
☐ **sodium nitroprusside (Nipride)**

other classes; most clients will require two or more antihypertensives for BP to be <140/90 mmHg or <130/90 for patients with kidney disease; if BP is more than 20/10 mmHg above goal BP, consider initiating two agents (one a thiazide diuretic); Motivation by the client makes antihypertensive therapy more successful."[2]

There are six classes of antihypertensives:

1. Adrenergic agents (including: alpha-adrenergic blockers, beta-blockers, centrally-acting adrenergic agents, peripherally acting adrenergic agents, and combined alpha-beta-blockers)

2. Calcium channel blockers (CCBs)

3. Diuretics

4. Angiotensin-converting enzyme (ACE) inhibitors

5. Angiotensin II receptor blockers

6. Vasodilators

Beta-blockers, CCBs, and diuretics will not be discussed in this chapter as they are covered in Chapters 40, 41, and 43.

It is imperative that the client also make lifestyle modifications to reduce coronary and stroke risk factors, which include proper diet, exercise, weight management, stress management, and smoking cessation.

Table 42-1 Antihypertensive Drugs

Prototype Drug	Related Drugs	Drug Classification
There is no prototype for this classification	carvedilol (Coreg) labetalol (Trandate, Normodyne)	Alpha$_1$ and beta-adrenergic blockers
prazosin (Minipress)	doxazosin (Cardura) terazosin (Hytrin)	Alpha$_1$-adrenergic blockers

Table 42-1 Antihypertensive Drugs (continued)

Prototype Drug	Related Drugs	Drug Classification
clonidine (Catapres)	guanabenz (Wytensin) guanfacine (Tenex) methyldopa (Aldomet)	Centrally-acting adrenergic agents (Alpha$_2$-agonists)
There is no prototype for this classification	guanadrel (Hylorel) guanethidine (Ismelin)	Peripherally-acting adrenergic neuronal blockers
	reserpine (Novoreserpine)	Also known as a Rauwolfia alkaloids
captopril (Capoten)	benazepril (Lotensin) enalapril (Vasotec) enalaprilat (Vasotec IV) fosinopril (Monopril) lisinopril (Prinivil) moexipril (Univasc) perindopril (Aceon) quinapril (Accupril) ramipril (Altace) trandolapril (Mavik)	ACE inhibitors
losartan (Cozaar)	candesartan (Atacand) eprosartan (Teveten) irbesartan (Avapro) olmesartan (Benicar) telmisartan (Micardis) valsartan (Diovan)	Angiotensin II receptor blockers
sodium nitroprusside (Nipride)	diazoxide (Hyperstat) hydralazine hydrochloride (Apresoline) minoxidil (Loniten, Rogaine)	Vasodilators

Diuretics, beta-blockers, and calcium channel blockers are indicated for the treatment of hypertension and were discussed in previous chapters. Note: There are many fixed combination antihypertensive drugs: (Thiazide with potassium diuretics, thiazide with beta-blockers, thiazide with ACE inhibitors, thiazide with angiotensin II receptor blockers, thiazide with alpha-blockers, and thiazide with centrally-acting adrenergics.)

ANTIHYPERTENSIVES CLIENT TEACHING

- Instruct clients on proper nutrition (decrease sodium intake, follow DASH diet), exercise, and managing stress.

- Do not abruptly stop taking medication as this can lead to rebound hypertension.
- Do not take OTC medications or herbal remedies without first consulting your health care provider.
- If a dose is missed, contact health care provider on what action to take.
- Do not strain when having a bowel movement since this can stimulate the Valsalva maneuver.
- Avoid alcohol due to its additive hypotension effect.
- Saunas, hot weather, hot showers, or baths and hot tubs may cause an additive hypotensive effect, causing dizziness. Sit or lie down until dizziness subsides.
- Monitor blood pressure.
- Contact health care provider if experiencing adverse effects, and do not stop taking medication without consulting health care provider.

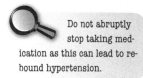

Instruct clients on proper nutrition (decrease sodium intake, follow DASH diet), exercise, and managing stress.

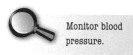

Do not abruptly stop taking medication as this can lead to rebound hypertension.

Monitor blood pressure.

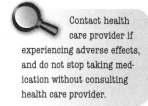

Contact health care provider if experiencing adverse effects, and do not stop taking medication without consulting health care provider.

- Instruct clients taking prazosin (Minipress) that the first dose will cause a drop in blood pressure. Clients should take the first dose at bedtime and lying down. Instruct clients that this disappears with time or after a reduction in dosage.
- Clients taking alpha-blockers and ACE inhibitors should monitor their weight and report changes to their health care provider.
- Clients taking rauwolfia alkaloids should report symptoms of mental depression to their health care provider.
- Drowsiness or dizziness is an adverse effect with many antihypertensives, and as a result clients should not take CNS depressants, and should use extra caution when operating heavy machinery until the personal effects of drug are known.
- Clients taking ACE inhibitors should report bruising, bleeding, infection, or weight gain or loss to health care provider.
- Clients taking ACE inhibitors should avoid using salt substitutes that contain potassium, as an adverse effect of these agents is hyperkalemia.

ACTION

Alpha$_1$- and Beta-Receptor Blockers

- Block alpha$_1$ receptors causing vasodilation and blocks beta receptors causing a decreased heart rate, cardiac output, and renin release from kidneys

Alpha-Adrenergic Blockers (Alpha$_1$-Blockers)

- Block stimulation of the sympathetic nervous system at the alpha$_1$-adrenergic receptor, which causes vasodilatation and reduces blood pressure

Centrally-Acting Adrenergic Agents (Alpha$_2$-Agonists)

- Work within the brainstem to suppress sympathetic outflow, by stimulating central alpha$_2$ receptors, to the heart and blood vessels, which results in vasodilatation and decreased cardiac output and reduces BP

Peripherally-Acting Adrenergic Neuronal Blockers and Rauwolfia Alkaloids

- These drugs work peripherally to inhibit the release of norepinephrine (guanadrel [Hylorel] and guanethidine [Ismelin]).
- Reserpine (Novoreserpine) causes norepinephrine depletion.
- All of these drugs decrease sympathetic stimulation of the heart and blood vessels which decreases BP. Reserpine is derived from the Rauwolfia serpentina plant.

Angiotensin-Converting Enzyme (ACE) Inhibitors

- Inhibit the angiotensin-converting enzyme, responsible for converting angiotensin I to angiotensin II, and inactivate bradykinin and other prostaglandins
- Reduce aldosterone levels causing vasodilatation and lower BP

Angiotensin II Receptor Blockers

* Block the vasoconstrictive and aldosterone-producing effects of Angiostensin II at the receptor sites, which causes vasodilatation and lowered BP

Vasodilators

* Directly act on arterial smooth muscle to cause vasodilatation and lower BP

USE

Alpha$_1$- and Beta-Adrenergic Blockers

* Treatment of hypertension may be used alone or with a diuretic or other antihypertensives.
* Carvedilol (Coreg) also used to treat CHF.

Alpha-Adrenergic Blockers (Alpha$_1$-Blockers)

* Treatment of hypertension may be used alone or with other anti-hypertensives.

Centrally-Acting Adrenergic Agents (Alpha$_2$-Agonists)

* Generally used as adjunct agents to treat hypertension or may be used with a diuretic or other antihypertensives
* Due to their side effects (drowsiness, orthostatic hypertension, dizziness), they are not usually prescribed as first-line antihypertensive agents.[3]

Clonidine (Catapres)

* Also has an unlabeled use to treat opioid and nicotine withdrawal[3]
* Epidural clonidine (Catapres) is indicated for treatment of cancer pain unresponsive to opioids.

Methylodopa (Aldomet)

- Also indicated to treat hypertension in pregnancy
- Peripherally-acting adrenergic neuronal blockers and rauwolfia alkaloids
- Used infrequently to treat hypertension due to their adverse effects and limited effectiveness. Indicated when other antihypertensives have not been effective and are primarily used for adjunctive antihypertensive therapy.[3] May be given with a diuretic to minimize fluid retention.

Angiotensin-Converting Enzyme Inhibitors

- Antihypertensive agents, used alone or in combination with other antihypertensives or diuretics, and also indicated as adjunct agents for CHF treatment[4]

Angiotensin II Receptor Blockers

- Treatment of hypertension; can be used alone or with other agents such as diuretics
- Also used to treat CHF

Vasodilators

- Treatment of severe hypertension; used alone or in combination with other antihypertensives

Diazoxide (Hyperstat)

- Also used as an antihypoglycemic when given orally[5]

Minoxidil (Loniten, Rogaine)

- Also used to treat baldness

Sodium Nitroprusside (Nipride) and Diazoxide (Hyperstat)

- Given IV for treatment of hypertensive emergencies
- Also used to treat CHF for controlled hypotension during anesthesia

ADVERSE EFFECTS AND SIDE EFFECTS

Alpha$_1$- and Beta-Adrenergic Blockers

- *Pregnancy category C*
- *CV:* Bradycardia, atrioventricular (AV) heart block
- *Resp:* Exacerbates asthma

Alpha-Adrenergic Blockers (Alpha1-Blockers)

- *Pregnancy category C*
- *CV:* First-dose orthostatic hypotension, palpitations, tachycardia, angina, and edema
- *CNS:* Dizziness, headache, weakness, drowsiness, depression, fatigue, depression
- *GI:* Nausea, vomiting, diarrhea, dry mouth, and abdominal cramps
- *GU:* Impotence, incontinence

Centrally-Acting Adrenergic Agents (Alpha$_2$-Agonists)

- *Pregnancy category C, although methylodopa (Aldomet) and guanfacine (Tenex) are pregnancy category B agents*
- *CV:* Bradycardia, palpitations
- *CNS:* Drowsiness, dizziness, severe rebound hypertension if abruptly discontinued, sleep disturbances
- *Derm:* Rash
- *GI:* Dry mouth, nausea, vomiting, and constipation
- *GU:* Impotence

Peripherally-Acting Adrenergic Neuron Blockers

- *Pregnancy category B*

Rauwolfia Alkaloids

- *Pregnancy category D*
- *CV:* Edema, chest pain, orthostatic hypotension, and bradycardia

- *CNS:* Dizziness, weakness, fainting, fatigue, headaches, and depression
- *EENT:* Visual disturbances, stuffy nose
- *GI:* Constipation, anorexia, dry mouth, diarrhea, indigestion
- *GU:* Impotence, nocturia, and urinary frequency
- *Resp:* Shortness of breath and cough

Angiotensin-Converting Enzyme (ACE) Inhibitors

- *Pregnancy category C (first trimester) and pregnancy category D (second and third trimesters)*
- *CV:* First-dose hypotensive effect
- *CNS:* Dizziness, fatigue, and headaches
- *Derm:* Rashes
- *F & E:* Hyperkalemia, angioedema
- *GI:* Taste disturbances, diarrhea, and nausea
- *GU:* Proteinuria, impotence, and renal failure
- *Hematologic:* Agranulocytosis, neutropenia
- *Resp:* Cough, which disappears when drug is discontinued

Angiotensin II Receptor Blockers

- *Pregnancy category B (first trimester) and pregnancy category C (second and third trimester)*
- *CNS:* Fatigue, dizziness, and headache, insomnia
- *F & E:* hyperkalemia
- *GI:* Diarrhea, heartburn
- *GU:* Impaired renal function
- *Resp:* Upper respiratory infection (although, this group of drugs does not cause cough)

Vasodilators

- *Pregnancy category C*

Diazoxide (Hyperstat)

- *CV:* Orthostatic hypotension, dysrhythmias
- *CNS:* Dizziness, headache
- *F & E:* Sodium and water retention

- *GI:* Nausea and vomiting
- *Other:* Acute pancreatitis, hyperglycemia in clients with diabetes mellitus

Hydralazine Hydrochloride (Apresoline)

- *CV:* Tachycardia, angina, edema, flushing
- *CNS:* Dizziness, headache
- *EENT:* Nasal stuffiness
- *GI:* Anorexia, nausea, vomiting, diarrhea
- *Hematologic:* Anemia, agranulocytosis
- *Other:* Hepatitis, systemic lupus erythematosus (SLE)-like syndrome, rash, peripheral neuritis

Minoxidil (Loniten, Rogaine)

- *CV:* Tachycardia, angina, flushing, and pericarditis
- *CNS:* Headache
- *GI:* Anorexia, nausea, and vomiting
- *Other:* Excessive hair growth

Sodium Nitroprusside (Nipride)

- *CV:* Tachycardia, hypotension, flushing
- *CNS:* Dizziness, headache, and anxiety
- *Hematologic:* Platelet aggregation
- *Other:* Possible cyanide toxicity, hypothyroidism, rash

CONTRAINDICATIONS

Alpha₁- and Beta-Adrenergic Blockers

- Hypersensitivity
- Asthma
- Severe CHF
- Bradycardia
- AV heart block

Alpha-Adrenergic Blockers (Alpha₁-Blockers)

- Hypersensitivity

Centrally-Acting Adrenergic Agents (Alpha$_2$-Agonists)

* Hypersensitivity

Peripherally-Acting Adrenergic Neuron Blockers

* Hypersensitivity
* Lactation
* Pheochromocytoma
* CHF, recent myocardial infarction
* Concurrent use of monoamine oxidase inhibitors (MAOIs)

Rauwolfia Alkaloids

* Hypersensitivity
* Mental depression
* Active peptic ulcer or ulcerative colitis

Angiotensin-Converting Enzyme (ACE) Inhibitors

* Hypersensitivity
* Angioedema
* Pregnancy

Angiotensin II Receptor Blockers

* Hypersensitivity
* Pregnancy or lactation

Vasodilators

* Hypersensitivity

Diazoxide (Hyperstat)

* Compensatory hypertension
* Functional hypoglycemia associated with coarctation or arteriovenous shunt hydralazine hydrochloride (Apresoline)
* Coronary artery disease
* Mitral valve or rheumatic heart disease

Minoxidil (Loniten, Rogaine)

* Pheochromocytoma

Sodium Nitroprusside (Nipride)

- Hypersensitivity
- Compensatory hypertension associated with coarctation or AV shunt
- Congenital Leber's optic atrophy
- Tobacco amblyopia
- Inadequate cerebral circulation

INTERACTIONS

Alpha₁- and Beta-Adrenergic Blockers

- None

Alpha-Adrenergic Blockers (Alpha₁-Blockers)

- Concurrent use of other antihypertensives, nitrates, and alcohol causes additive hypertension.

Centrally-Acting Adrenergic Agents (Alpha₂-Agonists)

- Concurrent use of alcohol, sedative-hypnotics, opioids, antihistamines, and anesthetics increases CNS depression.
- Concurrent use of alcohol, antihypertensives, and nitrates causes additive hypotension.
- Concurrent use with MAOIs, tricyclic antidepressants (TCAs), and amphetamines may decrease antihypertensive effects.
- Concurrent use of TCAs decreases antihypertensive effect.
- Concurrent use with beta-blockers may cause bradycardia and increase rebound hypertension for clients in clonidine withdrawal.

Peripherally-Acting Adrenergic Neuron Blockers and Rauwolfia Alkaloids

- Concurrent use of other antihypertensives and diuretics increases hypotensive effect.
- Concurrent use of TCAs decreases antihypertensive effect.
- MAOIs have additive effects and may cause hypertension and excitation.

- Increased CNS depression with alcohol, barbiturates, and other CNS depressants
- Decreased antihypertensive effects with phenothiazines and sympathomimetics

Angiotensin-Converting Enzyme (ACE) Inhibitors

- Concurrent use of other antihypertensives, diuretics, nitrates, and alcohol increases hypotensive effects.
- Aspirin and NSAIDs antagonize ACE inhibitors, decreasing antihypertensive effects.
- Concurrent use with lithium can cause lithium toxicity.
- Concurrent use of potassium-sparing diuretics or clients taking potassium supplements can cause increased hyperkalemia.

Angiotensin II Receptor Blockers

- Cimetadine may increase the effects of angiotensin II receptor blockers.
- Concurrent use of other antihypertensives and diuretics increases hypotensive effect.
- NSAIDs, phenobarbital, and rifampin decrease antihypertensive effect.
- Concurrent use with lithium can cause lithium toxicity.

Vasodilators

- Increased antihypertensive effects with alcohol, other antihypertensives, and nitrates

Diazoxide (Hyperstat)

- Concurrent use with oral anticoagulants increases anticoagulant effect.
- Concurrent use with sulfonylureas decreases hypoglycemic effect of sulfonylureas.

Hydralazine Hydrochloride (Apresoline)

- Concurrent use with adrenergics decreases antihypertensive effects.
- Concurrent use with MAOIs increases hypertension.

Minoxidil (Loniten, Rogaine)

- Concurrent use with guanethidine can cause severe hypertension.

Sodium Nitroprusside (Nipride)

- Concurrent use with ganglionic blocking agents increases hypertension.

NURSING IMPLICATIONS

All Antihypertensives

- Monitor vital signs, especially BP.
- Monitor I & O and daily weight.
- Monitor for edema or weight gain.
- Monitor electrolytes, especially potassium.
- Implement safety measures as initial use can cause drowsiness and dizziness.
- Antihypertensives should not be abruptly discontinued and should be resumed after treatment and surgery to avoid rebound hypertension.

Monitor vital signs, especially BP.

Implement safety measures as initial use can cause drowsiness and dizziness.

Antihypertensives should not be abruptly discontinued and should be resumed after treatment and surgery to avoid rebound hypertension.

Alpha$_1$- and Beta-Adrenergic Blockers

- Give PO.

Alpha$_1$-Adrenergic Blockers (Alpha$_1$ Blockers)

- Give PO.
- Report significant weight gain, edema, or BP changes.
- Monitor client for first-dose orthostatic hypotensive effects and implement safety measures to prevent injury.
- First dose orthostatic hypotensive effects may occur 30 to 90 minutes after first dose with symptoms of dizziness, weakness, or syncope.

Monitor client for first-dose orthostatic hypotensive effects and implement safety measures to prevent injury.

- Generally after the first dose, tolerance develops and orthostatic hypotensive effects diminish.

Centrally-Acting Adrenergic Agonists (Alpha₂-Agonists)

Clonidine (Catapress)

- Give PO, transdermally, and by epidural.
- Epidural use is indicated for management of cancer pain.

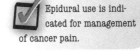
Epidural use is indicated for management of cancer pain.

- Transdermal use—reapply every 7 days. Rotate sites, use hairless sites, and avoid cuts or calluses; remove old patch before applying new patch; and wash area with soap and water before applying. Client can swim, bathe, or shower with application on. Monitor for skin reaction.

Encourage use of hard candy, rinsing mouth, and good oral hygiene to help decrease effects of dry mouth.

- Encourage use of hard candy, rinsing mouth, and good oral hygiene to help decrease effects of dry mouth.
- Assess for edema.
- Discontinue medication gradually over 2 to 4 days to prevent rebound hypertension.
- Implement safety measures as initial use can cause drowsiness and dizziness.

Guanabenz (Wytensin) and Guanfacine (Tenex)

- Give PO.

Methyldopa (Aldomet)

- Give PO and IV.

Peripherally-Acting Adrenergic Neuron Blockers and Rauwolfia Alkaloids

- Give PO.
- Assess for edema.
- Monitor bowel habits and report changes; excessive diarrhea may require a change in dose.

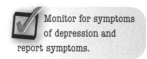

- Monitor for symptoms of depression and report symptoms.
- Implement safety measures as initial use can cause drowsiness and dizziness.

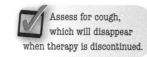

Monitor for symptoms of depression and report symptoms.

Angiotensin-Converting Enzyme (ACE) Inhibitors

- Give PO; enalaprilat (Vasotec IV) available IV.
- Captopril (Capoten) is given 1 hour before or 2 hours after meals.
- Assess for cough, which will disappear when therapy is discontinued.
- Periodically monitor blood urea nitrogen, creatinine, and electrolytes throughout therapy.
- Monitor complete blood count (CBC) periodically throughout therapy and for symptoms of agranulocytosis and neutropenia.
- Monitor for first-dose orthostatic hypotensive effect, especially the first 3 hours after initiating therapy, and may include treatment with IV fluids.[6]
- Implement safety measures as initial use can cause fatigue and dizziness.
- Notify health care provider immediately if client develops angioedema.

Assess for cough, which will disappear when therapy is discontinued.

Angiotensin II Receptor Blockers

- Give PO.
- Monitor for upper respiratory infection.
- Can be given without regard to meals.

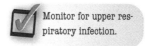

Monitor for upper respiratory infection.

Vasodilators

Diazoxide (Hyperstat)

- Give PO and administer IV for hypertensive emergencies
- Monitor for hyperglycemia and sodium and fluid retention.
- Onset of action is 1 minute after administering IV push.

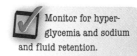

Monitor for hyperglycemia and sodium and fluid retention.

- Monitor BP every 5 minutes until stable with IV administration, then every hour throughout therapy.

> Monitor BP every 5 minutes until stable with IV administration, then every hour throughout therapy.

- Assess pulse before and during therapy.
- Keep client in a supine position for at least 30 minutes after administering.
- Monitor CBC, electrolytes, and glucose throughout therapy.
- Assess for extravasation during IV therapy.

Hydralazine Hydrochloride (Apresoline)

- Give PO, IM, or IV.
- Monitor CBC, electrolytes, SLE prep, and antinuclear antibody titer throughout therapy.
- Administer with food to enhance absorption.
- With IV administration, monitor BP and pulse frequently throughout therapy.

> With IV administration, monitor BP and pulse frequently throughout therapy.

- Monitor mental status and report anxiety or depression, which may indicate cerebral ischemia.[5]

Minoxidil (Loniten, Rogaine)

- Give PO or topically to treat baldness.
- Can be given without regard to food
- Monitor CBC, electrolytes, renal, and hepatic function throughout therapy.

Sodium Nitroprusside (Nipride)

- Give via IV infusion to treat hypertensive emergencies.
- Monitor for cyanide poisoning, which can occur if more than 500.0 mcg/kg is given faster than 2.0 mcg/kg/minute.

> Monitor for cyanide poisoning, which can occur if more than 500.0 mcg/kg is given faster than 2.0 mcg/kg/minute.

- Monitor thiocyanate levels every 24 to 48 hours; normal: less than 100.0 mcg thiocyante/mL or 3 μmol cyanide/mL.
- Protect drug from light and wrap bag in aluminum foil.
- Use an infusion pump to administer.
- Initially check BP every 5 minutes, then every 15 minutes.
- Use drug solution within 4 hours after preparing it.

Minoxidil (Loniten, Rogaine)

- Concurrent use with guanethidine can cause severe hypertension.

Sodium Nitroprusside (Nipride)

- Concurrent use with ganglionic blocking agents increases hypertension.

NURSING IMPLICATIONS

All Antihypertensives

- Monitor vital signs, especially BP.
- Monitor I & O and daily weight.
- Monitor for edema or weight gain.
- Monitor electrolytes, especially potassium.
- Implement safety measures as initial use can cause drowsiness and dizziness.
- Antihypertensives should not be abruptly discontinued and should be resumed after treatment and surgery to avoid rebound hypertension.

Monitor vital signs, especially BP.

Implement safety measures as initial use can cause drowsiness and dizziness.

Antihypertensives should not be abruptly discontinued and should be resumed after treatment and surgery to avoid rebound hypertension.

Alpha₁- and Beta-Adrenergic Blockers

- Give PO.

Alpha₁-Adrenergic Blockers (Alpha₁ Blockers)

- Give PO.
- Report significant weight gain, edema, or BP changes.
- Monitor client for first-dose orthostatic hypotensive effects and implement safety measures to prevent injury.
- First dose orthostatic hypotensive effects may occur 30 to 90 minutes after first dose with symptoms of dizziness, weakness, or syncope.

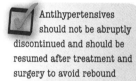

Monitor client for first-dose orthostatic hypotensive effects and implement safety measures to prevent injury.

- Generally after the first dose, tolerance develops and orthostatic hypotensive effects diminish.

Centrally-Acting Adrenergic Agonists (Alpha$_2$-Agonists)

Clonidine (Catapress)

- Give PO, transdermally, and by epidural.
- Epidural use is indicated for management of cancer pain.
- Transdermal use—reapply every 7 days. Rotate sites, use hairless sites, and avoid cuts or calluses; remove old patch before applying new patch; and wash area with soap and water before applying. Client can swim, bathe, or shower with application on. Monitor for skin reaction.
- Encourage use of hard candy, rinsing mouth, and good oral hygiene to help decrease effects of dry mouth.
- Assess for edema.
- Discontinue medication gradually over 2 to 4 days to prevent rebound hypertension.
- Implement safety measures as initial use can cause drowsiness and dizziness.

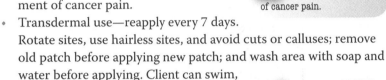

Epidural use is indicated for management of cancer pain.

Encourage use of hard candy, rinsing mouth, and good oral hygiene to help decrease effects of dry mouth.

Guanabenz (Wytensin) and Guanfacine (Tenex)

- Give PO.

Methyldopa (Aldomet)

- Give PO and IV.

Peripherally-Acting Adrenergic Neuron Blockers and Rauwolfia Alkaloids

- Give PO.
- Assess for edema.
- Monitor bowel habits and report changes; excessive diarrhea may require a change in dose.

REFERENCES

1. Lilley L, Harrington S, Snyder J. *Pharmacology and the Nursing Process,* 5th ed. St. Louis, MO: Mosby; 2007:368.

2. Chobanin AV, Bakris GL, Black HR, et al. The seventh report of the Joint National Committee on Prevention, Detection, Evaluation, and Treatment of High Blood Pressure: the JNC 7 report. *JAMA.* 2003; 289(19):2560–2572.

3. Lilley L, Harrington S, Snyder J. *Pharmacology and the Nursing Process,* 5th ed. St. Louis, MO: Mosby; 2007:373.

4. Karch A. *Focus on Nursing Pharmacology*, 4th ed. Philadelphia, PA: Wolters Kluwer/Lippincott, Williams & Wilkins; 2008:691.

5. Karch A. *Focus on Nursing Pharmacology*, 4th ed. Philadelphia, PA: Wolters Kluwer/Lippincott, Williams & Wilkins; 2008:701.

6. McKenry LM, Tessier E, Hogan M. Mosby's *Pharmacology in Nursing*, 22nd ed. St. Louis, MO: Mosby Elsevier; 2006:557.

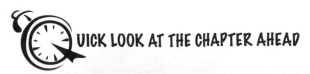

Diuretics work to prevent resorption of water and sodium and speed up urine formation. Diuretics are classified according to their sites of action, diuretic potency, and chemical structure. Diuretics decrease blood volume, venous pressure, arterial pressure, pulmonary and peripheral edema, and cardiac output.[1] They are indicated for clients with fluid overload and are used to treat hypertension, congestive heart failure (CHF), edema, and ascites.

43

Diuretic Drugs

TERMS
- ☐ acetazolamide (Diamox)
- ☐ furosemide (Lasix)
- ☐ hydrochlorothiazide (Esidrix, HydroDIURIL)
- ☐ mannitol (Osmitrol)
- ☐ spironalactone (Aldactone)

Table 43-1 Diuretic Drugs

Prototype Drug	Related Drugs	Drug Classification
acetazolamide (Diamox)	methazolamide (Glauc Tabs)	Carbonic anhydrase inhibitors (CAIs)
furosemide (Lasix)	bumetanide (Bumex) ethacrynic acid (Edecrin) torsemide (Demadex)	Loop diuretics
mannitol (Osmitrol)	glycerin (Osmoglyn) isosorbide (Ismotic) urea (Ureaphil)	Osmotic diuretics
spironalactone (Aldactone)	amiloride (Midamor) eplerenone (Inspra) triamterene (Dyrenium)	Potassium-sparing diuretics
hydrochlorothiazide (Esidrix, HydroDIURIL)	bendroflumethiazide (Nautretin) benzthiazide (Exna) chlorothiazide (Diuril) chlorthalidone (Hygroton) hydroflumethiazide (Saluron) indapamide (Lozol) methyclothiazide (Enduron) metolazone (Mykrox, Zaroxolyn) polythiazide (Renese-R) quinethazone (Hydromox) trichlormethiazide (Metahydrin, Naqua)	Thiazide and thiazide-like diuretics

DIURETIC DRUGS CLIENT TEACHING

- Avoid concurrent use of OTCs and herbal remedies without consulting with health care provider.
- Eat high potassium foods, except when taking potassium-sparing diuretics.
- Change positions gradually to prevent orthostatic hypotension.

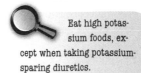
Eat high potassium foods, except when taking potassium-sparing diuretics.

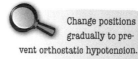
Change positions gradually to prevent orthostatic hypotension.

- Monitor weight and notify health care provider of a weight gain of 5 or more pounds in a week.
- Monitor and report symptoms of hypokalemia such as irregular heart rate, lethargy, or muscle weakness or cramping to health care provider.
- Follow up with laboratory and health care provider visits as indicated.
- Clients with diabetes mellitus need to monitor blood sugar levels as loop and thiazide diuretics can increase blood sugar.
- Notify health care provider of symptoms of fluid volume loss or hypotension, such as palpitations.
- Maintain fluid balance and notify health care provider if experiencing vomiting or diarrhea.
- Avoid alcohol, exercising in hot weather, barbiturates, or opioids to prevent orthostatic hypotension.
- Take diuretics in the morning.
- Clients taking cardiac glycosides with a diuretic should report symptoms of cardiac glycoside toxicity, such as visual changes, bradycardia, nausea, or anorexia.
- Wear sunscreen or protective clothing to prevent photosensitivity.

 Take diuretics in the morning.

ACTION

Carbonic Anhydrase Inhibitors (CAIs)

- Inhibit the enzyme carbonic anhydrase found in the eyes, kidneys, and other parts of the body
- Work primarily in the proximal tubule of the nephron and also decrease the aqueous humor in the eye[2]

Loop Diuretics

- Potent diuretics that act mainly in the ascending limb of the loop of Henle. They have a rapid onset of action and inhibit reabsorption of sodium and chloride.

Osmotic Diuretics

- Work in the proximal tubule and increase osmotic pressure of glomerular filtrate, which inhibits tubular reabsorption of water and electrolytes[3]
- Also decrease intraocular pressure

Potassium-Sparing Diuretics

- Block aldosterone receptors and work in the collecting ducts and distal convoluted tubules and interfere with sodium-potassium exchange. The result is excretion of sodium, but a retention of potassium.

Thiazide and Thiazide-Like Diuretics

- Thiazides are chemical derivatives of sulfonamides that inhibit tubular reabsorption of sodium and chloride ions in the ascending loop of Henle and in the early distal tubule.[4]

USE

Carbonic Anhydrase Inhibitors (CAIs)

- Used infrequently to treat fluid overload
- Primarily used to treat open-angle glaucoma
- Also used to treat acute altitude sickness, seizures, and edema

Loop Diuretics

- Edema related to CHF
- Hepatic or renal disease
- Hypertension
- Hypercalcemia

Osmotic Diuretics

- Acute renal failure
- Edema

- Genitourinary (GU) irrigant for transurethral procedures
- Increased intracranial or intraocular pressure (glaucoma)

Potassium-Sparing Diuretics

- Edema, hypertension, hyperaldosteronism
- Used frequently with diuretics (thiazides)

Thiazide and Thiazide-Like Diuretics

- Edema related to CHF, renal dysfunction, cirrhosis, glucocorticoid, and estrogen therapy
- Hypertension and diabetes insipidus

ADVERSE EFFECTS AND SIDE EFFECTS

Carbonic Anhydrase Inhibitors (CAIs)

- *Pregnancy category C*
- *CNS:* Drowsiness, depression, paresthesias
- *Derm:* Rash, photosensitivity, urticaria
- *F & E:* Acidosis, hypokalemia
- *GI:* Anorexia, metallic taste
- *Hematologic:* Leukopenia

Loop Diuretics

- *Furosemide (Lasix) and bumetanide (Bumex) are pregnancy category C; ethacrynic acid (Edecrin) is pregnancy category D; and torsemide (Demadex) is pregnancy category B.*
- *CNS:* Headache, dizziness, tinnitus, hearing loss, encephalopathy (especially with furosemide and bumetanide)
- *Derm:* Rash, photosensitivity
- *Endocrine:* Hyperglycemia
- *F & E:* Hypokalemia, dehydration, metabolic alkalosis
- *GI:* Nausea, vomiting, and diarrhea
- *Hematologic:* Blood dyscrasias

Osmotic Diuretics

* *Pregnancy category C*
* *CNS:* Headache, confusion, convulsions, blurred vision
* *CV:* Tachycardia, chest pain, pulmonary edema
* *Local:* Thrombophlebitis

Potassium-Sparing Diuretics

* *Spironalactone (Aldactone) and triamterene (Dyrenium) are pregnancy category D; amiloride (Midamor) and eplerenone (Inspra) are pregnancy category B.*
* *CNS:* Headache, dizziness
* *Derm:* Photosensitivity (triamterene [Dyrenium])
* *Endocrine:* Gynecomastia, irregular menses, or amenorrhea (spironaolactone [Aldactone])
* *F & E:* Hyperkalemia
* *GI:* Nausea, vomiting, diarrhea
* *GU:* Kidney stones (triamterene [Dyrenium])
* *Hematologic:* Dyscrasias (triamterene [Dyrenium] and spironolactone [Aldactone])

Thiazide and Thiazid-Like Diuretics

* *Hydrochlorothiazide (Esidrix), chlorothiazide (Diuril), indapamide (Lozol), methyclothiazide (Enduron), and metolazone (Mykrox, Zaroxolyn) are pregnancy category B; benzthiazide (Exna), polythiazide (Renese-R), and trichlormethiazide (Metahydrin, Naqua) are pregnancy category C; hydroflumethiazide (Saluron) is category D; and bendroflumethiazide (Nautretin), chlorthalidone (Hygroton), and quincthazone (Hydromox) are not classified in a pregnancy category.*
* *CNS:* Dizziness, drowsiness, decreased libido
* *Derm:* Rash, photosensitivity
* *Endocrine:* Hyperglycemia
* *F & E:* Hypokalemia, dehydration, hyperuricemia
* *GI:* Nausea, vomiting, and diarrhea; anorexia
* *Hematologic:* Blood dyscrasias, jaundice

CONTRAINDICATIONS

Carbonic Anhydrase Inhibitors (CAIs)

- Hypersensitivity and cross-sensitivity with sulfonamides. (CAIs are chemical derivatives of sulfonamide antibiotics.)

Loop Diuretics

- Hypersensitivity, cross-sensitivity with thiazides, and sulfonamides
- Clients with pre-existing electrolyte imbalance that has not been corrected
- Anuria, hepatic coma

Osmotic Diuretics

- Hypersensitivity, dehydration, anuria, and active intracranial bleeding

Potassium-Sparing Diuretics

- Hypersensitivity and hyperkalemia

Thiazide and Thiazide-Like Diuretics

- Hypersensitivity, cross-sensitivity with other thiazides or sulfon-amides, anuria, and lactation

INTERACTIONS

Carbonic Anhydrase Inhibitors (CAIs)

- Concurrent use with glucocorticoids may cause hypokalemia.
- Concurrent use with oral hypoglycemics, quinidine, and pro-cainamide may lead to toxicity with these drugs.
- May cause false-positive urine protein tests

Loop Diuretics

- Concurrent use with cardiac glycosides or corticosteroids may cause hypokalemia and increased cardiac glycoside toxicity.
- Concurrent use with antihypertensives, alcohol, or nitrates may cause additive hypotension.
- Concurrent use with aminoglycosides, vancomycin, phenylbutazone, chloroquine, or capremycin may increase neurotoxicity and ototoxicity.[5]
- Concurrent use with sulfonylureas may cause hyperglycemia.
- Lithium increases lithium toxicity due to decreased excretion of lithium.
- May increase glucose, creatinine, BUN, or uric acid levels

Osmotic Diuretics

- Concurrent use with cardiac glycosides increases risk of hypokalemia and cardiac glycoside toxicity.

Potassium-Sparing Diuretics

- Triamterene (Dyrenium) decreases effects of folic acid.
- Triamterene (Dyrenium) increases toxicity risk from amantadine.
- Concurrent use with alcohol, antihypertensives, and nitrates may cause additive hypotension.
- Concurrent use with angiotensin-converting enzyme inhibitors, indomethacin, potassium supplements, or cyclosporine increases risk of hyperkalemia.
- NSAIDs may decrease effectiveness of potassium-sparing diuretics.
- Concurrent use with lithium may result in lithium toxicity.

Thiazide Diuretics

- Concurrent use with other antihypertensives, alcohol, and nitrates increases additive hypotension.
- Lithium decreases lithium excretion.
- Concurrent use with cardiac glycosides increases hypokalemia and risk of cardiac glycoside toxicity.

- NSAIDs may decrease effectiveness of thiazide diuretics.
- Oral hypoglycemics antagonize effects of thiazides and decrease therapeutic effects of thiazides.
- Concurrent use with corticosteroids may cause additive hypokalemia.
- Excessive intake of licorice can cause additive hypokalemia.

℞ NURSING IMPLICATIONS

All Diuretics

- Monitor vital signs, daily weights, I & O, edema location, skin turgor, mucous membranes, lung sounds, and fluid and electrolyte balance—especially potassium.
- Observe for signs of hypokalemia.
- Observe for signs of hyperkalemia with potassium-sparing diuretics.

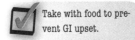

Monitor vital signs, daily weights, I & O, edema location, skin turgor, mucous membranes, lung sounds, and fluid and electrolyte balance—especially potassium.

Carbonic Anhydrase Inhibitors (CAIs)

- Give PO, IM, or IV.
- IM injection is painful and should be avoided.
- Take with food to prevent GI upset.
- Assess for allergy to sulfonamides or thiazides.

Take with food to prevent GI upset.

Loop Diuretics

- Give PO, IM, or IV.
- Assess for allergy to sulfonamides.
- Assess for tinnitus and hearing loss, especially with IV high dose therapy.
- Administer with food to decrease GI upset.
- When administering IV push, administer undiluted over 1 to 2 minutes.

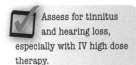

Assess for tinnitus and hearing loss, especially with IV high dose therapy.

Osmotic Diuretics

- Mannital is administered as an IV infusion or as a GU irrigant; urea (Ureaphil) is administered as an IV infusion, glycerin (Osmoglyn) and isosorbide (Ismotic) are given PO.
- Monitor neurological status with increased intracranial pressure.
- Monitor for eye pain or decreased visual acuity when monitoring for increased intraocular pressure.
- Monitor renal function studies during therapy.

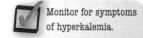
Monitor renal function studies during therapy.

Potassium-Sparing Diuretics

- Give PO.
- Administer with food to minimize GI upset.
- Triamterene (Dyrenium) capsules may be opened and mixed with food or fluids.
- Avoid salt substitutes as they contain potassium.
- Monitor for symptoms of hyperkalemia.

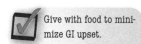
Monitor for symptoms of hyperkalemia.

Thiazide and Thiazide-Like Diuretics

- Give orally. Chlorothiazide (Diuril) can also be given IV.
- Give with food to minimize GI upset.

Give with food to minimize GI upset.

REFERENCES

1. Lehne RA. *Pharmacology for Nursing Care*, 6th ed. Philadelphia, PA: Saunders Elsevier; 2007:439.

2. Lilley L, Harrington S, Snyder J. *Pharmacology and the Nursing Process*, 5th ed. St. Louis, MO: Mosby; 2007:391.

3. Lilley L, Harrington S, Snyder J. *Pharmacology and the Nursing Process*, 5th ed. St. Louis, MO: Mosby; 2007:393.

4. Lilley L, Harrington S, Snyder J. *Pharmacology and the Nursing Process*, 5th ed. St. Louis, MO: Mosby; 2007:396.

5. Lilley L, Harrington S, Snyder J. *Pharmacology and the Nursing Process*, 5th ed. St. Louis, MO: Mosby; 2007:392.

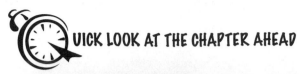

The antilipemic drugs are indicated to lower cholesterol and triglycerides levels. The National Cholesterol Education Program recommends that nondrug therapy such as diet, exercise, and reduction of other risk factors should be tried first, for at least 6 months, and if not effective, then drug therapy may be indicated.[1]

The 4 major classifications of antilipemics include: **bile acid sequestrants, fibric acid derivatives, HMG-CoA reduatase inhibitors,** also known as "statins," and cholesterol absorption inhibitors.

44

Antilipemic Drugs

TERMS
☐ atorvastatin (Lipitor)
☐ cholestyramine (Questran)
☐ ezetimibe (Zetia)

Table 44-1 Antilipemic Drugs

Prototype Drug	Related Drugs	Drug Classification
cholestyramine (Questran)	colestipol hydrochloride (Colestid) colesevelam (Welchol)	Bile acid sequestrants
There is no prototype for this classification	fenofibrate (Tricor) gemfibrozil (Lopid)	Fibric acid derivatives
atorvastatin (Lipitor)	fluvastatin (Lescol) lovastatin (Mevacor) pravastatin (Pravachol) rosuvastatin (Crestor) simvastatin (Zocor)	HMG-CoA reductase inhibitors (also called statins)
ezetimibe (Zetia)	There are no related drugs at this time	cholesterol absorption inhibitor
There is no prototype for this classification	niacin or nicotinic acid	Other/vitamin B_3
There is no prototype for this classification	Caduet (amlodipine and atorvastatin) Niacin extended release/ lovastatin (Advicor) Pravigard (buffered aspirin and pravastatin) Vytorin (ezetimibe and simvastatin)	Combination antilepemics

ANTILIPEMIC DRUGS CLIENT TEACHING

- Instruct client on proper nutrition and exercise.
- Notify health care provider of continuous gastrointestinal (GI) upset or distress, bleeding, yellow skin discoloration, decreased libido, or dysuria.
- Powder or granule preparations should be mixed with liquids or food.
- Do not change or stop medication without consulting with health care provider.
- Consult with health care provider before taking herbal remedies or OTC drugs.

> Notify health care provider of continuous gastrointestinal (GI) upset or distress, bleeding, yellow skin discoloration, decreased libido, or dysuria.

- Other drugs should be taken 1 hour before or 4 to 6 hours after bile acid sequestrants.
- Periodic laboratory and clinical monitoring are indicated.

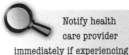
Notify health care provider immediately if experiencing muscle pain.

- Notify health care provider immediately if experiencing muscle pain.

ACTION

Bile Acid Sequestrants

- Combine with bile acids in the small intestine to form insoluble complexes excreted through stool, which reduces low-density lipoprotein (LDL) and serum cholesterol levels

Fibric Acid Derivatives

- Activate the enzyme lipoprotein lipase, which breaks down cholesterol, inhibit triglyceride synthesis in the liver, increase the secretion of cholesterol into bile, and suppress the release of fatty acid from adipose tissue[2]

HMG-CoA Reductase Inhibitors (Statins)

- Decrease the rate of cholesterol production by inhibiting HMG-CoA reductase
- They are potent and effective in decreasing LDL levels.

Cholesterol Absorption Inhibitors

- Inhibits cholesterol absorption in the small intestine

Other

Niacin: Vitamin B$_3$

- Unknown action but may prevent release of fatty acids from adipose tissue and decrease hepatic lipoprotein synthesis

USE

Bile Acid Sequestrants

- Type II hyperlipoproteinemia and for treatment of pruritus related to partial biliary obstruction

Fibric Acid Derivatives

- Decrease triglyceride levels and in type III, IV, and V, and some type IIb forms of hyperlipidemias[2]

HMG-CoA Reductase Inhibitors (Statins)

- Type IIa and IIb hyperlipidemias and effective in lowering LDL and increasing high-density lipoprotein (HDL) levels[3]

Cholesterol Absorption Inhibitors

- Homozygous sitosterolemia
- Hymozygous familial hypercholesterolemia

Other

Niacin: Vitamin B$_3$

- Decreases triglyceride levels, LDL, and total serum cholesterol levels, and increases HDL levels
- Type IIa, IIb, III, IV, and V hyperlipidemias

 ## ADVERSE EFFECTS AND SIDE EFFECTS

Bile Acid Sequestrants

- *Cholestyramine (Questran) is pregnancy category C, colestipol hydrochloride (Colestid) and colesevelam (Welchol) are pregnancy category B.*
- *GI:* Bloating, belching, constipation, nausea
- *Other:* Headache, bleeding

Fibric Acid Derivatives

- *Pregnancy category C*
- *GI:* Nausea, vomiting, diarrhea, and gallstones
- *Hematologic:* Increased prothrombin time, hematuria
- *Other:* Rash, pruitus, decreased libido, muscle aches, dizziness, and flu-like symptoms

HMG-COa Reductase Inhibitors (Statins)

- *Pregnancy category X*
- *GI:* Constipation, nausea, and diarrhea
- *Other:* Rash, muscle pain, headache, blurred vision, opthalmoplegia, insomnia, fatigue, and increased liver enzymes, myopathy rhabdomyolysis

Cholesterol Absorption Inhibitors

- *Pregnancy category C*
- *CNS:* Dizziness, fatigue, headache
- *GI:* Diarrhea, abdominal pain
- *Resp:* Cough, URI
- *Other:* Arthralgia, myalgias, back pain

Other

Niacin: Vitamin B$_3$

- *Pregnancy category C*
- *GI:* GI distress
- *Other:* Flushing, pruritus, blurred vision, glucose intolerance, hepatoxocity

CONTRAINDICATIONS

Bile Acid Sequestrants

- Biliary obstruction and hypersensitivity

Fibric Acid Derivatives

* Hypersensitivity, severe hepatic and renal disease

HMG-CoA Reductase Inhibitors

* Hypersensitivity, pregnancy or lactation, active liver disease

Cholesterol Absorption Inhibitors

* Hypersensitivity, hepatic disease

Other

Niacin: Vitamin B_3

* Hypersensitivity, heart block, blood pressure less than 90 mmHg

INTERACTIONS

Bile Acid Sequestrants

* Decrease absorption of fat-soluble vitamins
* Absorption of concurrently administered drugs is affected. Therefore, all drugs should be taken 1 hour before or 4 to 6 hours after administration of bile acid sequestrants.[4]

Fibric Acid Derivatives

* Oral anticoagulants: action-enhanced
* Concurrent use with HMA-CoA reductase inhibitors increases risk of myalgia and myositis.
* Fibric acid derivatives increase liver function studies and activated clotting time and decrease hemoglobin, hematacrit, and WBCs.

HMG-CoA Reductase Inhibitors

* Additive cholesterol lowering effects with concurrent use of bile acid sequestrants

- Increased anticoagulant action when taken with warfarin
- Increased risk of myopathy when taken with cyclosporine, erythromycin, gemfibrozil, and niacin
- May increase ACT, SGOT, and thrombocytopenia

Cholesterol Absorption Inhibitors

- Additive cholesterol lower effects with concurrent use of fenofibrate or gemfibrozil.
- Cholestyramine decreases ezetimibe levels.
- Concurrent use with fibric acid derivatives increases risk of cholethasis.
- Increased risk of toxicity if given with cyclosporine.[5]

Other

Niacin: B_3 Vitamin

- Increased risk of myopathy when taken concurrently with HMG-CoA reductase inhibitors
- Potentiates hypotensive effects of ganglionic blockers
- Concurrent use with alcohol may increase hypotensive effects.

 NURSING IMPLICATIONS

All Antilipemics

- With long-term use of antilipemics, clients may need to take supplemental fat-soluble vitamins.
- Encourage high-fiber diet, with fruits and vegetables, diet low in saturated fats, and adequate fluid intake.
- Monitor liver and renal function for adverse effects.
- Monitor serum cholesterol and triglyercide levels.
- Administer powder or granules in liquid (noncarbonated beverage) or food, and make sure that medication is mixed thoroughly.

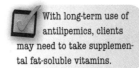
With long-term use of antilipemics, clients may need to take supplemental fat-soluble vitamins.

Encourage high-fiber diet, with fruits and vegetables, diet low in saturated fats, and adequate fluid intake.

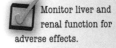
Monitor liver and renal function for adverse effects.

Bile Acid Sequestrants

* Should be taken before meals

Fibric Acid Derivatives

* Can be taken 30 minutes before eating or with meals

HMG-CoA Reductase Inhibitors (Statins)

* Generally taken in the evening

Cholesterol Absorption Inhibitors

* Can be given without regard to meals

Niacin

* Administer with food.

REFERENCES

1. Lilley L, Harrington S, Snyder J. *Pharmacology and the Nursing Process,* 5th ed. St. Louis, MO: Mosby; 2007:444.

2. Lilley L, Harrington S, Snyder J. *Pharmacology and the Nursing Process,* 5th ed. St. Louis, MO: Mosby; 2007:449.

3. Lilley L, Harrington S, Snyder J. *Pharmacology and the Nursing Process,* 5th ed. St. Louis, MO: Mosby; 2007:445.

4. Lilley L, Harrington S, Snyder J. *Pharmacology and the Nursing Process,* 5th ed. St. Louis, MO: Mosby; 2007:448.

5. Karch A. *Lippincott's Nursing Drug Guide.* Philadelphia, PA: Lippincott, Williams & Wilkins; 2007:500.

Anticoagulants are used to prevent intravascular thrombosis by decreasing blood coagulability.[1]

Anticoagulants suppress the production of fibrin by disrupting the coagulation cascade.

Parenteral anticoagulants include the natural anticoagulant heparin, low-molecular weight heparins (LMWHs), and thrombin inhibitors. Heparin is given IV or SC, and LMWHs are given SC. Antithrombin, argatroban, bivalirudin, and lepirudin are given IV; desirudin is given SC.

LMWHs have a longer half-life than heparin, require less laboratory monitoring than heparin, and are less likely to cause thrombocytopenia.[2,3]

Oral anticoagulants include warfarin sodium (Coumadin), the prototype Coumarin anticoagulant. Oral anticoagulants have a delayed onset of action and are indicated for long-term prophylaxsis.[4]

Oral anticoagulants interact with many drugs. Warfarin sodium is also available inravenously.

45

Anticoagulant Drugs

TERMS
- [ ] **enoxaparin (Lovenox)**
- [ ] **heparin (Hep-Lock)**
- [ ] **warfarin sodium (Coumadin)**

Table 45-1 Anticoagulant Drugs

Prototype Drug	Related Drugs	Drug Classification
enoxaparin (Lovenox)	ardeparin (Normiflo) dalteparin (Fragmin) danaparoid (Orgaran) tinzaparin (Innohep)	Low molecular weight heparin (LMWH)
Heparin (Hep-Lock)	antithrombin (Thrombate III) argatroban (Acova) bivalirudin (Angiomax) desirudin (Iprivask) lepirudin (Refludan)	Thrombin Inhibitor Natural anticoagulant
warfarin sodium (Coumadin)		Coumarin anticoagulant

ANTICOAGULANT DRUGS CLIENT TEACHING

- Use a soft toothbrush for brushing teeth and safety razor (electric) for shaving.
- Avoid concurrent use of OTC and herbal remedies without consulting with health care provider.
- Avoid taking aspirin and NSAIDs during therapy and read labels for OTC drugs that may contain these drugs.
- Report signs of bleeding or bruising (eg, nose, gums, emesis, sputum, stool, urine, bruising, severe headache).
- Notify health care provider if excessive bleeding occurs with menses.
- Notify health care provider, including dentist, if taking anticoagulants.
- Avoid activities (eg, contact sports) that may increase the risk of bleeding or injury

Use a soft toothbrush for brushing teeth and safety razor (electric) for shaving.

Avoid concurrent use of OTC and herbal remedies without consulting with health care provider.

Avoid taking aspirin and NSAIDs during therapy and read labels for OTC drugs that may contain these drugs.

Report signs of bleeding or bruising (eg, nose, gums, emesis, sputum, stool, urine, bruising, severe headache).

- Carry medication information and identification (eg, MedicAlert band).
- Avoid alcohol while on anticoagulant therapy.
- Avoid an increased intake of foods high in vitamin K (eg, green leafy vegetables and vitamin K supplements).
- Encourage client to stop tobacco use.

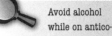 Avoid alcohol while on anticoagulant therapy.

 ## ACTION

Natural Anticoagulants

- With a short onset and short duration of action, prevent thrombus formation and extension of existing thrombi by binding with antithrombin III to inactivate thrombin, activated X, and activated IX factors.[5]
- Heparin works directly with antithrombin III, which promotes quick effects and is indicated for short-term or emergency therapy.

Low-Molecular Weight Heparin (LMWH)

- Similar to heparin but contains molecules that are shorter than unfractionated heparin and preferentially inactivates activated X, while less able to inactivate thrombin. LMWH has a high bioavailability and can be given on a fixed-dose schedule that requires less laboratory monitoring.[3,5]

Thrombin Inhibitors

- Antithrombin (Thrombate III) intereferes with the formation of thrombin from prothrombin. It is a naturally occurring anticoagulant.
- Argatroban (Acova), bivalirudin (Angiomax), desirudin (Iprivisk), and lepirudin (Refludan) inhibit thrombin by blocking the formation of thrombin from prothrombin.

Thrombin Inhibitors

- Antithrombin (Thrombate III) is used in clients who are anti-thrombin III deficient, undergoing obstetrical or surgical procedures that might put them at risk for thromboembolism.

Argatroban (Acova) and Lepirudin (Refludan)

- Heparin-induced thrombocytopenia

Bivalirudin (Angiomax)

- Clients undergoing percutaneous transluminal angioplasty who are receiving aspirin and have unstable angina

Desirudin (Iprivask)

- Prevention of deep vein thrombosis (DVT) in clients undergoing elective hip replacement

Coumarin Anticoagulant

- Has a slow onset and long duration of action
- Antagonizes vitamin K, which blocks vitamin K dependent factors

USE

All Anticoagulants

- For prevention and treatment of various thromboembolic disorders

Natural Anticoagulants

- Short-term or emergency use
- DVT
- Pulmonary embolism (PE)
- Disseminated intravasular coagulation
- Hemodialysis
- Myocardial infarction (MI)
- After coronary artery bypass graft surgery

Low-Molecular Weight Heparins (LMWH)

- Prophylaxis of DVT following orthopedic (total hip and total knee surgery) or abdominal surgery
- Unstable angina

Coumarin Anticoagulant

- Atrial fibrillation
- DVT
- PE
- Recurrent MI and transient ischemic attack
- Rheumatic heart disease
- Prophylaxis after major surgery, prosthetic heart valves, immobilization

ADVERSE EFFECTS AND SIDE EFFECTS

- All anticoagulant agents can cause bleeding.

Natural Anticoagulant and Thrombin Inhibitors

- *Pregnancy category C*
- *Hematologic:* Thromboctyopenia, hypersensitivity, rash, chills, and fever

Low-Molecular Weight Heparins (LMWH)

- *Pregnancy category B, although ardeparin (Normiflo) is pregnancy category C*
- *Hematologic:* Thrombocytopenia occurs less frequently; thrombosis erythemia or pain at injection site

Thrombin Inhibitors

- *Pregnancy category B*
- *Bleeding, bivalirudin (Angiomax)*
- Hypotension

Coumarin Anticoagulants

- *Pregnancy category X*
- *GI:* Abdominal cramps, nausea, vomiting, and diarrhea

CONTRAINDICATIONS

All Anticoagulants and Thrombin Inhibitors

- Hypersensitivity
- Open wounds
- Uncontrolled bleeding

Natural Anticoagulant, Coumarin Anticoagulant

- Severe thrombocytopenia, hypersensitivity

Coumarin Anticoagulant

- Crosses the placenta and is contraindicated in pregnancy
- Severe liver disease
- Conditions in which hemorrhage is possible (eg, peptic ulcer disease, spinal cord injury)

INTERACTIONS

All Anticoagulants and Thrombin Inhibitors

- Increased risk of bleeding with antiplatelets, NSAIDS, aspirin, alcohol, thrombolytics, garlic, ginger, ginkgo biloba, ginseng

Parenteral Anticoagulants

- Decreased anticoagulant effects when taken with digoxin (Lanoxin), antihistamines, or tetracycline
- Increased anticoagulant effects when taken with penicillin, cephalosporins, or quinidine

Coumarin Anticoagulant

- Increased anticoagulant effects when taken with high doses of acetaminophen (Tylenol), broad-spectrum antibiotics, furosemide (Lasix), mineral oil, sulfonamides, or vitamin E
- Decreased anticoagulant effects when taken with estrogen, oral contraceptives, or barbiturates
- Note: There are many interactions with oral anticoagulants.

 NURSING IMPLICATIONS

- Assess and monitor prothrombin time (PT) and international normalized ratio (INR) with oral anticoagulant use. PT time should be 1.5 to 2.5 times the control, and INR should be 2 to 3 times the control for oral anticoagulants. In some cases, the INR may be adjusted to 3 to 4.5 times the control.
- Assess and monitor activated partial prothromboplastin time with heparin therapy. Range is 1.5 to 2.5 times the control.
- Monitor for internal and external bleeding.
- Avoid IM injections.
- Monitor CBC and vital signs.
- Monitor for hypersensitivity reactions, especially with heparin and LMWH.
- When administering heparin or LMWH SC, use a tuberculin syringe, especially for small doses, inject at a 90-degree angle, do not aspirate, and do not massage or rub the skin. Any SC site may be used, but the abdomen is used most frequently.
- Continuous IV heparin must be given via an IV pump; follow agency protocols when administering as most agencies follow a heparin nomogram for dosing.

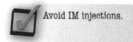

> Assess and monitor prothrombin time (PT) and international normalized ratio (INR) with oral anticoagulant use. PT time should be 1.5 to 2.5 times the control, and INR should be 2 to 3 times the control for oral anticoagulants. In some cases, the INR may be adjusted to 3 to 4.5 times the control.

> Assess and monitor activated partial prothromboplastin time with heparin therapy. Range is 1.5 to 2.5 times the control.

> Avoid IM injections.

- Intermittent infusions of heparin are given through an intermittent infusion lock and may be flushed with saline.
- Check IV or SC site for bleeding, and the IV site for infiltration.
- Administer oral anticoagulants at the same time daily to maintain blood levels.
- Oral anticoagulants may be administered concurrently during parenteral heparin therapy, as oral anticoagulants have a long onset (48 to 72 hours).

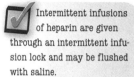 When administering heparin or LMWH SC, use a tuberculin syringe, especially for small doses, inject at a 90-degree angle, do not aspirate, and do not massage or rub the skin. Any SC site may be used, but the abdomen is used most frequently.

Intermittent infusions of heparin are given through an intermittent infusion lock and may be flushed with saline.

Antidotes

- Administer protamine sulfate for Heparin and LMWH. However, there is no antidote for danaparoid.
- Vitamin K is effective for coumarin anticoagulants.
- Lepirudin (Refludan) is given IV to treat a rare allergic reaction to heparin.

REFERENCES

1. McKenry LM, Tessier E, Hogan M. *Mosby's Pharmacology in Nursing*, 22nd ed. St. Louis, MO: Mosby Elsevier; 2006:602.

2. McKenry LM, Tessier E, Hogan M. *Mosby's Pharmacology in Nursing*, 22nd ed. St. Louis, MO: Mosby; 2003:606.

3. Lehne RA. *Pharmacology for Nursing Care*, 6th ed. Philadelphia, PA: Saunders Elsevier; 2007:591–592.

4. Lehne RA. *Pharmacology for Nursing Care*, 6th ed. Philadelphia, PA: Saunders Elsevier; 2007:594.

5. Lilley L, Harrington S, Snyder J. *Pharmacology and the Nursing Process*, 5th ed. St. Louis, MO: Mosby; 2007:421.

Antiplatelets are indicated for treatment of arterial thrombi as the composition of arterial thrombi is mainly platelet aggregates. There are three major groups of antiplatelets: **aspirin** (the prototype drug), **adenosine diphosphate** (ADP) **inhibitors,** and **glycoprotein** (GP) **IIb/IIIa inhibitors.** Other antiplatelet drugs include dipyridamole, dipyridamole plus aspirin, cilostazol, and anagrelide.

Aspirin and ADP inhibitors are limited in their antiplatelet effects as they affect one pathway of platelet activation. GP IIb/IIIa Inhibitors have strong antiplatelet effects as they block the final step in platelet activation.[1]

46

Antiplatelet Drugs

TERM
☐ aspirin

Table 46-1 Antiplatelet Drugs

Prototype Drug	Related Drugs	Drug Classification
aspirin	anagrelide (Agrylin) cilostazol (Pletal) dipyridamole (Persantine) dipyridamole plus aspirin (Aggrenox)	Antiplatelets
There is no prototype for this classification	clopidogrel (Plavix) ticlopidine (Ticlid)	ADP inhibitors
There is no prototype for this classification	abciximab (ReoPro) eptifibatide (Integrilin) tirofiban (Aggrastat)	GP IIb/IIIa inhibitors

ANTIPLATELET DRUGS CLIENT TEACHING

- See "Client Teaching" in Chapter 36.
- Use a soft toothbrush for brushing teeth and safety razor for shaving.
- Avoid concurrent use of OTC and herbal remedies without consulting with health care provider.
- Report signs of bleeding or bruising (eg, nose, emesis, sputum, stool, urine, petechiae).
- Report chest pain, edema, or palpitations to health care provider.
- Notify health care provider including the dentist if taking antiplatelets.
- Advise client that therapy is used for long-term prevention and treatment but is not a cure.
- Avoid alcohol and smoking while on antiplatelet therapy.

Ticlopidine (Ticlid)

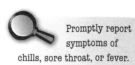

- Promptly report symptoms of chills, sore throat, or fever.
- Blood work (eg, complete blood count (CBC)) needs to be checked periodically.

ACTION

Aspirin

- Irreversibly inhibits the enzyme cyclooxygenase, which prevents synthesis of thromboxane A_2, thus suppressing vasoconstriction and platelet aggregation. It has irreversible antiplatelet effects.[2]

Anagrelide (Agrylin)

- Inhibits platelet aggregation and reduces platelet count

Cilostazol (Pletal)

- Phosphodiesterase III inhibitor increases deformity of erythrocytes, decreases blood viscosity, and promotes vasodilatation.

Dipyridamole (Persantine)

- Inhibits platelet aggregation by inhibiting ADP

ADP Inhibitors

- Inhibit ADP-mediated aggregation on the platelet surface with irreversible antiplatelet effects[3]

GP IIb/IIIa Inhibitors

- Cause irreversible blockade of GP IIb/IIIa receptors, which inhibits the final step of aggregation[4]

USE

Aspirin

- Prevention of myocardial infarction (MI) and reinfarction in clients who have had a MI, and cerebral vascular accident (CVA) in clients with a history of transient ischemic attacks (TIAs)

Anagrelide (Agrylin)

- Essential thrombocytopenic, to reduce blood counts

Cilostazol (Pletal)

- Intermittent claudication

Dipyridamole (Persantine)

- Administered after heart valve replacement therapy to prevent thromboembolism. It is given with coumadin.

Dipyridamole Plus Aspirin (Aggrenox)

- Prevents recurrent CVA in clients who have had a previous CVA or TIA.

ADP Inhibitors

Clopidogrel (Plavix)

- Causes fewer life-threatening hematologic events
- Prophylaxis of MI, thromboembolic stroke, vascular death

Ticlopidine (Ticlid)

- Prevention of thromboembolic CVA; is considered a second-line drug due to life-threatening adverse effects and cost

GB IIb/IIIa Inhibitors

- Acute coronary syndrome and percutaneous coronary intervention

ADVERSE EFFECTS AND SIDE EFFECTS

- All antiplatelet agents can cause bleeding.

Aspirin

- *Pregnancy category D (review Chapter 36 for other adverse effects and side effects)*

Anagrelide (Agrylin)

- *Pregnancy category C*
- Headache, dizziness, seizures, postural hypotension, thrombocytopenia, MI, nausea, vomiting, diarrhea

Cilostazol (Pletal)

- *Pregnancy category C*
- Headache, nausea, diarrhea, peripheral edema, palpitations

Dipyridamole (Persantine)

- *Pregnancy category B*
- Headache, hypertension, dizziness, GI upset, rash

ADP Inhibitors

- *Pregnancy category B*

Clopidogrel (Plavix)

- Similar to aspirin
- Does not have the life-threatening adverse effects of neutropenia or thrombocytopenia, but may cause thrombotic thrombocytopenic purpura (TTP)

Ticlopidine (Ticlid)

- *GI:* Nausea, diarrhea, and abdominal pain
- *Hematologic:* Life-threatening reactions—agranulocytosis, neutropenia, and TTP
- *Derm:* Rash

GP IIb/IIIa Inhibitors

- *Pregnancy category B*
- *Hematologic:* Bleeding is the primary adverse effect

CONTRAINDICATIONS

All Antiplatelets

- Contraindicated in clients with hematopoietic and hemostatic disorders, active bleeding such as intracranial bleeding, peptic ulcers, hypersensitivity, pregnancy, and hepatic dysfunction

INTERACTIONS

All Antiplatelets

- Increased risk of bleeding or antiplatelet effects with anticoagulants, NSAIDs, aspirin, thrombolytics, garlic, ginger, ginkgo biloba, ginseng
- Alcohol increases risk of hypotension.
- Nicotine in tobacco causes vasoconstriction.

NURSING IMPLICATIONS

All Antiplatelets

- Give PO (antiplatelets and ADP inhibitors).
- Assess and monitor clotting profiles including platelet counts and CBC.
- Monitor for internal and external bleeding.
- Monitor for hypersensitivity reactions.
- Administer ticlopidine (Ticlid) with food to decrease GI distress and monitor for symptoms of agranulocytosis or neutropenia (eg, fever, chills, sore throat).

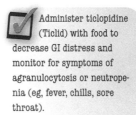

✓ Assess and monitor clotting profiles including platelet counts and CBC.

✓ Administer ticlopidine (Ticlid) with food to decrease GI distress and monitor for symptoms of agranulocytosis or neutropenia (eg, fever, chills, sore throat).

GP IIa/IIIb Inhibitors

- Give IV.

REFERENCES

1. Lehne RA. *Pharmacology for Nursing Care*, 6th ed. Philadelphia, PA: Saunders Elsevier; 2007:598.

2. Lilley L, Harrington S, Snyder J. *Pharmacology and the Nursing Process*, 5th ed. St. Louis, MO: Mosby; 2007:426.

3. Lehne RA. *Pharmacology for Nursing Care*, 6th ed. Philadelphia, PA: Saunders Elsevier; 2007:599.

4. Lehne RA. *Pharmacology for Nursing Care*, 6th ed. Philadelphia, PA: Saunders Elsevier; 2007:600.

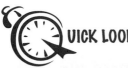

Thrombolytic drugs are administered in the hospital as close monitoring is indicated due to their toxic effects. Thrombolytic drugs dissolve clots, which may cause bleeding that is more severe and difficult to control than anticoagulants. They are used in treatment of acute thromboembolic disorders.[1]

It was discovered in 1933 that bacteria group **A beta-hemolytic streptococci** was capable of breaking down fibrin clots; this group became known as the drug streptokinase (Streptase, Kabikinase). In the 1980s, conclusive evidence demonstrated that myocardial infarctions (MIs) were coronary artery occlusions; as a result, using thrombolytics to treat early MI became popular.[2]

47

Thrombolytic Drugs

TERM
☐ streptokinase (Streptase, Kabikinase)

Table 47-1 Thrombolytic Drugs

Prototype Drug	Related Drugs	Drug Classification
streptokinase (Streptase, Kabikinase)	alteplase (Activase) anistreplase (Eminase) reteplase (Retavase) tenecteplase (TNKase) urokinase (Abbokinase)	Thrombolytic enzymes

 ## THROMBOLYTIC CLIENT TEACHING

- Close monitoring and bedrest with minimal activity/movement are indicated during therapy.
- Report symptoms of bleeding or hypersensitivity reactions.
- Avoid shaving and brushing teeth to minimize risk of bleeding during therapy.

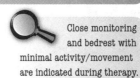
Close monitoring and bedrest with minimal activity/movement are indicated during therapy.

Avoid shaving and brushing teeth to minimize risk of bleeding during therapy.

 ## ACTION

- The thrombolytic enzymes convert plasminogen to plasmin. The enzyme plasmin dissolves fibrin clots.
- Streptokinase (Streptase, Kabikinase) and anistreplase (Eminase) indirectly activate plasminogen and are not clot specific, which means that clots can be broken down anywhere in the body.
- Alteplase (Activase), reteplase (Retavase), and tenecteplase (TNKase) directly activate plasminogen.
- Alteplase (Activase), reteplase (Retavase), and tenecteplase (TNKase) are clot specific, which does not cause a systemic lytic state.

 ## USE

- All thrombolytic enzymes: Treatment of acute arterial thrombus associated with acute MI

- Streptokinase (Streptase, Kabikinase), alteplase (Activase), urokinase (Abbokinase): Pulmonary embolism
- Streptokinase (Streptase, Kabikinase) and anistreplase (Eminase): Acute deep vein thrombosis
- Alteplase (Activase): Acute ischemic stroke
- Urokinase (Abbokinase): Pulmonary emboli, treat coronary thrombosis, and clear occluded intravenous catheters

ADVERSE EFFECTS AND SIDE EFFECTS

- *Pregnancy category C, except urokinase (Abbokinase), which is pregnancy category B*
- *CV:* Dysrhythmias, hypotension
- *Hematologic:* Hemorrhage major adverse effect: internal, intracranial, and superficial bleeding
- Hypersensitivity and anaphylaxis, especially with streptokinase (Streptase) and anistreplace (Eminase), and urokinase (Abbokenase)

CONTRAINDICATIONS

- In clients prone to hemorrhage (eg, hemophilia, recent surgery or trauma, liver disease, recent GI bleeding, renal disease intracranial disorders) or severe uncontrolled hypertension

INTERACTIONS

- Increased risk of hemorrhage when administered with anticoagulants and antiplatelets
- Herbals ginkgo, ginseng and garlic may potentiate bleeding.

NURSING IMPLICATIONS

- Administered IV.
- Follow manufacturer's directions for reconstitution and hospital protocols for administering.

- For treatment of acute MI and cerebral vascular accident, begin treatment as soon as possible after the onset of symptoms (ie, within 3 hours of onset of CVA, and 4–6 hours of acute MI).
- Assess and monitor clotting profiles and EKG.
- Assess and monitor vital signs frequently throughout therapy.
- Assess and monitor neurological status throughout therapy.
- Maintain bedrest throughout treatment and immediately after treatment.
- Continuously monitor for internal and external bleeding; if bleeding occurs notify health care provider.
- Monitor IV sites for bleeding.
- Avoid IM injections during treatment.
- Assess for hypersensitivity and anaphylaxis especially with streptokinase (Streptase, Kabikinase), anistreplase (Eminase), and urokinase (Abbokinase).

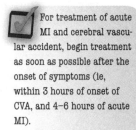
For treatment of acute MI and cerebral vascular accident, begin treatment as soon as possible after the onset of symptoms (ie, within 3 hours of onset of CVA, and 4–6 hours of acute MI).

Assess and monitor clotting profiles and EKG.

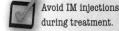
Avoid IM injections during treatment.

Antidote

Aminocaproic Acid (Amicar) and Tranexamic Acid (Cyklokapron)

- Antifibrinolytic drugs prevent the lysis of fibrin thus promoting clot formation. Both drugs are available PO or IV.

REFERENCES

1. McKenry LM, Tessier E, Hogan M. *Mosby's Pharmacology in Nursing*, 22nd ed. St. Louis, MO: Mosby Elsevier; 2006:616.

2. Lilley L, Harrington S, Snyder J. *Pharmacology and the Nursing Process*, 5th ed. St. Louis, MO: Mosby; 2007:430.

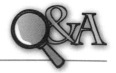

PART VI · QUESTIONS

1. Which of the following are common side effects of digoxin (Lanoxin, Lanoxicaps)?
   a. Constipation
   b. Colored vision
   c. Urinary retention
   d. Weight gain

2. Which of the following is a desired effect of digoxin (Lanoxin, Lanoxicaps)?
   a. Negative inotropic effect
   b. Negative chronotropic effect
   c. Positive dromotropic effect
   d. Decrease in stroke volume

3. Nursing considerations when administering digoxin (Lanoxin) to an adult include:
   a. Taking an apical pulse for 15 seconds.
   b. Encouraging the client to eat foods low in potassium.
   c. Reporting to the health care provider client complaints of anorexia, nausea, or vomiting.
   d. Notifying health care provider if the pulse is greater than 90 beats per minute.

4. Which of the following are indications for the use of Digoxin immune FAB (Digibind)?
   a. Cinchonism
   b. Severe hypokalemia
   c. Hyperthyroidism
   d. Severe digoxin (Lanoxin, Lanoxicaps) overdose

5. Which of the following is an adverse effect of procainamide (Pronestyl)?
   a. Cinchonism
   b. Systemic lupus erythematosus (SLE) syndrome
   c. Glaucoma
   d. Hypertension

6. Which of the following drugs may interact with Class I antidys-rhythmic drugs?
   a. Acetaminophen (Tylenol)
   b. Atropine
   c. Penicillin
   d. Psyllium (Metamucil)

7. Nursing considerations for a client taking lidocaine (Xylocaine) include:
   a. Monitoring neurological status.
   b. Administering lidocaine with food.
   c. Encouraging client to use sunscreen when exposed to sunlight.
   d. Not crushing enteric-coated tablets.

8. Of the following, which situation is adenosine (Adenocard) indicated?
   a. Converting paroxysmal supraventricular tachycardia (PSVT) to sinus rhythm
   b. Atrial fibrillation or atrial flutter
   c. Premature ventricular contractions (PVCs)
   d. Ventricular tachycardia (VT)

9. Which of the following is a common adverse effect of amiodarone (Cordarone)?
   a. Metallic taste
   b. Hypertension
   c. Corneal microdeposits
   d. Migraine headache

10. Of the following, which should be included in a teaching plan for a client taking nifedipine (Procardia) for angina?
    a. Encourage a diet high in fiber.
    b. Take hot showers to promote relaxation.
    c. Take with alcohol to enhance absorption of nifidepine.
    d. Encourage rigorous exercise.

11. Which of the following is correct concerning transdermal nitro-glycerin?
    a. Swimming or taking a bath should be avoided.
    b. A new patch should be applied if the old one falls off.
    c. The patch should be left on for 24 hours a day, before being replaced.
    d. The patch can be placed over skin folds or a hairy area.

12. Which is an adverse effect of nitroglycerin that may diminish with drug tolerance?
    a. Headache
    b. Flatulence
    c. Polyphagia
    d. Urinary retention

13. Which antihypertensive agent may cause a cough that will stop when the drug is discontinued?
    a. Clonidine (Catapres)
    b. Captopril (Capoten)
    c. Diazoxide (Hyperstat)
    d. Prazosin (Minipress)

14. A client is receiving transdermal clonidine (Catapres) for treatment of hypertension. Which of the following should the nurse include in teaching the client about care of a transdermal clonidine (Catapres) patch?
    a. Replace the patch every 24 hours.
    b. Remove the patch when swimming or bathing.
    c. Sites do not need to be rotated.
    d. Can be applied to any hairless site.

15. Which antihypertensive agent may cause cyanide poisoning?
    a. Diazoxide (Hyperstat)
    b. Hydralazine hydrochloride (Apresoline)
    c. Minoxidil (Loniten, Rogaine)
    d. Sodium nitroprusside (Nipride)

16. An increased risk of ototoxicity may occur when which diuretic drug is administered IV push too quickly?
    a. Furosemide (Lasix)
    b. Hydrochlorothiazide (Esidrix)
    c. Mannitol (Osmitrol)
    d. Spironolactone (Aldactone)

17. Which of the following diuretics is a potassium-sparing diuretic?
    a. Furosemide (Lasix)
    b. Hydrochlorothiazide (Esidrix)
    c. Mannitol (Osmitrol)
    d. Spironolactone (Aldactone)

18. Of the following, which diuretic is also used to treat acute open-angle glaucoma?
    a. Acetazolamide (Diamox)
    b. Bumetamide (Bumex)
    c. Metolazone (Mykrox)
    d. Triamterene (Dyrenium)

19. Which antilipemic agent may cause flushing?
    a. Atorvastatin (Lipitor)
    b. Cholestyramine (Questran)
    c. Gemfibrozil (Lopid)
    d. Niacin

20. Which of the following antilipemic drugs is used to treat type III and IV, V, and in some instances type IIb hyperlipidemias?
    a. Atorvastatin (Lipitor)
    b. Cholestyramine (Questran)
    c. Gemfibrozil (Lopid)
    d. Niacin

21. Which of the following antilipemics is contraindicated in pregnancy or lactation and is labeled as a pregnancy category X?
    a. Atorvastatin (Lipitor)
    b. Cholestyramine (Questran)
    c. Gemfibrozil (Lopid)
    d. Niacin

22. Which of the following is the antidote for severe heparin overdose?
    a. Protamine zinc
    b. Protamine sulfate
    c. Vitamin K
    d. Vitamin E

23. Which of the following adverse effects should the nurse monitor for a client who is receiving heparin therapy?
    a. Constipation
    b. Increased intraocular pressure
    c. Weight gain
    d. Thrombocytopenia

24. Of the following, which anticoagulant requires less laboratory monitoring and is often used to prevent deep vein thrombosis (DVT) following total knee or hip surgery?
    a. Antithrombin (Thrombate III)
    b. Enoxaparin (Lovenox)
    c. Heparin
    d. Warfarin sodium (Coumadin)

25. Which antiplatelet drug may cause life-threatening hematologic adverse effects?
    a. Clopidogrel (Plavix)
    b. Dipyridamole (Persantine)
    c. Tirofiban (Aggrastat)
    d. Ticlopidine (Ticlid)

26. Which drug inhibits ADP mediated aggregation that causes irreversible platelet effects?
    a. Abciximab (ReoPro)
    b. Clopidogrel (Plavix)
    c. Eptifibatide (Integrilin)
    d. Tirofiban (Aggrastat)

27. Client teaching for use of antiplatelets includes all of the following EXCEPT:
    a. Encouraging client to play contact sports.
    b. Using a safety razor when shaving.
    c. Using a soft toothbrush when brushing teeth.
    d. Wearing a MedicAlert identification band.

28. Which of the following drugs is an antidote for thrombolytic agents?
    a. Aspirin
    b. Aminocaproic acid (Amicar)
    c. Ibuprofen (Advil, Motrin, others)
    d. Clopidogrel (Plavix)

PART VI • ANSWERS

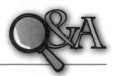

1. **The correct answer is b.** Colored vision, especially yellow-green, or halo vision are common side effects of digoxin (Lanoxin, Lanoxicaps). Diarrhea is also a common side effect of digoxin. Weight loss vs weight gain may be seen with digoxin due to the promotion of diuresis related to improved blood circulation.

2. **The correct answer is b.** Digoxin (Lanoxin, Lanoxicaps) has positive intotropic, negative chronotropic, and negative dromotropic effects, as well as increase in stroke volume.

3. **The correct answer is c.** Client complaints of anorexia, nausea, or vomiting may be signs of digoxin toxicity. Foods high in potassium to prevent hypokalemia should be encouraged, and the apical pulse should be taken for a full minute. The health care provider should be contacted if the pulse is less than 60 or greater than 120 beats per minute.

4. **The correct answer is d.** Digoxin immune FAB (Digibind) is the antidote for severe cardiac glycoside overdose (digoxin [Lanoxin, Lanoxicaps]), Cinchonism is an adverse effect of Quinidine, and digoxin immune FAB is not indicated for treatment of severe hypokalemia or hypothyroidism.

5. **The correct answer is b.** Procainamide (Pronestyl) may cause SLE syndrome. Cinchonism is an adverse effect of procainamide (Pronestyl) therapy. Glaucoma is not an adverse effect of procainamide. Procainamide may cause hypertension, not hypotension.

6. **The correct answer is b.** Atropine is an anticholinergic drug, which increases anticholinergic effects when administered with Class I antidysrhythmic drugs.

7. **The correct answer is a.** Due to the central nervous system effects of lidocaine (Xylocaine), the nurse should be monitoring the neurological status of the client. Lidocaine (Xylocaine) is only given parenterally and does not cause photosensitivity.

8. **The correct answer is a.** Adenosine (Adenocard) is indicated to convert PSVT to sinus rhythm especially when PSVT has not responded to verapamil. Adenosine (Adenocard) is contraindicated in clients with VT, atrial fibrillation or atrial flutter, and is not indicated to treat PVCs.

9. **The correct answer is c.** Corneal microdeposits are a common adverse effect seen in clients taking amiodarone (Cordarone). Clients may complain of dry eyes or halos.

10. **The correct answer is a.** Nifedipine (Procardia) can cause constipation, and a diet high in fiber should be encouraged. Hot showers and alcohol should be avoided as they promote vasodilatation and can cause hypotension. Rigorous exercise could trigger an anginal attack.

11. **The correct answer is b.** If a patch should fall off, it can be replaced with a new one. Swimming and bathing are not contraindicated, and the patch should be left off for at least 10 to 12 hours a day to prevent drug tolerance. The patch should not be placed over skin folds or a hairy area, as it may impair absorption of nitroglycerin.

12. **The correct answer is a.** Initially, headaches may occur, but they tend to diminish with drug tolerance. Headaches can be treated with analgesics. Flatulence, polyphagia, and urinary retention are not adverse effects of nitroglycerin.

13. **The correct answer is b.** Captopril (Capoten) is an ACE inhibitor that may cause a cough that will stop when the drug is discontinued.

14. **The correct answer is d.** Clonidine (Catapres) can be applied to any hairless site, while avoiding areas that may have cuts and calluses. The patch is replaced every 7 days and does not need to be removed when swimming or bathing. Sites should be rotated.

15. **The correct answer is d.** Sodium nitroprusside (Nipride) may cause cyanide poisoning. Sodium nitroprusside (Nipride) is converted to thiocyanate, and the client needs to be monitored for cyanide poisoning (tinnitus, blurred vision, and delirium).

16. **The correct answer is a.** Furosemide (Lasix) should be given IV push over 1 to 2 minutes to prevent an increased risk of ototoxicity.

17. **The correct answer is d.** Spironolactone (Aldactone) is a potassium-sparing diuretic.

18. **The correct answer is a.** Acetazolamide (Diamox) is a carbonic anhydrase inhibitor (CAI) that is mainly used to treat acute open-angle glaucoma. Carbonic anhydrase is an enzyme that is found in the eyes and kidneys, as well as other parts of the body.

19. **The correct answer is d.** Niacin may cause flushing, especially in the face, neck, and ears.

20. **The correct answer is c.** Fibric acid derivatives, such as gemfibrozil (Lopid) are indicated to treat type III and IV, V, and in some instances type IIb hyperlipidemias.

21. **The correct answer is a.** HMG-CoA reductase inhibitors such as atorvastatin (Lipitor) are contraindicated in pregnancy or lactation and are labeled as a pregnancy category X agent.

22. **The correct answer is b.** Protamine sulfate is a protein that when combined with heparin counteracts the heparin-antithrombin III complex, which reduces the anticoagulant effects of heparin.

23. **The correct answer is d.** The nurse should monitor the client for thrombocytopenia.

24. **The correct answer is b.** Enoxaparin (Lovenox) is a LMWH that requires less laboratory monitoring and is often used to prevent DVT following total knee or hip surgery.

25. **The correct answer is d.** Ticlopidine (Ticlid) may cause life-threatening agranulocytosis, neutropenia, and TTP.

26. **The correct answer is b.** Clopidogrel (Plavix) and ticlopidine (Ticlid) are ADP inhibitors.

27. **The correct answer is a.** Clients should avoid contact sports as bruising or bleeding may occur. Encourage noncontact sports such as swimming and walking.

28. **The correct answer is b.** Aminocaproic acid (Amicar) is an antifibrinolytic agent used to control bleeding and is the antidote for thrombolytic agents.

VII

Endocrine System Drugs

Marilyn J. Herbert-Ashton, MS, RN, BC

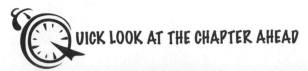

Drugs that affect the anterior and posterior pituitary gland are generally used for replacement therapy for hormone deficiency, diagnosis to determine if there is hypofunction or hyperfunction of pituitary hormones, and drug therapy for specific disorders to produce a therapeutic hormonal response.[1]

Anterior pituitary hormones include: **adrenocorticotropic hormone** (ACTH), **follicle stimulating hormone**, **growth hormone** (GH), **lutenizing hormone**, **melanocyte-stimulating hormone**, **prolactin**, and **thyroid-stimulating hormone**. Posterior pituitary hormones include: **antidiuretic hormone** (ADH) and **oxytocin.**

ACTH, GH, and ADH are discussed in this chapter. Other drugs that affect the pituitary gland are discussed in Chapter 58.

The **parathyroid hormone** (PTH) is secreted by the parathyroid gland when calcium levels are low. Calcitonin is a hormone released by specialized cells of the thyroid gland in humans when serum calcium levels increase and there is a reduction of PTH secretion.[2] Calcitonin decreases serum calcium by inhibiting bone resorption and, with PTH, assists in finely regulating serum calcium levels.[2]

48

Pituitary and Parathyroid Hormones

TERMS
- ☐ **bromocriptine mesylate (Parlodel)**
- ☐ **corticotropin (Acthar, HP)**
- ☐ **somatrem (Protropin)**
- ☐ **vasopressin (Pitressin)**

Table 48-1 Pituitary and Parathyroid Hormones

Prototype Drug	Related Drugs	Drug Classification
		Anterior Pituitary Hormones
bromocriptine mesylate (Parlodel)	octreotide (Sandostatin) pegvisomant (Somavert)	GH Antagonist
corticotropin (Acthar, HP)	cosyntropin (Cortrosyn)	**Adrenocorticotropic Hormone (ACTH)**
somatrem (Protropin)	somatropin (Humatrope, Nutropin, Saizen)	Growth hormone (GH)
		Posterior Pituitary Hormones
vasopressin (Pitressin)	desmopressin acetate (DDAVP) lypressin (Diapid)	Antidiuretic hormone (ADH hormone)
There is no prototype at this time	calcitonin-human (Cibacalcin) calcitonin-salmon (Calcimar, Miacalcin) teriparatide (Forteo)	**Parathyroid Hormones**

PITUITARY AND PARATHYROID HORMONES CLIENT TEACHING

Adrenocorticotropic Hormone (ACTH)

- Notify other health care providers, including dentist or specialist if taking ACTH.

Avoid vaccines during therapy.

- Do not take OTC or herbal remedies without consulting health care provider.
- Avoid vaccines during therapy.
- Avoid alcohol during therapy.

Do not discontinue abruptly.

- Do not discontinue abruptly.
- Notify health care provider if signs of infection or muscular pain occur.
- Carry MedicAlert identification.

Growth Hormone (GH)

- Keep a journal of growth measurements.
- Maintain follow-up care with health care provider that includes laboratory testing and bone age determinations.

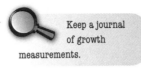

Keep a journal of growth measurements.

GH Antagonists

- Rotate injection sites.
- Report symptoms of hyper- or hypoglycemia or irritation at injection site to health care provider.
- May take at bedtime or between meals to minimize GI effects.

May take at bedtime or between meals to minimize GI effects.

Antiduretic Hormones (ADH)

- Report symptoms of water intoxication to health care provider and hold medication if symptoms occur.
- Take as directed and maintain follow-up care with health care provider.
- Clients with diabetes insipidus should carry MedicAlert identification.
- Do not take OTC or herbal remedies without consulting health care provider.
- Avoid alcohol while taking ADH.

Report symptoms of water intoxication to health care provider and hold medication if symptoms occur.

Lypressin (Diapid) for Treatment of Nocturia

- Administer 1 to 2 sprays intranasally when urinary frequency increases.
- Bedtime dose can be taken if daily dose doesn't control nocturia.
- Do not inhale medication.

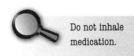

Do not inhale medication.

Parathyroid Hormones

- Take at bedtime to avoid nausea and flushing.

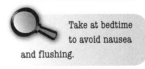

Take at bedtime to avoid nausea and flushing.

Nasal Spray: Calcitonin-Salmon (Miacalcin, Calcimar)

- Blow nose before using nasal spray and do not inhale while spraying.
- Follow manufacturer's instructions in assembling and storage of pump.

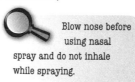

Blow nose before using nasal spray and do not inhale while spraying.

ACTION

Adrenocorticotropic Hormone (ACTH)

Corticotropin (Acthar, HP) and Cosyntropin (Cortrosyn)

- The physiologic effects are similar to cortisone. The adrenal cortex is stimulated to secrete mineralcorticoids, glucocorticoids, and androgens.

Growth Hormone (GH)

Somatrem (Protropin) and Somatropin (Humatrope, Saizen, Nutropin)

- Promote growth through stimulating the anabolic processes that cause growth[3]

GH Antagonists

- Antagonize the effects of natural GH, by inhibiting release of GH[3]
- Bromocriptine mesylate (Parlodel) is also a dopamine agonist, which increases the release of somatostatin from the hypothalamus.

Antiduretic Hormones (ADH)

Vasopressin (Pitressin) and Related Drugs

- Have ADH hormone effects, increase water resorption, concentrate urine, and have vasoconstricting effects
- Increase water, concentrate urine, and resorption in the distal tubules and collecting ducts of the kidneys[3]

Parathyroid Hormones

- Decrease serum calcium through direct effects on the bone, GI tract, and kidneys, and promote excretion of calcium

 USE

Adrenocorticotropic Hormone (ACTH)

Corticotropin (Acthar, HP) and Cosyntropin (Cortrosyn)

- Used to diagnose adrenocortical insufficiency
- Corticotropin (Acthar, HP) is also used to treat multiple sclerosis, myasthenia gravis, and corticotropin insufficiency caused by long-term corticosteroid use.

Growth Hormone (GH)

Somatrem (Protropin) and Somatropin (Humatrope, Saizen, Nutropin)

- Pituitary dwarfism

GH Antagonists

- Treatment of acromegaly
- Octreotide (Sandostatin) is also used to treat metastatic carcinoid tumors.

Antidiuretic Hormones (ADH)

- Diabetes insipidus

Vasopressin (Pitressin)

- Also used to treat postoperative abdominal distention, and diagnostic x-ray study of abdomen

Desmopressin Acetate (DDAVP)

- Nocturnal enuresis, hemophilia A, type 1 von Willebrand's disease

Parathyroid Hormones

- Used to treat hypercalcemia, postmenopausal osteoporosis, and Paget's disease

Teriparatide (Forteo)

- Used to prevent and treat osteoporosis.

ADVERSE EFFECTS AND SIDE EFFECTS

Adrenocorticotropic Hormone (ACTH)

- *Corticotropin (Acthar, HP) and cosyntropin (Cortrosyn) are pregnancy category C.*
- *CNS:* Headache, depression, dizziness, insomnia, euphoria, and nervousness
- *Endocrine:* Acne, Cushing's syndrome, and hyperpigmentation
- *F & E:* Hypokalemia, sodium, and water retention
- *GI:* Nausea and vomiting, peptic ulcer perforation
- *Musculoskeletal:* Muscle atrophy, myalgia, and weakness
- *Other:* Hypersensitivity

Growth Hormone (GH) and GH Antagonists

- *Somatrem (Protropin), somatropin (Humatrope, Saizen, Nutropin), and bromocriptine mesylate (Parlodel) are pregnancy category C; octreotide (Sandostatin) and pegvisomant (Somavert) are category B.*
- *CNS:* Headache
- *Derm:* Flushing, rash, urticaria
- *Endocrine:* Hyperglycemia, hypothyroidism
- *F & E:* Edema
- *GI:* Nausea, vomiting, and diarrhea
- *GU:* Hypercalciuria
- *Other:* Pain at injection site, development of antibodies

Antiduretic Hormones (ADH)

- *Vasopressin (Pitressin) is pregnancy category C; desmopressin acetate (DDAVP) and lypressin (Diapid) are pregnancy category B.*

- *CV:* Chest pain, myocardial infarction, hypertension
- *CNS:* Drowsiness, dizziness, and headache
- *Derm:* Sweating
- *GI:* Nausea, vomiting, diarrhea, and cramps
- *GU:* Uterine cramping
- *Other:* Water intoxication, allergic reaction, nasal irritation, and congestion

Parathyroid Hormones

- *Pregnancy category C*
- *CNS:* Headaches
- *EENT:* Rhinitis (nasal Miacalcin), nasal irritation, and epistaxis
- *GI:* Anorexia; nausea, vomiting and diarrhea
- *Musculoskeletal:* Back pain and muscle pain (nasal Miacalcin)
- *Other:* Allergic reactions, facial flushing, tingling, pain, or swelling at injection site

INTERACTIONS

Adrenocorticotropic Hormone (ACTH)

- Concurrent use with Amphotericin B or diuretics may produce an additive potassium-lowering effect.

Growth Hormone (GH) and GH Antagonists

- Insulin or oral hypoglycemics may need to be adjusted.
- Concurrent use with glucocorticoids or ACTH with somatrem and somatropin can oppose the effects of GH.
- Erythromycin increases serum bromocriptine levels.

Antiduretic Hormones (ADH)

Vasopressin (Pitussin) and Desmopressin (DDAVP)

- Decrease ADH effects when given concurrently with alcohol, lithium, demeclocyclin, heparin, or norepinephrine
- Increase effects of desmopressin (DDAVP) when given concurrently with carbamazepine, chlorpropamide, and clofibrate

Parathyroid Hormones

* Concurrent use with bisphosphonates may decrease response to calcitonin.

 CONTRAINDICATIONS

Adrenocorticotropic Hormone (ACTH)

* Hypersensitivity
* Congestive heart failure
* Peptic ulcer disease
* Hypertension
* Cushing's syndrome
* Scleroderma
* Osteoporosis
* Clients who have undergone recent surgery

Growth Hormone (GH) and GH Antagonists

* Hypersensitivity

Somatrem (Protropin) and Somatropin (Humatrope, Saizen, Nutropin)

* In individuals who have closed epiphyses or in clients who have an active tumor

Antiduretic Hormones (ADH)

* Hypersensitivity

Desmopressin Acetate (DDAVP) and Lypressin (Diapid)

* Nephrogenic diabetes insipidus

Vasopressin (Pitressin)

* Chronic renal failure

Parathyroid Hormones

* Hypersensitivity to salmon protein or gelatin diluent
* Pregnancy or lactation

NURSING IMPLICATIONS

Adrenocorticotropic Hormone (ACTH)

Corticotropin (Acthar, HP)

- Give IV, IM, or SC, also repository form give IM or SC.
- Give deep IM.
- Monitor for hypersensitivity.
- Monitor glucose and electrolytes throughout therapy.
- Monitor I & O and weight throughout therapy.
- Monitor vital signs throughout therapy.
- Monitor for and report signs of infection.

 Monitor for hypersensitivity.

 Monitor glucose and electrolytes throughout therapy.

Cosyntropin (Cortrosyn)

- Give IV, IM, or IV infusion.
- Monitor plasma cortisal levels before and after administration.

Growth Hormones (GH)

Somatrem (Protropin) and Somatropin (Humatrope, Saizen, Nutropin)

- Give Somatrem SC, IM, or IV; give somatropin SC or IM.
- Use sterile water to mix drug and don't shake vial.
- Do not use if solution is cloudy.
- Monitor height, weight, and head circumference.
- Monitor for symptoms of hypothyroidism and report symptoms to health care provider.
- Obtain baseline and monitor throughout therapy thyroid function studies, bone age determinations, and anti-growth hormone antibodies.
- Monitor for noncompliance or antibody formation, hypothyroidism, or malnutrition if growth rate does not exceed pretreatment rate of 2.0 cm per year.[4]
- Monitor for pain at injection site.

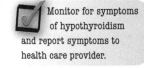 Monitor height, weight, and head circumference.

Monitor for symptoms of hypothyroidism and report symptoms to health care provider.

GH Antagonists

Bromocriptine Mesylate (Parlodel)

- Give PO with food.
- Monitor kidney and liver function throughout therapy.

Octreotide (Sandostatin)

- Give SC, IM, or IV.
- Give between meals and at bedtime to minimize GI effects.

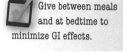
Give between meals and at bedtime to minimize GI effects.

- Report symptoms of hypoglycemia or hyperglycemia to health care provider and monitor blood glucose levels.
- Monitor pain at injection site.
- Administer drug at room temperature, rotate injection sites; do not use if solution is cloudy.

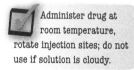
Administer drug at room temperature, rotate injection sites; do not use if solution is cloudy.

- Obtain baseline and monitor vital signs throughout therapy.
- Monitor fluid and electrolyte balance (I & O).
- Assess for gallbladder disease; monitor ultrasound tests before and periodically throughout long-term therapy.

Pegvisomant (Semavert)

- Give SC.
- Monitor glucose and liver function throughout therapy.
- Rotate injection sites.

All ADH Drugs

- Obtain baseline and monitor vital signs, especially blood pressure, weight, and I & O throughout therapy.
- Monitor for signs of water intoxication, discontinue drug temporarily until polyuria occurs, and report symptoms to health care provider.

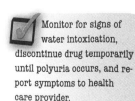
Monitor for signs of water intoxication, discontinue drug temporarily until polyuria occurs, and report symptoms to health care provider.

- Monitor specific gravity of urine periodically throughout therapy.
- Monitor electrolytes periodically throughout therapy.

Vasopressin (Pitressin) and Desmopressin Acetate (DDAVP)

- Monitor electrocardiogram periodically throughout therapy.

Desmopressin Acetate (DDAVP)

- For treatment of hemophilia A or von Willebrand's disease, monitor factor. VIII coagulant concentrations and other bleeding factors

Antiduretic Hormones (ADH)

Vasopressin (Pitressin)

- Give SC, IM, IV, or intra-arterially.

Desmopressin Acetate (DDAVP)

- Give PO, intranasally, or IV.

Lypressin (Diapid)

- Give intranasally.

Parathyroid Hormones

Calcitonin

- Give SC, IM, and intranasally.
- Monitor for signs of hypersensitivity and keep epinephrine, antihistamine, and oxygen nearby in case of a reaction.
- Perform skin testing to determine sensitivity to calcitonin before therapy is started.
- Monitor for symptoms of hypocalcemia and monitor calcium and alkaline phosphatase levels throughout therapy.
- Perform periodic urine (24 hours) hydroxyproline testing for Paget's disease.
- Rotate injection sites and monitor for pain, redness, or edema.
- Do not use discolored solutions.

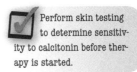
Perform skin testing to determine sensitivity to calcitonin before therapy is started.

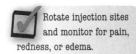
Rotate injection sites and monitor for pain, redness, or edema.

Teriparatide (Forteo)

- Give SC.

REFERENCES

1. McKenry LM, Tessier E, Hogan M. *Mosby's Pharmacology in Nursing,* 22nd ed. St. Louis, MO: Mosby Elsevier; 2006:824.

2. Lehne RA. *Pharmacology for Nursing Care,* 6th ed. St. Louis, MO: Saunders/Elsevier; 2007:849.

3. Lilley L, Harrington S, Snyder J. *Pharmacology and the Nursing Process,* 5th ed. St. Louis, MO: Mosby; 2007:459.

4. McKenry LM, Tessier E, Hogan M. *Mosby's Pharmacology in Nursing,* 22nd ed. St. Louis, MO: Mosby Elsevier; 2006:826.

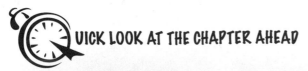
Thyroid agents are used to treat hypothyroidism. Hypothyroidism is called myxedema in adults and cretinism in children. Goiter may also occur in some forms of hypothyroidism and results in an enlarged thyroid gland. Synthetic thyroid agents are usually more prescribed as they are more stable and standardized than desiccated or natural thyroid.[1]

Treatment of hypothyroidism is aimed at eliminating symptoms so that normal hormonal balance is restored.

49

Thyroid Drugs

TERM

☐ **levothyroxine (Synthroid)**

Table 49-1 Thyroid Drugs

Prototype Drug	Related Drugs	Drug Classification
levothyroxine (Synthroid)		Synthetic thyroid hormone (T_4)
	liothyronine (Cytomel)	Synthetic thyroid hormone (T_3)
	liotrix (Euthroid, Thyrolar)	Synthetic T_3/T_4 Thyroid hormone combination
	thyroid (S-P-T)	Desiccated thyroid gland

THYROID DRUGS CLIENT TEACHING

- Consult with health care provider before taking other OTC medications or herbal remedies.
- Do not stop taking without consulting with health care provider.
- Do not change brands unless approved by health care provider, as this can affect bioavailability.

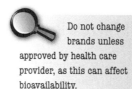

Do not change brands unless approved by health care provider, as this can affect bioavailability.

- If a dose is missed, take as soon as remembered unless almost time for next dose.
- Thyroid drugs do not cure hypothyroidism, and therapy is lifelong.
- Take exactly as ordered, at the same time daily (preferably in the morning) to prevent insomnia.

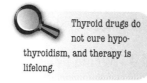

Thyroid drugs do not cure hypothyroidism, and therapy is lifelong.

- Report chest pain, palpitations, weight loss, insomnia, headache, nervousness, excessive perspiration, heat intolerance, or any other unusual symptoms to health care provider.
- Thyroid function studies are performed at least yearly, and follow-up examinations are indicated.

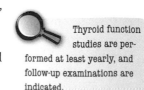

Thyroid function studies are performed at least yearly, and follow-up examinations are indicated.

- Check pulse before taking drug. If pulse is greater than 100 beats per minute in adults, or if pulse rate is elevated in children, hold and notify health care provider.
- Inform health care provider or dentist if taking thyroid preparations.
- Carry MedicAlert identification.

 ## ACTION

All Thyroid Drugs

- Increase metabolic rate of body tissues; stimulate the cardiovascular system; increase body temperature, oxygen consumption, and blood volume; promote glyconeogenesis; increase utilization and mobilization of glycogen stores; stimulates protein synthesis; and promote cell growth and differentiation

 ## USE

All Thyroid Drugs

- Replacement therapy for hypothyroidism
- Prevention and treatment of goiter
- Prevention and treatment of thyroid carcinoma
- Thyroid function diagnostic tests

 ## ADVERSE EFFECTS AND SIDE EFFECTS

All Thyroid Drugs

- *Pregnancy category A*
- *CV:* Palpitations, tachycardia, hypertension chest pain, dysrhythmias, angina, and cardiac arrest
- *CNS:* Insomnia, headache, irritability, and nervousness
- *Derm:* Hair loss in children (usually temporary) and sweating
- *Endocrine:* Thyroid storm, heat intolerance, menstrual irregularities, weight loss
- *GI:* Nausea, vomiting, diarrhea, and cramps

INTERACTIONS

All Thyroid Drugs

- Concurrent use with bile acid sequestrants decreases absorption of orally administered thyroid agents.
- May increase insulin or oral hypoglycemic agent requirements
- Concurrent use with warfarin may increase effects of warfarin; therefore warfarin doses may need to be decreased.
- Additive cardiovascular effects with adrenergic agents

CONTRAINDICATIONS

All Thyroid Drugs

- Hypersensitivity
- Recent myocardial infarction
- Adrenal insufficiency
- Thyrotoxicosis

NURSING IMPLICATIONS

- Give PO as a single daily dose.
- Monitor thyroid function tests.
- Elderly are more prone to adverse effects and are more sensitive to the effects of thyroid agents. Therefore therapy should be individualized, and dose may be reduced.
- Check apical pulse before giving, and hold if pulse is greater than 100 beats per minute; in children if pulse rate is elevated, hold and notify health care provider.
- Dosage is increased gradually based on thyroid function studies.

 Monitor thyroid function tests.

Check apical pulse before giving, and hold if pulse is greater than 100 beats per minutes; in children if pulse rate is elevated, hold and notify health care provider.

- Side effects are usually dose related.
- Report symptoms of hyperthyroidism to health care provider.

Levothyroxine (Synthroid)

- Give IM or IV.

Liothyronine (Cytomel)

- Give IV.
- Has a rapid onset of action and side effects may be seen more quickly

REFERENCE

1. Lilley L, Harrington S, Snyder J. *Pharmacology and the Nursing Process*, 5th ed. St. Louis, MO: Mosby; 2007:467.

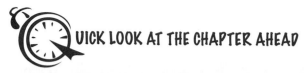

Antithyroid drugs are used to treat hyperthyroidism. There are different types of hyperthyroidism, and the most common form of hyperthyroidism is Graves' disease.

Antithyroid drugs decrease the basal metabolic rate by interfering with the action, formation, or release of thyroid hormones.[1] Iodides, radioactive iodine, and thioamide derivatives treat the underlying cause of hypothyroidism, and beta-blockers treat the symptoms.[2] A subtotal thyroidectomy is also used to treat hyperthyroidism.

50

Antithyroid Drugs

TERMS
- ☐ **Strong iodine solution (Lugol's solution)**
- ☐ **Propylthiouracil (PTU)**

Table 50-1 Antithyroid Drugs

Prototype Drug	Related Drugs	Drug Classification
Strong iodine solution (Lugol's solution)	potassium iodine (SSKI, Thyro-Block)	Iodides
There is no prototype for this classification	sodium iodide (1^{131} Iodotope)	Radioactive iodine
Propylthiouracil (PTU)	methimazole (Tapazole)	Thioamide derivatives

ANTITHYROID DRUGS CLIENT TEACHING

All Antithyroid Drugs

- Consult with health care provider before taking other OTC medications (as some contain iodine) or herbal remedies.
- Continue follow-up care with health care provider so that periodic blood counts and thyroid function testing may be done.
- Provide teaching about hypothyroidism and hyperthyroidism.
- Take as prescribed, do not skip or double dose, and avoid missing doses to prevent thyroid storm.
- Notify health care provider if pregnant or breast-feeding.
- Carry MedicAlert identification.
- Avoid eating foods high in iodine such as soybeans, seafood, and iodized salt.
- Maintain a journal to document therapy responses, such as weight, pulse, or mood, and report changes to health care provider.[3]

Consult with health care provider before taking other OTC medications (as some contain iodine) or herbal remedies.

Continue follow-up care with health care provider so that periodic blood counts and thyroid function testing may be done.

Avoid eating foods high in iodine such as soybeans, seafood, and iodized salt.

Iodides

- Discontinue and contact health care provider if you experience symptoms of iodism such as fever, skin rash, or metallic/brassy taste; symptoms of a cold; neck and throat swelling; severe GI distress; or burning soreness in gums and teeth.[4]

- Dilute liquid iodines in water or fruit juice and use a straw when taking to prevent staining of teeth.

Dilute liquid iodines in water or fruit juice and use a straw when taking to prevent staining of teeth.

Radioactive Iodines

- Teach clients to avoid radiation contamination by double flushing the toilet after use (urine and stool), and hand washing after toilet use.
- Avoid extended contact with people for 1 week.
- Report redness, sore throat, or swelling as this may indicate dyscrasias.
- Void frequently during treatment to prevent irradiation of gonads.
- Avoid coughing or expectoration for the first 24 hours as saliva and vomitus are radioactive for 6 to 8 hours after dose taken.
- For the first 48 hours, increase fluids up to 3 to 4 L/day to help excrete agent.

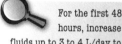

Teach clients to avoid radiation contamination by double flushing the toilet after use (urine and stool), and hand washing after toilet use.

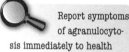

For the first 48 hours, increase fluids up to 3 to 4 L/day to help excrete agent.

Thioamide Derivatives

- Report symptoms of agranulocytosis immediately to health care provider such as sore throat, fever, or malaise.

- Take with food to decrease GI upset.

Report symptoms of agranulocytosis immediately to health care provider such as sore throat, fever, or malaise.

℞ ACTION

Iodides

- Decrease the vascularity of the thyroid gland and inhibit the release and synthesis of thyroid hormones. Effects are noted in 24 hours with maximum effects within 10 to 14 consecutive days of therapy.

Radioactive Iodine

• Selectively damages or destroys thyroid tissue

Thioamide Derivatives

• Inhibit the incorporation of iodide into tyrosine and inhibit the coupling of Iodotyrosines[5]

Propylthiouracil (PTU)

• Inhibits the conversion of T_4 to T_3, making it more effective to treat thyrotoxicosis or thyroid storm[5]

 USE

All Antithyroid Drugs

• Hyperthyroidism (Graves' disease)

Iodides

• Adjunct with other antithyroid drugs in preparation for thyroidectomy
• Radiation protectant before and after administration of radioactive iodine or in radiation emergencies
• Thyrotoxicosis
• Iodine replacement therapy

Radioactive Iodine

• Thyroid carcinoma

Thioamide Derivatives

• Used before thyroidectomy or radiotherapy

Propylthiouracil (PTU)

• Adjunct in treatment of thyrotoxicosis or thyroid storm

ADVERSE EFFECTS AND SIDE EFFECTS

Iodides

- *Potassium iodide (SSKI, Thyro-Block) is pregnancy category A; strong iodine solution (Lugol's solution) is pregnancy category UK.*
- *Endocrine:* Hypothyroidism
- *F & E:* Hyperkalemia with potassium iodide
- *GI:* GI irritation, diarrhea
- *Other:* Iodism, hypersensitivity

Radioactive Iodine

- *Pregnancy category X*
- *EENT:* Sore throat, temporary loss of taste
- *Endocrine:* Hypothyroidism, hyperthyroid adenoma
- *GI:* Nausea, vomiting, and diarrhea
- *Hematologic:* Blood dyscrasias, anemia

Thioamide Derivatives

- *Pregnancy category D*
- *CNS*: Dizziness, fever
- *Derm*: Skin rash
- *GI*: Nausea, vomiting, diarrhea, jaundice, hepatitis, and loss of taste
- *Hematologic*: Agranulocytosis, leukopenia

INTERACTIONS

All Antithyroid Drugs

- Concurrent use with lithium: additive hypothyroidism

Iodides

Potassium Iodide (SSKI, Thyro-Block)

- Concurrent use with potassium-sparing diuretics, potassium supplements, or angeotensin-converting enzyme inhibitors causes additive hyperkalemia.

Radioactive Iodine

- Concurrent use with other antithyroid drugs causes a decreased uptake.

Thioamide Derivatives

- Concurrent use with bone marrow suppressants increases risk of agranulocytosis.
- Concurrent use with anticoagulants increases anticoagulant effects.

 ## CONTRAINDICATIONS

Iodides

- Hypersensitivity

Radioactive Iodine

- Under age 30
- Pregnant and lactating women
- Recent myocardial infarction

Thioamide Derivatives

- Pregnant women in their third trimester

 ## NURSING IMPLICATIONS

All Antithyroid Drugs

- Monitor vital signs, daily weights, I & O
- Monitor thyroid function.
- Monitor for symptoms of hypothyroidism such as cold intolerance, weight gain, constipation.
- Monitor and report symptoms of thyroid storm such as palpitations, tachycardia, fever, CNS changes, and peripheral edema.

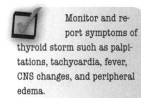

Monitor and report symptoms of thyroid storm such as palpitations, tachycardia, fever, CNS changes, and peripheral edema.

Iodides

- Give PO (IV as a nutritional supplement).
- Assess for symptoms of iodism and report symptoms to health care provider.
- Monitor for and report hypersensitivity reactions.
- Monitor potassium levels.
- Discard brownish-yellow solutions.

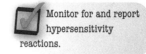
Monitor for and report hypersensitivity reactions.

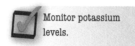
Monitor potassium levels.

Radioactive Iodine

- Give PO.
- Administer only after discontinuing other antithyroid drugs for 5 to 7 days.
- Administer after nothing by mouth overnight—food slows absorption of drug.
- Administer the first few days after the onset of menses in women with child-bearing potential.
- Monitor CBC for blood dyscrasias.

Administer after nothing by mouth overnight—food slows absorption of drug.

Thioamide Derivatives

- Give PO.
- Monitor CBC
- Monitor for agranulocytosis, such as a sore throat, fever, and malaise.

REFERENCES

1. McKenry LM, Tessier E, Hogan M. *Mosby's Pharmacology in Nursing*, 22nd ed. St. Louis, MO: Mosby Elsevier; 2006:843.

2. Lilley L, Harrington S, Snyder J. *Pharmacology and the Nursing Process*, 5th ed. St. Louis, MO: Mosby; 2007:469.

3. Lilley L, Harrington S, Snyder J. *Pharmacology and the Nursing Process*, 5th ed. St. Louis, MO: Mosby; 2007:471.

4. McKenry LM, Tessier E, Hogan M. *Mosby's Pharmacology in Nursing*, 22nd ed. St. Louis, MO: Mosby Elsevier; 2006:844.

5. McKenry LM, Tessier E, Hogan M. *Mosby's Pharmacology in Nursing*, 22nd ed. St. Louis, MO: Mosby Elsevier; 2006:846.

The adrenal cortex produces corticosteroid hormones, which include glucocorticoids, mineralocorticoids, and androgens. The androgens are discussed in Chapter 61.

The glucocorticoids increase carbohydrate, protein, and fat metabolism. The mineralocorticoids include the steroid hormone aldosterone and affect homeostasis and electrolyte balance. At high levels, the glucocorticosteroid hormones cortisol and hydrocortisone also have mineralocorticoid effects. Systemic glucocorticoids are classified as short acting, intermediate-acting, or long-acting.

Adrenal steroid inhibitors suppress or inhibit the function of the adrenal cortex.

51

Corticosteroids

TERMS
- ☐ fludrocortisone (Florinef)
- ☐ hydrocortisone (Cortef, Hydrocortone, Solu-Cortef)
- ☐ prednisone (Orasone, Deltasone)

425

Table 51-1 Corticosteroids

Prototype Drug	Related Drugs	Drug Classification
hydrocortisone (Cortef, Hydrocortone, Solu-Cortef)	cortisone (Cortone)	**Glucocorticoids** (Systemic) Short-acting glucocorticoid
prednisone (Orasone, Deltasone)	methylprednisolone (A-Methapred, Medrol, Solu-Medrol) prednisolone (Articulose, Delta-Cortef) triamcinolone (Amcort, Kenalog, Aristocort)	Intermediate-acting glucocorticoid
There is no prototype for this classification	betamethasone (Celestone) budesonide (Entocort EC, Rhinocort) dexamethasone (Cortastat, Decadron, others)	Long-acting glucocorticoid
fludrocortisone (Florinef)		Mineralocorticoid
There is no prototype for this classification	aminoglutethimide (Cytadren)	Adrenal corticosteroid inhibitors

CORTICOSTEROIDS CLIENT TEACHING

Glucocorticosteroids and Mineralocorticosteroids

- Wear or carry MedicAlert identification.
- Notify other health care providers, including dentists and specialists, of drug therapy.
- Continue follow-up care with health care provider. Periodic bloodwork including electrolyte levels is indicated throughout therapy.
- Restrict sodium intake and eat high potassium foods.

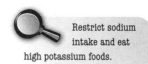
Restrict sodium intake and eat high potassium foods.

- Monitor weight daily and report sudden weight gain to health care provider.
- Do not take over-the-counter drugs or herbal remedies without consulting a health care provider.

Glucocorticoids

- Report symptoms of infection to health care provider.
- Avoid individuals with infections.
- Do not receive immunizations while on therapy.
- Do not take with grapefruit juice.
- Take drug exactly as prescribed at the same time and do not abruptly stop taking.
- Take drug with food to minimize gastrointestinal (GI) distress.
- Avoid alcohol, aspirin, caffeine, or other agents that cause GI bleeding or irritation.
- A single daily dose is usually taken in the morning.
- Report changes in mental status including depression or euphoria.
- Report symptoms of bleeding, abdominal pain, or visual changes.

> Report symptoms of infection to health care provider.

> Do not receive immunizations while on therapy.

> Report changes in mental status including depression or euphoria.

Topical Glucocorticoids

- Take triamcinolone (Amcort, Aristocort, Kenalog), betamethasone (Celastone), and dexamethasone (Decadron) exactly as directed. Apply to a clean and dry area.
- Apply sparingly.

Intra-Arterial Injection

- Rest joint for 24 to 48 hours after administration of hydrocortisone (Cortef), methylprednisolone (Medrol), triamcinolone (Amcort, Aristocort, Kenalog) and do not overuse joint.

Ophthalmic

- Take hydrocortisone (Cortef), prednisolone (Delta-Cortef, Articulose), and dexamethasone (Decadron) exactly as prescribed
- Do not abruptly discontinue without consulting health care provider.

- Maintain follow-up care with health care provider.
- To prevent risk of infection, avoid wearing contact lenses during therapy and for a period of time after therapy.
- Shake suspension before administering.
- Stinging may occur temporarily after administering.

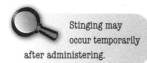

Stinging may occur temporarily after administering.

Anorectal Glucocorticoids

- Call health care provider if bleeding or protrusion occurs, or if symptoms do not improve in 7 days.
- Maintain normal bowel function.

Adrenal Corticosteroid Inhibitors

- Change positions slowly to minimize orthostatic hypotension.
- Wear or carry MedicAlert identification.
- Notify other health care providers, including dentists and specialists, of drug therapy.
- Contact health care provider if infection, injury, or illness occurs.
- Due to the adverse effects of the drug, avoid driving or operating heavy machinery until response to drug is known.

Contact health care provider if infection, injury, or illness occurs.

 ACTION

Glucocorticoids

- Glucocorticoids have anti-inflammatory effects; maintain blood pressure; increase carbohydrate, protein, and fat metabolism; suppress the immune response; and in stressful situations, release cortisol to maintain homeostasis.

Mineralocorticoids

- Promote sodium and water reabsorption, maintain control of normal blood pressure, and influence serum potassium levels and pH
- Have weak glucocorticoid effects

Adrenal Steroid Inhibitors

- Inhibit the conversion of cholesterol into adrenal corticosteroids

 USE

Glucocorticoids

- Glucocorticoids are used in replacement therapy for adrenocortical insufficiency, treatment of anaphylactic reactions not responsive to other treatments, asthma, severe allergic reactions, collagen and rheumatic disorders, shock, cerebral edema, eye diseases, dermatologic disorders, topical and systemic inflammation, hematologic disorders, and adjunct treatment in neoplastic disease.

Mineralocorticoids

- Replacement therapy for adrenocortical insufficiency (eg, Addison's disease)

Adrenal Corticosteroid Inhibitors

- Treatment of Cushing's syndrome, adrenal cancer, and metastatic breast cancer

 ADVERSE EFFECTS AND SIDE EFFECTS

Glucocorticoids

- *Pregnancy category C*
- *CV:* Congenital heart failure, hypertension
- *CNS:* Mood swings, depression, insomnia, nervousness, headache, convulsions, and vertigo
- *Derm:* Petechiae, poor wound healing, urticaria, hirsutism, ecchymoses, and fragile skin
- *Endocrine:* Cushing's syndrome, growth suppression, hyperglycemia, and menstrual irregularities

- *F & E:* Hypokalemia, fluid retention
- *GI:* nausea, vomiting, diarrhea, and peptic ulcers with possible perforation
- *Hematologic:* Thromboembolism
- *Musculoskeletal:* Muscle wasting, osteoporosis
- *Other:* Glaucoma, increased intraocular pressure, cataracts, weight gain

Mineralocorticoids

- *Pregnancy category C*
- *CV:* Hypertension, dysrhythmias, congenital heart failure
- *CNS:* Headache, dizziness
- *Endocrine:* Adrenal suppression, weight gain
- *F & E:* Hypokalemia
- *GI:* Anorexia, nausea
- *Musculoskeletal:* Muscular weakness, arthralgia
- *Other:* Hypersensitivity

Adrenal Corticosteroid Inhibitors

- *Pregnancy category D*
- *CV:* Hypotension
- *CNS:* Drowsiness, headache, dizziness, uncontrolled eye movements
- *Derm:* Rash, hirsutism
- *GI:* Nausea, vomiting, anorexia, and hepatotoxicity
- *Hematologic:* Agranulocytosis, leukopenia

 # INTERACTIONS

Glucocorticoids

- Concurrent use with loop or thiazide diuretics, amphotericin B, or Digoxin may cause increased hypokalemia.
- May increase need for insulin or oral hypoglycemics
- Concurrent use of aspirin (NSAIDs) increases GI effects.
- Aloe or licorice may prolong or enhance corticosteroid effects.

- Concurrent use with barbituates, phenytoin, rifampin, salicylates, cholestyramine increases metabolism of glucocorticoids.
- Concurrent use with immunizing biological agents inhibits immune response to biological.
- Avoid taking with grapefruit juice as it increases serum levels of glucocorticoids.
- Increased sodium retention occurs when eating foods high in sodium.
- Avoid immunizations during therapy as immunization effect may be reduced as the antibody response is inhibited and may cause neurological complications.
- May suppress reactions to allergy skin tests

Mineralocorticoids

- Increased sodium retention when eating foods high in sodium
- Concurrent use with loop or thiazide diuretics, amphotericin B, mezlocillin, or piperacillin may cause increased hypokalemia.
- Hypokalemia can increase risk of digoxin toxicity.

Adrenal Corticosteroid Inhibitors

- Increases metabolism of dexamethasone

CONTRAINDICATIONS

Glucocorticoids

- Hypersensitivity
- Bacterial or fungal infections
- Lactation
- Mineralocorticoids
- Hypersensitivity

Adrenal Corticosteroid Inhibitors

- Hypersensitivity
- Hypothyroidism
- Pregnancy

NURSING IMPLICATIONS

Glucocorticoids

- Give PO, intranasal, respiratory inhalant ophthalmic, topical, intra-articular injection, IV, IM, or rectally.
- Monitor I & O and daily weight.
- Monitor vital signs, especially blood pressure.
- Check stool for occult blood.
- Monitor glucose and electrolyte levels throughout therapy.
- Avoid immunizations during therapy as immunization effect may be reduced as the antibody response is inhibited and may cause neurological complications.
- For long-term use, assess for ophthalmic, CNS, Cushing's syndrome hypertension, hyperglycemia, hypokalemia effects.
- For long-term use, HPA axis suppression test should be performed to assess suppression.
- Periodic eye exams are indicated for clients taking glucocorticoids for longer than 6 weeks.
- A daily dose should be given in the early morning.
- Discontinuing therapy should be done slowly and with monitoring, using tapered doses to prevent adrenal insufficiency.
- Give IM suspensions deep in the gluteal muscle.

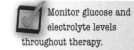
Monitor glucose and electrolyte levels throughout therapy.

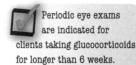
Avoid immunizations during therapy as immunization effect may be reduced as the antibody response is inhibited and may cause neurological complications.

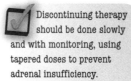
Periodic eye exams are indicated for clients taking glucocorticoids for longer than 6 weeks.

Discontinuing therapy should be done slowly and with monitoring, using tapered doses to prevent adrenal insufficiency.

Mineralocorticoids

Fludrocortisone (Florinef)

- Give PO.
- Monitor vital signs, especially blood pressure, and lung sounds for edema (eg, crackles).

- Monitor I & O and weight, and report significant changes.
- Monitor electrolytes, especially potassium, for hypokalemia throughout therapy.

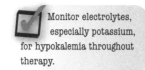
Monitor electrolytes, especially potassium, for hypokalemia throughout therapy.

- Report increases in blood pressure, edema, or significant weight gain to health care provider.

Adrenal Corticosteroid Inhibitors

Aminoglutethimide (Cytadren)

- Give PO.
- Monitor vital signs, especially blood pressure.

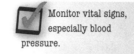
Monitor vital signs, especially blood pressure.

- Monitor I & O.
- Monitor and obtain baseline thyroid function studies, electrolytes, hematologic, and liver function studies throughout therapy.
- For adrenal disorders, monitor plasma cortisol or 24-hour urinary 17-hydroxycorticosteroid concentrations to determine if steroid supplementation is required.

QUICK LOOK AT THE CHAPTER AHEAD

Insulin and oral hypoglycemics are used to treat diabetes mellitus (DM) by preventing hyperglycemia. Insulin is used to treat Type I (insulin-dependent-diabetes mellitus IDDM). Insulin can be extracted from domesticated animals or synthesized in the laboratory using recombinant DNA technology.[1] Recombinant or human insulin is identical to insulin produced by the pancreas.[1]

There are five categories of insulin, including **rapid-acting, short-acting, intermediate-acting, long-acting,** and **combination** insulin. The dose of insulin is based on individual client needs.

Oral antidiabetics are used to treat Type 2 (non-insulin-dependent-diabetes mellitus NIDDM). Diet and exercise are also included in treating NIDDM and, when needed, insulin. The three categories of oral antidiabetics include **first-** and **second-generation sulfonylureas** and **miscellaneous** group, which include alpha-glucosidase inhibitors, biguanides, meglitinides, and thiazolidinediones. Two new injectable drugs include pramlintide acetate (Symlin), anmylin mimetic, and exenatide (Byetta), an incretin mimetic.

52

Antidiabetics

TERMS
☐ **acarbose (Precose)**
☐ **chlorpropamide (Diabenese)**
☐ **glyburide (Diabeta, Micronase)**
☐ **insulin injection, regular**

Table 52-1 Antidiabetics

Prototype Drug	Related Drugs	Drug Classification
acarbose (Precose)	miglitol (Glyset)	Alpha-glucosidase inhibitor
chlorpropamide (Diabenese)	acetohexamide (Dymelor) tolazamide (Tolinase) tolbutamide (Orinase)	Oral antidiabetics: First-generation sulfonylureas
glyburide (Diabeta, Micronase)	glimepiride (Amaryl) glipizide (Glucotrol) glyburide micronized (Glynase)	Second-generation sulfonylureas
insulin injection, regular	(Humulin R)	Short-acting insulin
There is no prototype for this classification	insulin glulisine (Apidra) insulin lispro (Humalog)	Rapid-acting insulin
There is no prototype for this classification	Insulin detemir (Levemir) isophane insulin suspension (NPH Insulin, Humulin N, Novolin N)	Intermediate-acting insulin
There is no prototype for this classification	extended insulin zinc suspension (Humulin U Ultralente) glargine insulin (Lantus)	Long-acting insulin
There is no prototype for this classification	isophane human insulin (70%) and human insulin (30%) (Humulin 70/30, Novolin 70/30) isophane human insulin 50% and human insulin 50% (Humulin 50/50) 70% insulin protamine/ 30% insulin aspart (Novolog Mix 70/30) 75% insulin lispro protamine/25% insulin lispro (Humalog mix 75/25) Inhalational (Exubera)	Combination insulin

continues

Table 52-1 Antidiabetics (continued)

Prototype Drug	Related Drugs	Drug Classification
There is no prototype for this classification	metformin (Glucophage)	Biguanides
There is no prototype for this classification	nateglinide (Starlix) repaglinide (Prandin)	Meglitinide
There is no prototype for this classification	pioglitazone (Actos) rosiglitazone (Avandia)	Thiazolidinediones
There is no prototype for this classification	exenatide (Byetta) glipizide/metformin (Metaglip) glyburide/metformin (Glucovance) pioglitazone/metformin (Actoplusmet) pramlintide acetate (Symlin) rosiglitazone/glimepiride (Avandaryl) rosiglitazone/metformin (Avandamet)	Incretin mimetics Combination/ oral agents Amylin mimetics

℞ ANTIDIABETICS CLIENT TEACHING

Insulin and Oral Agents

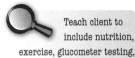
Teach client to include nutrition, exercise, glucometer testing, and type of diabetes with specific management.

- Carry medical identification and MedicAlert identification.
- Teach client to include nutrition, exercise, glucometer testing, and type of diabetes with specific management.
- Maintain follow-up care with health care provider, which may include periodic laboratory testing.
- Carry a supply of glucose in case of hypoglycemic reaction.
- Avoid alcohol, as it can cause hypoglycemia.
- Do not take over-the-counter or herbal medications without consulting with health care provider.
- Notify dentist, specialists, and other health care providers of disease.
- Teach symptoms of hypoglycemia and hyperglycemia.

- Notify health care provider if you experience jaundice, dark urine, sore throat, bruising or unusual bleeding, secondary illness, inability to eat, or inability to control glucose levels.
- If ill, more frequent testing of glucose is indicated.

Insulin

- Teach client about rotating injection sites, syringe disposal, storage of insulin, checking expiration date, type and administration of insulin, and when mixing insulin not to shake the vial but to gently agitate vial.
- Runners and walkers should be aware that exercise accelerates absorption, especially in the injected limb.

 Runners and walkers should be aware that exercise accelerates absorption, especially in the injected limb.

 # ACTION

Insulin

Decreases hyperglycemia and controls the storage and metabolism of carbohydrates, protein, and fat that bind to receptor sites on cellular plasma membrane.[1]

Oral Antidiabetics

First- and Second-Generation Sulfonylureas

- Stimulate insulin release from beta cells in the pancreas
- Second-generation sulfonylureas have fewer adverse effects than first-generation sulfonylureas and have a longer duration of action.
- The miscellaneous agents may be used in combination with the sulfonylureas.

Alpha-Glucosidase Inhibitor

- Inhibit alpha-glucosidase and delay glucose absorption

Biguanides

- Decrease the production of glucose and increase its uptake, and do not produce hypoglycemia as seen in the sulfonylureas

Meglitinides

- Rapid-acting drugs that act like the sulfonylureas to increase insulin release

Thiazolidinediones

- Decrease insulin resistance and enhance glucose uptake and storage

 ## USE

Insulin

- Used to treat Type 1 IDDM and Type 2 NIDDM not responsive to treatment with oral antidiabetics or diet
  Pramlintide (Symlin) type 1 IDDM to supplement mealtime insulin
- Type 2 NIDDM, in combination with insulin or oral agents

Oral Antidiabetics

- Used to treat Type 2 NIDDM
  Exenatide (Byetta) adjunctive therapy for Type 2 NIDDM

 ## ADVERSE EFFECTS AND SIDE EFFECTS

Insulin

- *Pregnancy category B; glargine insulin (Lantus) and insulin aspart (Novolog) are category C.*
- *Derm:* Urticaria, rash, lipodystrophy, anaphylaxis
- *Endocrine:* Hypoglycemia, Somogyi effect

Pramlintide (Symlin) and Exenatide (Byetta)

- *Pregnancy Category C*
- *Endocrine:* hypoglycemia
- *GI:* Nausea
- Other injection site reaction

Table 52-2 Overview of Onset, Peak, and Duration of Insulin

	Onset	Peak	Duration
Short-Acting Insulin			
insulin injection regular (Humulin R)	30 to 60 minutes	1 to 5 hours	6 to 10 hours
Rapid-Acting Insulin			
insulin aspart (Novolog)	10 to 20 minutes	1 to 3 hours	3 to 5 hours
insulin lispro (Humalog)	15 to 30 minutes	0.5 to 2.5 hours	3 to 6 hours
insulin glulisine (Apidra)	10 to 15 minutes	1 to 1.5 hours	3 to 5 hours
Intermediate-Acting Insulin			
isophane insulin suspension (NPH insulin, Humulin N, Novolin N)	1 to 2 hours	6 to 14 hours	18 to 24 hours
Insulin detemir (Levemir)	—	6 to 8 hours	12 to 24 hours
Long-Acting Insulin			
Extended insulin zinc suspension (Humulin U Ultralente)	4 to 8 hours	10 to 30 hours	20 to 36 hours
glargine Insulin (Lantus)	70 minutes	none	24 hours
Combination Insulin			
isophane human insulin (70%) and human insulin (30%) (Humulin 70/30, Novolin 70/30)	30 to 60 minutes	1.5 to 16 hours	up to 24 hours
isophane human insulin (50%) and human insulin (50%) (Humulin 50/50)	30 to 60 minutes	2 to 5.5 hours	up to 24 hours
70% insulin aspart protamine/ 30% insulin aspart (NovoLog Mix 70/30)	Rapid	1 to 4 hours	up to 24 hours
75% insulin lispro protamine/ 25% insulin lispro (Humalog mix 75/25)	Rapid	1 to 6.5 hours	up to 24 hours
Inhalational (Exubera)	10 to 20 minutes	2 hours	6 hours

Adapted from Lehne RA. *Pharmacology for Nursing Care,* 6th ed. St. Louis, MO: Saunders Elsevier; 2007:652–656.

Oral Antidiabetics

- *Acarbose (Precose), glyburide (Diabeta, Micronase), and metformin (Glucophage) are pregnancy category B; chlorpropamide (Diabenese) is pregnancy category D; all other oral antidiabetics are pregnancy category C.*

First- and Second-Generation Sulfonylureas

- *CV:* Potential for increased risk of cardiac death, especially with first-generation sulfonylureas
- *CNS:* Headache
- *Derm:* Photosensitivity and rash
- *Endocrine:* Hypoglycemia
- *GI:* Anorexia, flatus, nausea, vomiting, diarrhea, constipation, jaundice
- *Hematologic:* Agranulocytosis, thrombocytopenia

Miscellaneous

Alpha-Glucosidase Inhibitors

- *GI:* Flatus, abdominal discomfort, and diarrhea; elevated liver enzymes at high doses

Biguanides

- *GI:* abdominal discomfort, nausea, vomiting, diarrhea, bloating

Meglitinides

- Similar to sulfonylureas

Repanglinide (Prandin)

- May cause hypertension or dysrhythmias

Thiazolidinediones

- Edema, fluid retention, weight gain
- Newer drugs are not associated with severe hepatotoxicity, but client should still be monitored for liver function changes.
- Monitor for signs of heart failure.

INTERACTIONS

Insulin

* Alcohol, NSAIDs, salicylates oral hypoglycemic agents, monoamine oxidase inhibitors (MAOIs), anabolic steroids, guanethidine, and warfarin can increase hypoglycemic effects of insulin.
* Beta-blockers may block some symptoms of hypoglycemia.
* Corticosteroids, thiazide diuretics, estrogens, nicotine, thyroid preparations, rifampin, diltazem, dobutamine, and protease inhibitor antivirals antagonize the hypoglycemic effects of insulin and increase insulin requirements.

First- and Second-Generation Sulfonylureas

* Alcohol may cause a disulfiram-like reaction.
* Alcohol, beta-blockers, NSAIDs, salicylates, chloramphenicol, sulfonamides, MAOIs, anabolic steroids, guanethidine, and warfarin can increase hypoglycemic effects of sulfonylureas.
* Adrenergics, corticosteroids, thiazide diuretics, estrogens, nicotine, thyroid preparations, phenytoin, and isoniazid decrease the hypoglycemic effect of sulfonylureas.

Alpha-Glucosidase Inhibitors

* Decreased effects by concurrent administration of intestinal adsorbents or digestive enzyme preparations

Biguanides

* Increased effects of biguanides, with cimetidine, furosemide, and nifedipine

Meglitinides

* See sulfonylureas.

Thiazolidinediones

* Rosiglitazone (Avandia): None known
* Pioglitazone (Actos): Increased pioglitazone (Actos) levels with concurrent use of ketoconazole

Pramlintide (Symlin)

- Delayed absorption of oral drugs
- Combined effects of gastric emptying if given with anticholinergics or with drugs that slow absorption of nutrients

Exenatide (Byetta)

- Delayed absorption of oral drugs
- Reduced absorption with antibiotics or oral contraceptives

 ## CONTRAINDICATIONS

Insulin

- Hypersensitivity to a particular type of insulin (ie, beef or pork, additives or preservatives)

Oral Antidiabetics

- Hypersensitivity to sulfonylureas
- Type 1 diabetes IDDM
- Ketoacidosis
- Uncontrolled infection or trauma
- Severe hepatic or thyroid disease
- Pregnancy
- Lactation

Miscellaneous

Alpha-Glucosidase Inhibitors

- Hypersensitivity
- Ketoacidosis
- Cirrhosis
- Impaired renal function
- Pregnancy
- Lactation

Biguanides

- Alcoholism
- Hypersensitivity

- Hepatic or renal disease
- Cardiopulmonary disease
- Meglitinides
- Hypersensitivity
- Pregnancy
- Lactation
- Ketoacidosis
- Type 1 diabetes IDDM

Thiazolidinediones

- Hypersensitivity
- Pregnancy
- Lactation
- Children under age 18
- Hepatic disease
- Type 1 diabetes IDDM
- Ketoacidosis

Pramlintide (Symlin) and Exenatide (Byetta) Hypersensitivity

 ## NURSING IMPLICATIONS

Insulin

- Give SC; regular insulin also available IV and via an insulin pump (delivers regular insulin over a 24-hour period).
- Dosing of insulin is based in units.
- Insulin pump: check for battery failure and defects in tubing.
- Monitor blood glucose levels and glycosylated hemoglobin throughout therapy.
- Certain religions may have dietary codes that include the avoidance of pork (ie, Jewish or Islamic clients), and therefore may prefer not to use pork insulin.
- Teach client about injection, site rotation, glucose testing, diet, foot care, exercise, and DM management

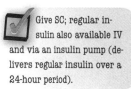
Give SC; regular insulin also available IV and via an insulin pump (delivers regular insulin over a 24-hour period).

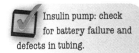
Insulin pump: check for battery failure and defects in tubing.

- Do not shake vial, but gently rotate, check expiration date, and use insulin syringes to draw up dose.
- When mixing insulin, draw up rapid or short-acting first.

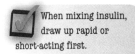
When mixing insulin, draw up rapid or short-acting first.

- Use caution when mixing types of insulin. NPH is the only insulin appropriate for mixing short-acting insulin.
- Insulin can be stored in a cool place and does not have to be refrigerated, but do not freeze.

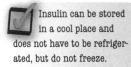
Insulin can be stored in a cool place and does not have to be refrigerated, but do not freeze.

- Exubera is given by inhalation and contains regular insulin.

Sliding-Scale Insulin

- Give SC with regular and lispro (Humalog) or aspart (Novolog) insulin.
- Dose is based on glucose results.
- Usually given to hospitalized DM clients whose insulin requirements may vary drastically[2]

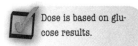
Dose is based on glucose results.

Oral Antidiabetics

- Give PO.
- Monitor during illness, infection, pregnancy, and stress as client may need to be switched to insulin coverage.
- Monitor glucose and glycosylated hemoglobin throughout therapy.
- Administer as prescribed to be taken with meals.
- Monitor for symptoms of hypoglycemia and hyperglycemia.

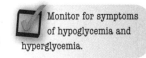
Monitor for symptoms of hypoglycemia and hyperglycemia.

- Stress the importance of following diet and exercising.

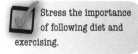
Stress the importance of following diet and exercising.

Miscellaneous

Biguanides

- Monitor renal function throughout therapy.

Thiazolidinediones

- Monitor liver function studies
- Monitor for signs of heart failure.

> Monitor liver function studies.

Pramlintide (Symlin) and Exenatide (Byetta)

- Give SC.

REFERENCES

1. Lilley L, Harrington S, Snyder J. *Pharmacology and the Nursing Process,* 5th ed. St. Louis, MO: Mosby; 2007:479.

2. Lilley L, Harrington S, Snyder J. *Pharmacology and the Nursing Process,* 5th ed. St. Louis, MO: Mosby; 2007:483.

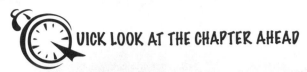

Hyperglycemic drugs are indicated for the treatment of severe hypoglycemia.

Glucagon is effective when liver glycogen is available and is ineffective in chronic hypoglycemia, adrenal insufficiency, and starvation.[1]

Oral diazoxide is indicated for the treatment of hypoglycemia caused by hyperinsulinism and is not indicated for treatment of functional hypoglycemia.[1]

53
Hyperglycemic Drugs

TERM
☐ **glucagon (GlucaGen)**

Table 53-1 Hyperglycemic Drugs

Prototype Drug	Related Drugs	Drug Classification
glucagon (GlucaGen)	diazoxide (Proglycem)	Hyperglycemic

HYPERGLYCEMIC DRUGS CLIENT TEACHING

- Instruct about the importance of diet, exercise, blood glucose testing, and regular follow-up care with health care provider.
- Monitor blood sugar and report signs of hypo- or hyperglycemia to health care provider.
- Change positions gradually to avoid light-headedness.
- Take oral glucose as soon as symptoms of hypoglycemia occurs.
- Check expiration date frequently and replace outdated drug as soon as possible.

Monitor blood sugar and report signs of hypo- or hyperglycemia to health care provider.

Change positions gradually to avoid light-headedness.

Glucagon (GlucaGen)

- Reserved for when client cannot swallow due to decreased level of consciousness or is unconscious
- Instruct how to mix and inject.
- Give SC at a 90-degree angle.
- If nausea and vomiting occur for more than 1 hour, thus preventing eating after taking, contact health care provider.

Reserved for when client can not swallow due to decreased level of consciousness or is unconscious

ACTION

Glucagon (GlucaGen)

- Stimulates hepatic production of glucose from glycogenolysis (glycogen stores)

Diazoxide (Proglycem)

- Increases blood sugar by inhibiting the release of pancreatic insulin

USE

Glucagon

- Severe hypoglycemia when use of glucose not feasible
- Facilitation of GI radiograph

Diazoxide (Proglycem)

- Hypoglycemia caused by hyperinsulism
- IV use for hypertensive emergency

ADVERSE EFFECTS AND SIDE EFFECTS

Glucagon (GlucaGen)

- *Pregnancy category B*
- *GI:* Nausea and vomiting
- *Other:* Allergic reaction

Diazoxide (Proglycem)

- *Pregnancy category C*
- *Derm:* Hirsutism
- *Endocrine:* Hyperglycemia, ketoacidosis
- *GI:* anorexia, nausea, vomiting, constipation, abdominal pain, taste alterations
- *GU:* Decreased urine output, edema, weight gain

 ## INTERACTIONS

Glucagon

- None significant

Diazoxide (Proglycem)

- Concurrent use with alcohol, antihypertensives, diuretics, beta-blockers, calcium channel blockers, and peripheral vasodilators increases hypotensive effects.
- Concurrent use with phenytoin decreases effects of phenytoin.

CONTRAINDICATIONS

Glucagon (GlucaGen)

- Hypersensitivity including hypersensitivity to thiazides or other sulfonamide medications
- Pheochromocytoma

Diazoxide (Proglycem)

- Hypersensitivity
- Functional hypoglycemia

 # NURSING IMPLICATIONS

All Hyperglycemics

- Assess for signs of hypoglycemia.
- Monitor blood sugar throughout hypo-glycemic episode.
- Assess neurological status throughout therapy and institute safety precautions.

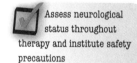

Monitor blood sugar throughout hypo-glycemic episode.

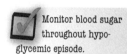

Assess neurological status throughout therapy and institute safety precautions

Glucagon (GlucaGen)

- Give SC, IV, and IM.
- Assess for nausea and vomiting after administration.
- Keep suction nearby and keep client in a side-lying position to prevent aspiration.
- A second dose of glucagon can be administered if client doesn't respond to first dose in 5 to 20 minutes. (If client is at home, health care provider should be notified and client should be admitted to the Emergency Department).
- IV glucose should be given if client doesn't respond to second dose of glucagon.
- Glucagon and glucose can be given at the same time.

Assess for nausea and vomiting after administration.

Keep suction nearby and keep client in a side-lying position to prevent aspiration.

Diazoxide (Proglycem)

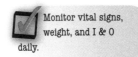
Monitor vital signs, weight, and I & O daily.

- Give PO.
- Monitor vital signs, weight, and I & O daily.
- Report signs of edema, decreased urinary output, and weight gain to health care provider.
- Diuretics may be indicated to treat fluid retention.
- Monitor for symptoms of hyperglycemia.

REFERENCE

1. McKenry LM, Tessier E, Hogan, M. *Mosby's Pharmacology in Nursing*, 22nd ed. St. Louis, MO: Mosby Elsevier; 2006:884.

PART VII • QUESTIONS

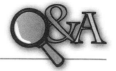

1. Which of the following is a therapeutic response to calcitonin?
   a. Decreased serum calcium
   b. Increased rate of bone turnover
   c. Control of bleeding
   d. Suppression of inflammation

2. Which of the following is an adverse effect of vasopressin (Pitressin)?
   a. Hypernatremia
   b. Hypotension
   c. Water intoxication
   d. Yellow vision

3. Which of the following should the nurse include in a teaching plan for a client taking somatrem (Protopin)?
   a. A cloudy or discolored solution is safe to use.
   b. Keep a journal of growth measurements.
   c. Mix drug with normal saline.
   d. Take oral somatrem with food to minimize GI effects.

4. An adult taking a thyroid agent should hold the drug if the apical pulse rate is over:
   a. 85 beats per minute.
   b. 90 beats per minute.
   c. 95 beats per minute.
   d. 100 beats per minute.

5. Which of the following are adverse effects of thyroid agents?
   a. Bradycardia
   b. Constipation
   c. Palpitations
   d. Urinary retention

6. Which of the following should the nurse include when teaching a client about thyroid agents?
   a. Take thyroid agent before going to bed.
   b. Thyroid agents can be taken at different times during the day.
   c. Check pulse before taking.
   d. Thyroid agents are used short term as they cure hypothyroidism.

7. Of the following, which drug should be taken with a straw to prevent tooth discoloration?
   a. Sodium Iodide (I^{131} Iodotrope)
   b. Methimazole (Tapazole)
   c. Propylthiouracil (PTU)
   d. Potassium Iodide (SSKI)

8. Which of the following drugs should be given in the morning to a client who is NPO overnight?
   a. Sodium Iodide (I^{131} Iodotrope)
   b. Methimazole (Tapazole)
   c. Propylthiouracil (PTU)
   d. Potassium Iodide (SSKI)

9. Which of the following is an adverse effect of Propylthiouracil (PTU)?
   a. Agranulocytosis
   b. Cyanosis
   c. Green halos in eyes
   d. Urinary retention

10. Of the following, which drug is used to treat Cushing's syndrome?
    a. Aminoglutethimide (Cytadren)
    b. Dexamethasone (Decadron, Cortastat, others)
    c. Fludrocortisone (Florinef)
    d. Hydrocortisone (Cortef, Hydrocrotone)

11. Which of the following are adverse effects of fludrocortisone (Florinef)?
    a. Hyperkalemia
    b. Increased muscle strength
    c. Urinary frequency
    d. Weight gain

12. What time of day should once-a-day dosing glucocorticosteroids be taken?
    a. Between 6:00 AM and 9:00 AM
    b. Noon
    c. Between 3:00 PM and 6:00 PM
    d. At bedtime

13. When mixing insulin, which insulin should be drawn up first?
    a. Regular
    b. NPH
    c. Humulin 70/30
    d. Glargine insulin (Lantus)

14. Of the following, which insulin can be given IV?
    a. Regular
    b. NPH
    c. Insulin detemir (Levemir)
    d. Glargine insulin (Lantus)

15. Liver function studies should be monitored with which of the following group of oral antidiabetics?
    a. Alpha-glucosidase inhibitors
    a. Biguanides
    a. Meglitinides
    a. Thiazolidinediones

16. Which of the following adverse effects should the nurse monitor for a client taking glucagon?
    a. Nausea and vomiting
    b. Development of cataracts
    c. Weight loss
    d. Urinary retention

PART VII • ANSWERS

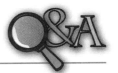

1. **The correct answer is a.** Calcitonin is used to treat hypercalcemia and decreases serum calcium. Calcitonin is also used to treat Paget's disease and decreases the rate of bone turnover. ADH hormones are used to control bleeding in hemophilia A or type 1 von Willebrand's disease, and ACTH or corticosteroids suppress inflammation.

2. **The correct answer is c.** Hypertension, water intoxication, and hypernatremia are adverse effects of vasopressin (Pitressin). An adverse effect of digoxin is yellow vision.

3. **The correct answer is b.** The client should keep a journal of growth measurements, as the effect of the drug is to promote growth. If the solution is cloudy or discolored, it should not be used. Somatrem (Protopin) should be mixed with sterile water and is not available for oral use.

4. **The correct answer is d.** An adult taking a thyroid agent should hold the drug if the pulse rate is over 100 beats per minute. Adverse effects of thyroid agents include tachycardia and palpitations. These symptoms should be reported to the health care provider.

5. **The correct answer is c.** Palpitations and tachycardia are adverse effects of thyroid agents. Adverse effects are often dose related and may cause symptoms of hyperthyroidism.

6. **The correct answer is c.** The pulse should be taken before taking, and if the pulse is greater than 100 beats per minute, hold and contact health care provider. Thyroid agents do not cure hypothyroidism and are used lifelong. Thyroid agents should be taken in the morning to prevent insomnia and should be taken exactly as prescribed at the same time each day.

7. **The correct answer is d.** Potassium Iodide (SSKI) is a liquid preparation and should be taken with a straw to prevent tooth discoloration.

8. **The correct answer is a.** Sodium Iodide (I^{131} Iodotrope) should be taken when the client has been NPO overnight. Food decreases the absorption of the sodium iodide.

9. **The correct answer is a.** Agranulocytosis may occur too rapidly to be tested by periodic blood testing. Symptoms of agranulocytosis may include fever, sore throat, and malaise.

10. **The correct answer is a.** Aminoglutethmide (Cytadren) is an adrenal steroid inhibitor used to treat Cushing's syndrome.

11. **The correct answer is d.** Fludrocortisone (Florinef) is a mineral-corticoid and may cause weight gain, edema, hypokalemia, hypertension, and muscle weakness. It doesn't cause urinary frequency.

12. **The correct answer is a.** Once-a-day dosing of glucocorticosteroids should be taken in the early morning, between 6:00 AM and 9:00 PM to minimize adrenal suppression.

13. **The correct answer is a.** Regular insulin is clear and should be drawn up first to prevent contamination of the regular insulin vial.

14. **The correct answer is a.** Regular insulin is clear and is the only insulin that is available IV.

15. **The correct answer is d.** Clients taking thiazolidinediones should have liver function studies monitored throughout therapy. The first drug in this group, troglitazone, was removed from the market as it caused severe liver toxicity. The other drugs have not been associated with severe liver toxicity, but clients should be monitored for liver toxicity.

16. **The correct answer is a.** Nausea and vomiting are adverse effects of glucagon, that may be related to hypoglycemia or overdose of glucagon.

VIII

Female Reproductive System Drugs

Marilyn J. Herbert-Ashton, MS, RN, BC

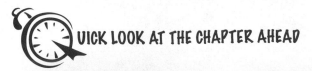

Estrogen is primarily secreted by the ovary and produced by the cells of the developing graafian follicle. Some estrogen is secreted by the adrenal glands, corpus luteum, placenta, and testes.[1] Estrogens are important in the development and maintenance of primary and secondary female sex characteristics. There are three endogenous or natural estrogens: **estradiol, estrone**, and **estriol.** They have the structure of a steroid and are synthesized by cholesterol in the ovarian follicles.[2] Natural estrogens are also called steroid hormones, and most are inactivated by the liver are not effective orally. Synthetic estrogens do not have the steroid structure and can be given orally.

54

Estrogens

TERMS

☐ estradiol (Estrace,
   Estraderm, Alora,
   Climara, Menostar,
   Esclim, Vivelle,
   Vivelle-Dot)

Table 54-1 Estrogens

Prototype Drug	Related Drugs	Drug Classification
estradiol (Estrace, Estraderm, Alora, Climara, Menostar, Esclim, Vivelle, Vivelle-Dot)	conjugated estrogens (Premarin) conjugated synthetic estrogens (Cenestin) esterified estrogens (Menest, Estratab) ethinyl Estradiol (Estinyl) estradiol valerate (Delestrogen)	Steroidal estrogens
There is no prototype for this classification	estropipate (Ogen, Ortho-Est)	(Stabilized estrone)
There is no prototype for this classification	chlorotrianisene (TACE) dienestrol (DV) diethylstilbestrol (DES, Stilphostrol)	Synthetic nonsteroidal estrogen
There is no prototype for this classification	conjugated estrogens/ medroxyprogesterone (Prempro, Premphase) estradiol/norethindrone (CombiPatch) estradiol/norgestimate (Prefest) ethinyl estradiol/ etonogestrel (NuvaRing) norethindrone acetate/ ethinyl estradiol (Femhrt)	Estrogen-progesten combinations

FEMALE REPRODUCTIVE SYSTEM DRUGS CLIENT TEACHING

All Estrogens

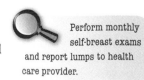

Perform monthly self-breast exams and report lumps to health care provider.

- Perform monthly self-breast exams and report lumps to health care provider.
- Continue regular follow-up care with health care provider.

- Use sunscreen and protective clothing to prevent changes in skin pigmentation.
- Advise other health care providers (eg, specialist, surgeon, dentist) about medication use before surgery or treatment.

Advise other health care providers (eg, specialist, surgeon, dentist) about medication use before surgery or treatment.

- If pregnancy is suspected, stop taking and notify health care provider.
- Report symptoms of headache, blurred vision (stroke), chest pain, pain, swelling, tenderness in extremities, shortness of breath (thromboembolism), weight gain, edema in ankles/feet (fluid retention), depression, severe abdominal pain, jaundice (hepatic dysfunction), and changes in vaginal bleeding.
- Bleeding occurs when estrogen is withheld.

Bleeding occurs when estrogen is withheld.

- Avoid smoking as smoking increases risk of serious side effects, especially in women over 35.
- Consult with health care provider before taking herbal preparations such as St. John's wort.
- Diabetics should report increased glucose levels to health care provider as dosage adjustments to oral hypoglycemic or insulin may be necessary.
- Maintain good oral hygiene and maintain preventive dental care to minimize gingival hyperplasia.
- Read package insert carefully for directions and contact health care provider with questions.

Oral Estrogen

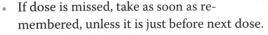

Take with food or immediately after eating to decrease nausea.

- Take with food or immediately after eating to decrease nausea.
- If dose is missed, take as soon as remembered, unless it is just before next dose.
- Do not take double doses.

Transdermal estrogen

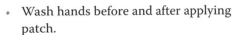

Wash hands before and after applying patch.

- Wash hands before and after applying patch.
- Apply to intact, hairless site on abdomen.

- Press disc to site for 10 seconds and check to make sure edges are secure.
- Avoid application to waistline or breasts as clothing can loosen the disc.
- Rotate sites and do not reuse site for 7 days.
- Disc may be reapplied if it falls off.

Vaginal

- Stay in a recumbent position for at least 30 minutes after inserting.

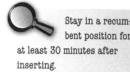
Stay in a recumbent position for at least 30 minutes after inserting.

- Do not use tampons, but sanitary napkins may be used to protect clothing.
- If dose is missed (do not use missed dose), wait until next regularly scheduled dose.
- Use provided applicator to insert vaginal cream or tablet.
- Wash applicator with mild soap and water after each use.

Vaginal Ring

- To insert, press ring into oval and insert into upper third of the vagina.
- No discomfort should be felt.
- If discomfort occurs, ring may not be inserted high enough and can be gently pushed into vagina.

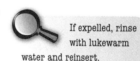
If expelled, rinse with lukewarm water and reinsert.

- Leave in place for 90 days.
- If expelled, rinse with lukewarm water and reinsert.
- Ring can be expelled by pulling out with a finger.
- Ring does not interfere with sexual intercourse.

ACTION

All Estrogens

- Stimulate synthesis of DNA and RNA and protein and promote growth and development of female sex organs and maintain secondary sex characteristics

USE

All Estrogens

- Atrophic vaginitis
- Vasomotor symptoms
- Dysmenorrhea
- Hypogonadism
- Palliative treatment of breast or prostate cancer
- Oral contraception
- Ovariectomy
- Primary ovarian failure
- Prevention of postpartum lactation
- Postmenopausal osteoporosis
- Uterine bleeding

Diethylstilbestrol (DES, Stilphostrol)

- Used primarily for palliative treatment of breast or prostate cancer

ADVERSE EFFECTS AND SIDE EFFECTS

- *Pregnancy category X*
- *CV:* Edema, thromobphlebitis, thromboembolic disorders, hypertension
- *CNS:* Headache, depression
- *GI:* Abdominal pain, nausea, vomiting, diarrhea, constipation, jaundice
- *GU:* Amenorrhea, breakthrough bleeding, dysmenorrhea, decreased libido, and impotence (men)
- *Other:* Breast tenderness, chloasma, fluid retention, weight gain, hyperglycemia, gynecomastia (in men, this disappears after therapy is discontinued), urticaria, and intolerance to contact lenses

INTERACTIONS

- Concurrent use of barbiturates or rifampin decreases effectiveness of estrogen.

- Concurrent use with oral anticoagulants or antihyperglycemics may decrease the effectiveness of oral anticoagulants or antihyperglycemics.
- Concurrent use with bromocriptine may interfere with the effects of bromocriptine.
- Concurrent use with St. John's wort may decrease estrogen levels.
- Tobacco increases the risk of cardiovascular adverse effects.
- Grapefruit juice increases the effects of estrogen.

CONTRAINDICATIONS

- Hypersensitivity
- Pregnancy
- Lactation
- History of thromboembolic disorders
- Undiagnosed vaginal bleeding
- Breast cancer
- Estrogen-dependent neoplasms (endometrial cancer)

NURSING IMPLICATIONS

- Give PO, IM, IV, transdermally, or intravaginally.
- Give IM injections slowly into a large muscle.
- Give IV estrogens slowly to minimize vaginal burning.
- Start transdermal application 1 week after last PO dose.
- Monitor blood pressure and report changes throughout therapy.
- Monitor I & O and weight, and report changes.
- Monitor hepatic function studies throughout therapy.
- Encourage client to undergo physical examination every 6 to 12 months to include mammogram, breast and pelvic exam, and pap smear.

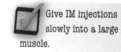

Give IM injections slowly into a large muscle.

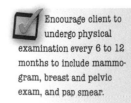

Encourage client to undergo physical examination every 6 to 12 months to include mammogram, breast and pelvic exam, and pap smear.

- Monitor and report adverse
  effects. (See "Client Teaching" on
  pages 459–460 for list of adverse
  effects.)

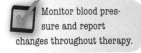

Monitor blood pressure and report changes throughout therapy.

REFERENCES

1. McKenry LM, Tessier E, Hogan M. *Mosby's Pharmacology in Nursing,* 22nd ed. St. Louis, MO: Mosby Elsevier; 2006:899.

2. Lilley L, Harrington S, Snyder J. *Pharmacology and the Nursing Process,* 5th ed. St. Louis, MO: Mosby Elsevier; 2007:507.

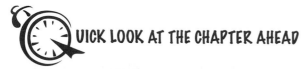

Progesterone is the hormone of pregnancy and is produced primarily by the corpus luteum and by the placenta during pregnancy. Progesterone is a natural progestational hormone. When progesterone is taken orally, it is quickly inactivated. Parenteral progesterone causes local reactions and pain. Consequently, synthetic derivatives, known as progestins, were developed. These are more effective when administered orally and are more potent and sustained.[1]

55
Progestins

TERM
☐ levonorgestrel (Norplant system, Prev, Plan B)

Table 55-1 Progestins

Prototype Drug	Related Drugs	Drug Classification
levonorgestrel (Norplant system, Prev, Plan B)	hydroxyprogesterone (Hylutin) levonorgestrel-releasing intrauterine system (Mirena) medroxyprogesterone (Provera, Depo-Provera) megestrol (Megace) norethindrone acetate (Aygestin, Micronor, Nor-QD) norgestrel (Ovrette) progesterone (Gesterol, Progestasert) progesterone, micronized (Prometrium)	Progestins

$\mathbf{R_x}$ PROGESTERONE PROGESTINS CLIENT TEACHING

- Perform monthly self-breast exams and report lumps to health care provider.
- Continue regular follow-up care with health care provider.
- Use sunscreen and protective clothing to prevent photosensitivity reactions.
- Advise other health care providers (eg, specialist, surgeon, dentist) about medication use before surgery or treatment.
- If pregnancy is suspected, stop taking and notify health care provider.
- Report symptoms of headache, blurred vision (stroke), chest pain, pain, swelling, tenderness in extremities, shortness of breath (thromboembolism), weight gain, edema in ankles/feet (fluid retention), depression, severe abdominal pain, jaundice, pruritus, dark urine or light-colored stools (hepatic dysfunction), changes in vaginal bleeding, or spotting.

 Perform monthly self-breast exams and report lumps to health care provider.

 Use sunscreen and protective clothing to prevent photosensitivity reactions.

 If pregnancy is suspected, stop taking and notify health care provider.

- Diabetics should report changes in glucose levels to health care provider as progestins may cause glucose intolerance, and adjustment to oral hypoglycemic or insulin may be necessary.
- If taking for contraceptive purposes, take at the same time daily, every day throughout the year.
- Keep oral medication in the original packaging.
- Read package insert carefully for directions and contact health care provider with questions.

Diabetics should report changes in glucose levels to health care provider as progestins may cause glucose intolerance, and adjustment to oral hypoglycemic or insulin may be necessary.

ACTION

All Progesterone/Progestins

- Progesterone and progestins produce secretion changes in the endometrium for preparation of implantation and nourishment of the embryo.
- Other functions include suppressing of ovulation during pregnancy, supplementing the action of estrogen in its effects on the uterus and mammary glands, increasing basal body temperature, causing relaxation of smooth uterine muscle, and inhibiting in large doses the secretion of the lutenizing hormone from the anterior pituitary gland.[2]

USE

All Progesterone/Progestins

- Amenorrhea
- Dysmenorrhea
- Dysfunctional uterine bleeding caused by hormonal imbalance
- Endometriosis
- Infertility
- Threatened abortion
- Contraception

- Premenstrual syndrome
- Adjunct or palliative treatment for some carcinomas

ADVERSE EFFECTS AND SIDE EFFECTS

All Progesterone/Progestins

- *Pregnancy category X, although progesterone (Micronized) and (Gesterol, Progestasert) and hydroxyprogesterone (Hylutin) are pregnancy category D.*
- *CV:* Edema, thrombophlebitis, thromboembolic disorders, hypertension
- *CNS:* Anxiety, headache, depression, and insomnia
- *GI:* Abdominal pain, nausea, vomiting, diarrhea, constipation, and hepatitis
- *GU:* Amenorrhea, breakthrough bleeding, changes in menstrual flow
- *Other:* Breast tenderness, chloasma, fluid retention, weight gain, glucose intolerance, and rashes

INTERACTIONS

All Progesterone/Progestins

- Concurrent use of aminoglutethimide (Cytadren), rifampin, phenytoin, and carbamazepine increases metabolism of medroxyprogesterone or norethindrone.
- Concurrent use with bromocriptine may decrease effectiveness of bromocriptine.

CONTRAINDICATIONS

- Hypersensitivity
- Pregnancy (Congenital anomalies reported in the first 4 months of pregnancy)
- Lactation (progestins are secreted in breast milk)
- History of thromboembolic disorders

- History of thrombophlebitis
- Undiagnosed vaginal bleeding
- Pre-existing breast or endometrial cancer
- Cardiac disease
- Cerebrovascular disease
- Liver disease

 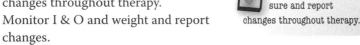

NURSING IMPLICATIONS

All Progesterones/Progestins

- Monitor blood pressure and report changes throughout therapy.
- Monitor I & O and weight and report changes.
- Monitor hepatic function studies, baseline and periodically throughout therapy.
- Monitor and report adverse effects. (See "Client Teaching" for list of adverse effects.)

> ✓ Monitor blood pressure and report changes throughout therapy.

Progesterone (Gesterol)

- Used to treat amenorrhea. Give PO, IM (give deep IM), or vaginally.
- Vaginal gel should not be used concurrently with other vaginal agents.
- If concurrent vaginal use is indicated, wait at least 6 hours before or after vaginal gel to administer.
- Discontinue if menses occurs while receiving the injection series.

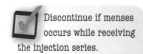

> ✓ Discontinue if menses occurs while receiving the injection series.

Progesterone (Progestasert) and Levonorgestrel-Releasing Intrauterine System (Mirena)

- Used as a contraceptive, available as an intrauterine device
- Usually indicated for women who have at least 1 child, are involved in a monogamous relationship, and who do not have a history of pelvic inflammatory disease[3]

- Progesterone should be replaced after 1 year; copper T380A (Paragard) and levonorgestrel-releasing intrauterine system (Mirena) are replaced after 5 years.

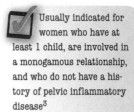
Usually indicated for women who have at least 1 child, are involved in a monogamous relationship, and who do not have a history of pelvic inflammatory disease[3]

Megestrol (Megace)

- Used in treatment of breast cancer or endometrial cancer, and in management of anorexia and weight loss in clients with Acquired Immune Deficiency Syndrome
- Give PO.
- Evaluate effectiveness after 2 months of therapy.

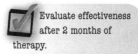
Used in treatment of breast cancer or endometrial cancer, and in management of anorexia and weight loss in clients with Acquired Immune Deficiency Syndrome (AIDS)

Hydroxyprogesterone (Hylutin)

- Used to treat amenorrhea and uterine bleeding
- Available IM (give deep IM)

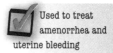
Evaluate effectiveness after 2 months of therapy.

Levonorgestrel (Norplant System)

- Used as a contraceptive implant
- Subdermal implant: 6 capsules implanted subdermally during first 7 days of menses or immediately after abortion, and replaced every 5 years[4]
- Capsules implanted in the midportion of the upper arm
- Monitor insertion site for symptoms of infection.
- Due to manufacturing problems, the Norplant system is no longer available.

Used to treat amenorrhea and uterine bleeding

Monitor insertion site for symptoms of infection.

Levonorgestrel (Prev, Plan B)

- Give PO for emergency contraception.

Medroxyprogesterone (Provera, Depo-Provera)

- Give PO or IM. (Give deep IM.)

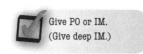
Give PO or IM. (Give deep IM.)

- Used to treat amenorrhea, uterine bleeding, and endometrial or renal cancer; prevent endometrial cancer caused by estrogen replacement; and as a contraceptive

Norethindrone (Norlutin)

- Give PO.
- Used to treat amenorrhea, uterine bleeding, and as a contraceptive

Norgestrel (Ovrette)

- Give PO.
- Used as a contraceptive

Norethindrone (Aygestin, Micronor, Nor-QD)

- Give PO.
- Used to treat amenorrhea or used in combination oral contraceptives

Progesterone micronized (Prometrium)

- Give PO, IM, intrauterine system, or gel. Intrauterine device can remain in place for 1 year for contraception. Gel is used to treat infertility.

REFERENCES

1. Lilley L, Harrington S, Snyder J. *Pharmacology and the Nursing Process,* 5th ed. St. Louis, MO: Mosby; 2007:509.

2. McKenry LM, Tessier E, Hogan M. *Mosby's Pharmacology in Nursing,* 22nd ed. St. Louis, MO: Mosby Elsevier; 2006:905.

3. McKenry LM, Tessier E, Hogan M. *Mosby's Pharmacology in Nursing,* 22nd ed. St. Louis, MO: Mosby Elsevier; 2006:911.

4. Skidmore-Roth L. *Mosby's Nursing Drug Reference.* St. Louis, MO: Mosby Elsevier. 2007:602.

Oral contraceptives that contain both estrogen and progestin are known as combination oral contraceptives; those that contain progestin only are also called progestin-only oral contraception, also known as the "mini-pill." The combination oral contraceptives are more widely used than progestin only.

The combination oral contraceptives have three subgroups: **monophasic, biphasic,** and **triphasic.** The monophasic form contains the same daily amount of estrogen and progestin. The biphasic form contains the same daily amount of estrogen, but the progestin dose is increased in the second half of the cycle. The triphasic form contains estrogen and progestin dosage changes for each phase of the cycle in two regimens.

56

Oral Contraceptives

TERMS
☐ biphasic
☐ monophasic
☐ triphasic

Table 56-1 Oral Contraceptives

Prototype Drug	Related Drugs	Drug Classification
There is no prototype for this classification	Alesse-28 Demulen 1/35 LoOvral Necon 1/35 Ortho-Cyclen Yasmin	Oral contraceptives (OCs) (Monophasic)
There is no prototype for this classification	Mircette Nelova 10/11 Necon 10/11 Ortho-Novum 10/11	(Biphasic)
There is no prototype for this classification	Ortho-Tricyclen 21 & 28 Triphasil 21 & 28 Trivora-28	(Triphasic)

ORAL CONTRACEPTIVES CLIENT TEACHING

* Take exactly as prescribed at the same time each day and in proper sequence.
* Keep an extra month's supply available.
* When beginning to use oral contraceptives, use an additional form of birth control for the first cycle.
* If one dose is missed, take as soon as remembered.
* If 2 consecutive days are missed, take 2 tablets a day for the next 2 days. Continue with regular dosing schedule, and use an additional method of contraception for the rest of the cycle.
* If 3 consecutive days are missed, discontinue and use another form of contraception until menses begins or pregnancy is ruled out.
* If nausea occurs, drug may be taken with food.

Take exactly as prescribed at the same time each day and in proper sequence.

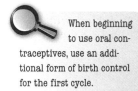

When beginning to use oral contraceptives, use an additional form of birth control for the first cycle.

If one dose is missed, take as soon as remembered.

- Perform monthly self-breast exams, and report lumps to health care provider.
- Continue regular follow-up gynecological exams with health care provider, including pap smears.
- Use sunscreen and protective clothing to prevent changes in skin pigmentation.

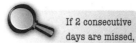

If 2 consecutive days are missed, take 2 tablets a day for the next 2 days. Continue with regular dosing schedule, and use an additional method of contraception for the rest of the cycle.

- Advise other health care providers (eg, specialist, surgeon, dentist) about medication use before surgery or treatment.
- Report symptoms of headache, blurred vision (stroke), chest pain, swelling, tenderness in extremities, shortness of breath (thromboembolism), weight gain, edema in ankles/feet (fluid retention), depression, severe abdominal pain, jaundice (hepatic dysfunction), or changes in vaginal bleeding.
- Bleeding occurs when oral contraceptives are suddenly stopped.
- Avoid smoking, as smoking increases risk of serious side effects, especially in women over 35.
- Consult with health care provider before taking herbal preparations such as St. John's wort.
- If pregnancy is suspected, stop taking, and contact health care provider.

℞ ACTION

- Inhibit ovulation by increasing serum estrogen and progestins, which inhibit the secretion of the follicle stimulating hormone and lutenizing hormone from the pituitary gland[1]
- There are also endometrial changes that impair implantation of the ova. An increase in cervical mucus prevents the passage of sperm.

℞ USE

- Oral contraception
- Treatment of hypermenorrhea

- Postcoital emergency contraception, taken with 72 hours of un-protected intercourse, or known or suspected contraceptive failure, with follow-up dose 12 hours after first dose

ADVERSE EFFECTS AND SIDE EFFECTS

All Oral Contraceptives

- *Pregnancy category X*
- *CV:* Edema, thrombophlebitis, thromboembolic disorders, hypertension
- *CNS:* Headache, depression, stroke
- *GI:* Abdominal pain, nausea, vomiting, diarrhea, constipation, jaundice, weight gain, cramps
- *GU:* Amenorrhea, breakthrough bleeding, dysmenorrhea
- *Other:* Breast tenderness, melasma, fluid retention, hyperglycemia, rash, and intolerance to contact lenses

INTERACTIONS

- Concurrent use of antibiotics, barbiturates, mineral oil, griseofulvin, rifampin, and St. John's wort decreases effectiveness of oral contraceptives.
- Concurrent use with oral anticoagulants, anticonvulsants, beta-blockers, caffeine, corticosteroids, theophylline, tricyclic antidepressants, or antihyperglycemics may decrease the effectiveness of these drugs.
- Concurrent use with bromocriptine may interfere with the effects of bromocriptine.
- Tobacco increases the risk of cardiovascular adverse effects.

CONTRAINDICATIONS

- Pregnancy
- Lactation

- History of thromboembolic disorders
- Coronary disease
- Cerebrovascular disease
- Liver tumors
- Undiagnosed vaginal bleeding
- Breast cancer
- Estrogen-dependent neoplasms (endometrial cancer)

NURSING IMPLICATIONS

- Give PO.
- Monitor blood pressure, and report changes throughout therapy.
- Monitor hepatic function studies, baseline and periodically throughout therapy.
- Monitor and report adverse effects. (See client teaching on page 474 for list of adverse effects.)

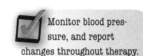

Monitor blood pressure, and report changes throughout therapy.

REFERENCE

1. McKenry LM, Tessier E, Hogan M. *Mosby's Pharmacology in Nursing*, 22nd ed. St. Louis, MO: Mosby Elsevier; 2006:908–909.

Selective estrogen receptor modulators (SERMs) work on estrogen receptors and are indicated for the prevention of postmenopausal osteoporosis. Raloxifene (Evista) is indicated for the treatment and prevention of osteoporosis. Tamoxifen (Nova-dex) is an antineoplastic, used as an adjunct in the treatment of breast cancer, after surgery or radiation, and in the prevention of breast cancer in high-risk clients.

Bisphosphonates are also known as bone resorption inhibitors and are used to treat or prevent osteoporosis. Alendronate (Fosamax) is the first bisphosphonate in its class.

57

Selective Estrogen Receptor Modulators and Bisphosphonates

TERMS
☐ alendronate (Fosamax)
☐ raloxifene (Evista)

Table 57-1 Tetracyclines

Prototype Drug	Related Drugs	Drug Classification
raloxifene (Evista)	fulvestrant (Faslodex) tamoxifen (Novadex) toremifene (Fareston)	Selective estrogen receptor modulators SERMs) (bone resorption inhibitors) (antineoplastic)
alendronate (Fosamax)	ibandronate sodium (Boniva) etidronate disodium (Didronel) pamidronate disodium (Aredia) risedronate sodium (Actonel) tiludronate (Skelid) zoledronic acid (Zometa)	Bisphosphonates (bone resorption inhibitors) (hypocalcemics)

SELECTIVE ESTROGEN RECEPTOR MODULATORS AND BISPHOSPHONATES CLIENT TEACHING

Selective Estrogen Receptor Modulators (SERMs)

- Periodic laboratory testing CBC with a differential and platelets is indicated.
- For oral SERMs, antacids may help reduce GI distress.
- Teach client to assess for symptoms of thrombophlebitis and to immediately report symptoms to health care provider.
- Make client aware that she may experience hot flashes or flushing.
- Take exactly as prescribed.
- Advise other health care providers (eg, specialist, surgeon, dentist) about medication use before surgery or treatment.

Periodic laboratory testing CBC with a differential and platelets is indicated.

For oral SERMs, antacids may help reduce GI distress.

Teach client to assess for symptoms of thrombophlebitis and to immediately report symptoms to health care provider.

Raloxifene (Evista)

- Can be taken without regard to meals
- Notify health care provider if pregnancy is suspected as raloxifene may have teratogenic effects.

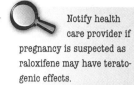

Notify health care provider if pregnancy is suspected as raloxifene may have teratogenic effects.

- Encourage regular weight bearing exercise such as walking.
- Teach client which foods are high in calcium and vitamin D.
- Consult with health care provider about calcium and vitamin D supplements.
- Encourage client to stop smoking and limit alcohol intake.

Tamoxifen (Novadex)

- Take with food if GI distress occurs.
- Omit dose if missed.
- Do not take an antacid within 1 to 2 hours after taking an enteric-coated tablet.
- Monitor weight weekly and report weight gain or edema to health care provider.
- Report bone pain to health care provider as analgesics may be ordered to control pain.
- Bone pain usually is relieved over time and is an indication of the drug's effectiveness.

Bone pain usually is relieved over time and is an indication of the drug's effectiveness.

- Use nonhormonal contraception during therapy and for at least 1 month after surgery as the drug may have teratogenic effects and may also stimulate ovulation.

Toremifene (Fareston)

- If you are childbearing age, use barrier contraceptives.
- Do not take if pregnant.
- Take without regard to food.

Take without regard to food.

Bisphosphonates

- Continue regular follow-up care with health care provider, which may also include laboratory testing.

Continue regular follow-up care with health care provider, which may also include laboratory testing.

- Advise other health care providers (eg, specialist, surgeon, dentist) about medication use before surgery or treatment.
- Take with 6 to 8 ounces of water.
- Do not double doses; if missed, omit and resume the next day.

Take with 6 to 8 ounces of water.

- Encourage regular weight bearing exercise such as walking.
- Teach client which foods are high in calcium and vitamin D.
- Consult with health care provider about calcium and vitamin D supplements.
- Do not stop taking without consulting with health care provider.
- Encourage client to stop smoking and limit alcohol intake.
- Notify health care provider if pregnancy is suspected.

Aldendronate (Fosamax) and Ibandronate (Boniva)

- Take first thing in the morning after rising, with 6 to 8 ounces of water on an empty stomach, and do not eat or lie down for 30 minutes after taking.

Take first thing in the morning after rising, with 6 to 8 ounces of water on an empty stomach, and do not eat or lie down for 30 minutes after taking.

Other Bisphosphonates

- Take with 6 to 8 ounces of water 2 hours before or after food—
especially foods high in calcium such as milk or milk products, antacids, or medications high in iron or other mineral supplements.

 ## ACTION

SERMs

- Stimulate estrogen receptors on bone and block estrogen receptors on the breast
- Additionally, raloxifene (Evista) also blocks estrogen receptors of the uterus.[1]

Bisphosphonates

- Inhibit the normal and abnormal resorption of bone, by inhibiting osteoclast activity

USE

SERMs

Raloxifene (Evista)

- Treatment and prevention of postmenopausal osteoporosis

Toremifene (Fareston) and Fulvestrant (Faslodex)

- Are also used as an antineoplastic to treat advanced breast cancer in postmenopausal women, who are estrogen receptor-positive.

Tamoxifen (Novadex)

- Treatment and prevention of breast cancer

Bisphosphonates

- Prevention and treatment of osteoporosis in men and post-menopausal women
- Paget's disease

Etidronate disodium (Didronel)

- Is used to treat Paget's disease and hypercalcemia associated with malignancies

Zoledronic acid (Zometa)

- Is used to treat hypercalcemia associated with malignancies.

ADVERSE EFFECTS AND SIDE EFFECTS

SERMs

- *Raloxifene (Evista) is pregnancy category X; tamoxifen (Novadex), toremifene (Fareston), and fulvestrant (Faslodex) are pregnancy category D.*
- Dizziness
- Hot flashes, skin rash
- Leg cramps

- Increased risk of thromboembolism
- Teratogenic effects
- Nausea, vomiting

Bisphosphonates

- *Pregnancy category C, although oral etidronate disodium (Didronel) is pregnancy category B and intravenous etidronate is pregnancy category C; zoledronic acid (Zometa) is pregnancy category D.*
- *CNS:* Headache
- *GI:* Nausea, vomiting, diarrhea, constipation, abdominal distention, dyspepsia, flatulence, esophageal ulcer, acid, regurgitation, and metallic taste
- *Derm:* Rash
- *Musculoskeletal:* Musculoskeletal pain

INTERACTIONS

SERMs

- Concurrent use with warfarin may alter effects of warfarin.

Raloxifene (Evista)

- Cholestyramine decreases the absorption of raloxifene.

Tamoxifen (Novadex)

- Increased risk of thromboembolic effects when administered with other antineoplastics

Fulvestrant (Faslodex)

- No known interactions

Toremifene (Fareston)

- Increased risk of bleeding if taken with oral anticoagulants

Bisphosphonates

- Food, calcium, antacids, caffeine, orange juice, mineral supplements, mineral water, iron, and other oral medications decrease absorption of biphosphonates (biphosphonates should be taken with plain water).

- Food that decreases absorption of biphosphonates includes caffeine, orange juice, and mineral water.

CONTRAINDICATIONS

SERMs

- Hypersensitivity
- Childbearing potential
- Pregnancy
- Lactation
- History of thromboembolic disease

Bisphosphonates

- Hypersensitivity
- Renal insufficiency
- Pregnancy
- Lactation

Etidronate disodium (Didronel)

- Hypercalcemia due to hyperparathyroidism

NURSING IMPLICATIONS

SERMs

Raloxifene (Evista)

- Give PO.
- Assess bone mineral density results, baseline and periodically throughout therapy.
- May cause a decrease in platelets and decrease in calcium and phosphate levels

> May cause a decrease in platelets and decrease in calcium and phosphate levels

- May cause decreased low-density lipoprotein and total cholesterol levels
- May need calcium supplements if calcium intake is inadequate

Tamoxifen (Novadex)

- Give PO.
- Assess for bone pain and consult with health care provider for analgesia.
- Bone pain usually resolves even with continued therapy.
- Monitor CBC, calcium, and platelets before and during therapy.
- Monitor liver function studies and T_4 periodically throughout therapy.
- If vomiting occurs after taking, check with health care provider to determine whether or not to repeat dose. (Nausea is a common adverse effect of tamoxifen.)

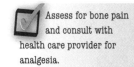
Assess for bone pain and consult with health care provider for analgesia.

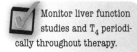
Monitor liver function studies and T_4 periodically throughout therapy.

Fulvestrant (Faslodex)

- Give IM.
- Give deep IM monthly.

Toremifene (Fareston)

- Give PO.
- Monitor CBC and platelets.
- Monitor for bleeding and allergic reactions.
- Give with an antacid, after evening meal, before bedtime.

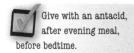
Give with an antacid, after evening meal, before bedtime.

Bisphosphonates

- Give PO.
- Etidronate disodium (Didronel) andibandronate sodium (Boniva) are also available IV.
- Assess and monitor serum calcium before and periodically throughout therapy.

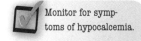
Monitor for symptoms of hypocalcemia.

- Monitor for symptoms of hypocalcemia.
- Paget's disease: monitor serum alkaline phosphatase before and periodically throughout therapy.
- Assess and monitor for bone pain and weakness before and throughout therapy.
- Consult with health care provider about use of analgesics.

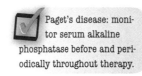

Paget's disease: monitor serum alkaline phosphatase before and periodically throughout therapy.

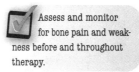

Assess and monitor for bone pain and weakness before and throughout therapy.

REFERENCE

1. Lilley L., Harrington S, Snyder J. *Pharmacology and the Nursing Process,* 5th ed. St. Louis, MO: Mosby; 2007:513.

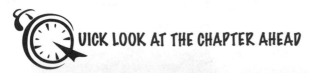

Oxytocics, ergot alkaloids, and prostaglandins stimulate uterine contractions. The uterus is a very vascular and muscular organ with smooth muscle fibers extending vertically, horizontally, and obliquely.[1] Oxytocin is a hormone secreted by the posterior pituitary gland, causing uterine contractions and labor, and facilitates milk ejection during lactation. Pitocin is a synthetic form of oxytocin. The ergot alkaloids increase the frequency and force of uterine contractions and have potent oxytocic effects. The prostaglandins are natural hormones involved in regulating the myometrium and may be responsible for the natural induction of labor and stimulation of Braxton Hicks contractions, seen in the final week of labor.[2]

58

Uterine Stimulants

TERMS
- ☐ dinoprostone (Prepidil Gel, Prostin E$_2$)
- ☐ oxytocin (Pitocin, Syntocinon)
- ☐ methylerogonovine (Methergine)

Table 58-1 Uterine Stimulants

Prototype Drug	Related Drugs	Drug Classification
oxytocin (Pitocin, Syntocinon)	There are no related drugs at this time	Oxytocics
methylergonovine (Methergine)	ergonovine maleate (Ergotrate)	Ergot alkaloids
dinoprostone (Prepidil Gel, Prostin E₂)	carboprost tromethamine (Hemabate) mifepristone (RU-486)	Prostaglandins, abortifacient oxytocic

UTERINE STIMULANTS CLIENT TEACHING

Oxytocics

- Instruct clients when administering nasal spray to clear nasal passages, sit upright, hold the container upright, insert into nostril, and squeeze solution into nostril on inspiration.
- Nasal spray should be used before breast-feeding or pumping breasts.
- Contractions will occur after administration of oxytocin.

Instruct clients when administering nasal spray to clear nasal passages, sit upright, hold the container upright, insert into nostril, and squeeze solution into nostril on inspiration.

Nasal spray should be used before breast-feeding or pumping breasts.

Ergot Alkaloids

- Avoid smoking as nicotine increases the effects of ergot derivatives (vasoconstriction).
- Ergot alkaloids may cause discomfort from uterine contractions.
- Do not double up on missed dose. Omit and resume normal dosage schedule.

Avoid smoking as nicotine increases the effects of ergot derivatives (vasoconstriction).

Prostaglandins

- Notify health care provider if experiencing fever, chills, foul-smelling vaginal discharge, increased bleeding, or lower abdominal pain.

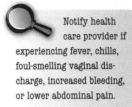

Notify health care provider if experiencing fever, chills, foul-smelling vaginal discharge, increased bleeding, or lower abdominal pain.

 ACTION

All Uterine Stimulants

- Stimulate uterine smooth muscle contractions, producing uterine contractions

Oxytocics

Oxytocin (Pitocin, Syntocinon)

- Synthetic oxytocin also stimulates the smooth muscle of the mammary gland, facilitating lactation.
- Also has antidiuretic and vasopressor effects

Ergot Alkaloids

- Directly stimulate uterine and vascular smooth muscle, which also causes vasoconstriction

Prostaglandins

- Also stimulate GI smooth muscle
- Uterus, in early pregnancy, is more responsive to prostaglandins' ability to stimulate contractions, which is why they are used to induce abortion.
- Cervical dilation and softening

USE

Oxytocics

Oxytocin (Pitocin, Syntocinon)

- Induction of labor
- Control postpartum or postabortion hemorrhage
- Intranasal: stimulation of lactation

Ergot Alkaloids

- Prevention and treatment of postpartum or postabortion hemorrhage caused by uterine atony or subinvolution

Prostaglandins

- Intravaginally to induce abortion from 12 to 20 weeks gestation (Carboprost tromethamine [Hemabate] given from 13 to 20 weeks)
- Management of nonmetastatic gestational trophoblastic disease (benign hydatidiform mole)
- Cervical gel: Ripens cervix near term when induction of labor is indicated
- Treatment of incomplete abortion, fetal death within the uterus

 ## ADVERSE EFFECTS AND SIDE EFFECTS

Oxytocics

- *Oxytocin (Pitocin, Syntocinon) is pregnancy category X when given intranasally; however, it is pregnancy UK if given IM or IV.*
- *CV:* Tachycardia, hypertension or hypotension (maternal), dysrhythmias
- *CNS:* Maternal: seizures; fetal: intracranial hemorrhage
- *F & E:* Hyponatremia, prolonged use can cause water intoxication (antidiuretic effects).
- *GI:* Nausea and vomiting
- *Other:* Hypersensitivity

Ergot Alkaloids

- *Ergonovine maleate (Ergotrate) is pregnancy category X; methyl-ergonovine (Methergine) is pregnancy category C.*
- *CV:* Hypertension or hypotension, dysrhythmias, palpitations, chest pain
- *CNS:* Dizziness, headache
- *EENT:* Tinnitus
- *GI:* Nausea and vomiting
- *GU:* Cramps
- *Resp:* Dyspnea
- *Other:* Diaphoresis, pruritus

Prostaglandins

- *Pregnancy category C, mifepristone (RU-486) pregnancy category X*
- *CV:* Hypertension or hypotension
- *CNS:* Headache, drowsiness
- *GI:* Nausea, vomiting, and diarrhea
- *GU:* Uterine rupture, uterine/vaginal pain
- *Resp:* Dyspnea
- *Other:* Allergic reactions including anaphylaxis, fever, chills, blurred vision

 ## INTERACTIONS

All Uterine Stimulants

- Concurrent use with sympathomimetic (vasopressors) can cause severe hypertension.

 ## CONTRAINDICATIONS

All Uterine Stimulants

- Hypersensitivity

Ergot Alkaloids

* Due to their potent effects these drugs should not be used to induce labor or with spontaneous threatened abortion.
* Should not be given before delivery of the placenta; could cause placental entrapment

Prostaglandins

* Pelvic inflammatory disease
* Cervical stenosis
* Uterine fibrosis

NURSING IMPLICATIONS

Oxytocics

Oxytocin (Pitocin, Syntocinon)

* Give IM, IV, or intranasally.
* Intranasal use for promotion of milk letdown
* Assess character, frequency, and duration of contractions frequently throughout administration.
* Monitor maternal vital signs frequently throughout administration.
* Use fetal monitoring and assess fetal heart rate continuously throughout administration.
* Monitor maternal electrolytes.
* Monitor I & O.
* Monitor for symptoms of water intoxication such as headache, anuria, drowsiness, and confusion. Notify health care provider if symptoms occur.
* Have magnesium sulfate available if needed to treat severe contractions.

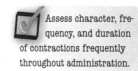

Assess character, frequency, and duration of contractions frequently throughout administration.

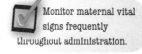

Monitor maternal vital signs frequently throughout administration.

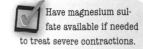

Have magnesium sulfate available if needed to treat severe contractions.

- Notify health care provider if symptoms of fetal distress occur or if contractions increase in frequency or duration.
- Use an infusion pump when administering IV and should be connected via a Y-site so that oxytocin can be disconnected while maintaining vein access.
- Clients receiving parenteral oxytocin should be under medical supervision and in a hospital setting.

Ergot Alkaloids

- Give PO, IM, or IV.
- PO and IM routes are preferred.
- IV use is for emergency use only.
- Monitor vital signs, fundus (location and tone), and vaginal drainage frequently throughout administration.
- Notify health care provider if uterine relaxation is prolonged or if there are changes in vaginal bleeding.
- Check calcium levels if client doesn't respond to drug; effectiveness is decreased with hypocalceimia.
- Assess for ergotism: headache, nausea, vomiting, paresthesias, chest pain, peripheral ischemia, and report symptoms to health care provider.

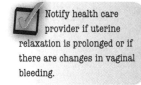

Notify health care provider if uterine relaxation is prolonged or if there are changes in vaginal bleeding.

Prostaglandins

Carboprost thromethamine (Hemabate)

- Give deep IM.

Dinoprostone (Prepidil Gel, Prostin E$_2$)

- Available as a vaginal suppository or cervical gel
- Monitor vital signs throughout treatment.
- Osculate lungs and assess for wheezing or chest tightness and report to health care provider as these could be signs of anaphylaxis.
- Monitor for nausea, vomiting, and diarrhea. Premedicate with an antiemetic and antidiarrheal.
- Fever may occur in 15 to 45 minutes after insertion of vaginal suppository but temperature returns to normal 2 to 6 hours after discontinuation of therapy.[1]

- Monitor for hemorrhage and assess vaginal discharge.
- Report signs of hemorrhage to health care provider.

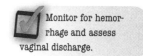

Monitor for hemorrhage and assess vaginal discharge.

Abortifacients

- Provide emotional support before and after abortion.
- Wear gloves when touching vaginal suppository to prevent skin absorption.[3]
- Have client lay supine for 10 minutes after insertion of suppository.[1]
- Insert at room temperature.[1]

Wear gloves when touching vaginal suppository to prevent skin absorption.[3]

Vaginal Insert

- Use water-soluble lubricant sparingly as too much can impede the release of the drug.[1]
- Make sure insert has a retrieval system.[1]
- Have client lay supine for 2 hours after insertion, then may ambulate.[1]
- Drug can be delivered up to 12 hours. Remove after 12 hours or at onset of active labor.[1]

Make sure insert has a retrieval system.[1]

Cervical Gel

- Avoid contact with skin, wash hands thoroughly after insertion.[3]
- Administer at room temperature.[1]
- Use a speculum to visualize the cervix with the client in a dorsal position.[1]
- Keep client in a supine position for 15 to 30 minutes after insertion of drug.[1]

Cervical Ripening

- Fetal monitoring is indicated; monitor uterine activity and dilation and effacement of cervix throughout treatment.[1]

Mifepristone (RU-486)

- Give PO.
- Menses begins within 5 days of treatment lasting 1–2 weeks.

REFERENCES

1. McKenry LM, Tessier E, Hogan M. *Mosby's Pharmacology in Nursing*, 22nd ed. St. Louis, MO: Mosby; 2006:921.

2. Lilley L, Harrington S, Snyder J. *Pharmacology and the Nursing Process*, 5th ed. St. Louis, MO: Mosby; 2007:516.

3. McKenry LM, Tessier E, Hogan M. *Mosby's Pharmacology in Nursing*, 22nd ed. St. Louis, MO: Mosby; 2006:922.

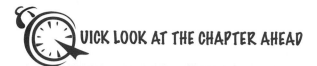

Uterine relaxants, also called tocolytics, are used to treat preterm labor. Preterm labor occurs before the thirty-seventh week of pregnancy. Uterine relaxants are generally used between the twentieth and thirty-seventh week of pregnancy. They work by relaxing the smooth muscles of the uterus and preventing contractions and labor induction. This action increases the chances of fetal survival.[1] Other treatment of preterm labor includes bedrest, hydration, and sedation. Although Terbutaline (Brethine) is prescribed to treat preterm labor, its use is considered off-label as the United States drug labeling does not recognize it for this use.[1] Magnesium sulfate can be used to treat preterm labor but is used primarily as an anticonvulsant in pregnancy-induced hypertension. Note, nifedipine, a calcium channel blocker, and the nonsteroidal anti-inflammatory drug indomethacin may be used to treat preterm labor.

59

Uterine Relaxants (Tocolytics)

TERM
☐ ritodrine (Yutopar)

495

Table 59-1 Uterine Relaxants (Tocolytics)

Prototype Drug	Related Drugs	Drug Classification
ritodrine (Yutopar)	terbutaline (Brethine)	Beta$_2$-adrenergic agonists
There is no prototype for this classiication	magnesium sulfate	Mineral and electrolyte replacements/ supplements (magnesium salts)

 ## UTERINE RELAXANTS (TOCOLYTICS) CLIENT TEACHING

- Instruct client on the importance of following treatment including bed rest.
- Contact health care provider if membranes rupture or if contractions resume or if there is loss of fetal activity.

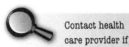 Contact health care provider if membranes rupture or if contractions resume or if there is loss of fetal activity.

 ## ACTION

All Uterine Stimulants

- All uterine stimulants relax the smooth muscle of the uterus, preventing the uterus from contracting.

 ## USE

All Uterine Stimulants

- Inhibit contractions in preterm labor, usually after the 20th week of gestation

Terbutaline (Brethine)

- Also used as a bronchodilator to treat asthma

Magnesium Salts

Magnesium Sulfate
- Also used as an anticonvulsant in severe preeclampsia (pregnancy-induced hypertension [PIH])
- Other uses: Treatment of torsades de pointes and treatment/ prevention of hypomagnesemia

ADVERSE EFFECTS AND SIDE EFFECTS

Beta$_2$-Adrenergic Agonists

- *Pregnancy category B*
- *CV:* Palpitations, tachycardia, hypertension, altered maternal and fetal heart rate/blood pressure, and chest pain
- *CNS:* Anxiety, dizziness, headache, tremors, and restlessness
- *GI:* Anorexia, nausea, vomiting, diarrhea, and constipation
- *Resp:* Hyperventilation, dyspnea
- *Other:* Hyperglycemia, hypokalemia, glycosuria, and rash[2]

Magnesium Salts

Magnesium Sulfate

- *Pregnancy category D*
- *CV:* Dysrhythmias, hypotension, bradycardia
- *CNS:* Drowsiness
- *GI:* Diarrhea
- *Resp:* Decreased respiratory rate
- *Other:* Hypothermia, flushing, sweating

INTERACTIONS

Beta$_2$-Adrenergic Agonists

- Concurrent use with other adrenergics has additive adrenergic effects.

- Concurrent use with beta-blockers antagonizes beta$_2$-adrenergic effects.
- Concurrent use with ephedra increases stimulant effects.

Magnesium Salts

Magnesium Sulfate

- Potentiates neuromuscular blocking agents

 ## CONTRAINDICATIONS

Beta$_2$-Adrenergic Agonists

- Hypersensitivity
- Hyperthyroidism
- Cardiovascular disorders
- Dysrhythmias
- Eclampsia, severe eclampsia
- Pulmonary hypertension
- Magnesium salts
- Magnesium sulfate
- Heart block
- Hypermagnesemia
- Hypocalcemia
- Anuria

 ## NURSING IMPLICATIONS

All Uterine Stimulants

- Frequent monitoring and baseline assessment of vital signs, uterine activity, and fetal heart rate
- Monitor I & O.
- Notify health care provider if symptoms of fetal distress occur or if contractions increase in frequency or duration.

 Frequent monitoring and baseline assessment of vital signs, uterine activity, and fetal heart rate

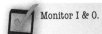 Monitor I & O.

- Use an infusion pump when administering IV.

Beta₂-Adrenergic Agonists

Nitrodrine (Yutopar)

- Give PO or IV.

Terbutaline (Brethine)

- Give PO, SC, or IV.
- Monitor lung sounds and assess for symptoms of pulmonary edema and notify health care provider.
- Monitor maternal and newborn glucose, and monitor for hypoglycemia.
- Monitor maternal electrolytes, and monitor for hypokalemia.
- Monitor and report adverse effects to health care provider.
- When giving IV, avoid using sodium chloride (increases risk of pulmonary hypertension).
- Keep client on left side to minimize hypotension.
- If labor persists after administration of maximum dose, drug may be discontinued.

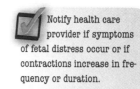

Notify health care provider if symptoms of fetal distress occur or if contractions increase in frequency or duration.

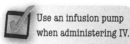

Use an infusion pump when administering IV.

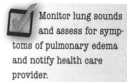

Monitor lung sounds and assess for symptoms of pulmonary edema and notify health care provider.

Magnesium Salts

Magnesium Sulfate

- Give IM or IV.
- For IM administration, give deep IM into gluteal muscle.
- Monitor ECG and neurological status before and throughout therapy.
- Implement seizure precautions.
- Check patellar reflex before each dose. If absent, do not administer additional doses as respiratory center failure may occur.[3]
- Monitor magnesium levels and renal function throughout therapy.
- When administered as an anticonvulsant, IV rate is not to exceed 3 mL/minute.
- Monitor newborn for hyporeflexia, hypertension, and respiratory depression.

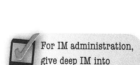

For IM administration, give deep IM into gluteal muscle.

REFERENCES

1. Lilley L, Harrington S, Snyder J. *Pharmacology and the Nursing Process,* 5th ed. St. Louis, MO: Mosby; 2007:518.

2. Lilley L, Harrington S, Snyder J. *Pharmacology and the Nursing Process,* 5th ed. St. Louis, MO: Mosby; 2007:519.

3. Karch A. *Lippincott's Nursing Drug Guide.* Philadelphia, PA: Lippincott, Williams & Wilkins; 2007:725.

Fertility agents are also called ovulation stimulants. Fertility agents stimulate follicle development and ovulation in functioning ovaries and are combined with human chorionic gonadotropin to maintain the follicles once ovulation has occurred.[1] Gonadorelin (Factrel), a synthetic gonadotropin-releasing hormone, is a diagnostic agent used to diagnose hypogonadism in men and women. It is administered SC or IV. Chorionic gonadotropin alpha (Ovidrel) and chorionic gonadotropin (Chorex, Pregnyl) are drugs that stimulate ovulation. Clomiphene (Clomid), an ovulation stimulant, and follitropin beta (Follistim), follitropin alfa (Gonal-F), menotropins (Pergonal), lutropin alfa (Luveris), urofollitropin (Metrodin), and urofollitropin purified (Bravelle) are human pituitary gonadotropins that promote follicular maturation. Cetrorelix (Cetrotide) and ganirelix (Antagon) are gonadotropin-releasing hormone (GnRH) antagonists used to prevent premature ovulation.[2]

60

Fertility Agents

TERM

☐ clomiphene (Clomid)

501

Table 60-1 Fertility Agents

Prototype Drug	Related Drugs	Drug Classification
There is no prototype for this classification	gonadorelin (Factrel)	Gonadotropin-Releasing Hormone
There is no prototype for this classification	chorionic gonadotropin alpha (Ovidrel) chorionic gonadotropin (Chorex, Pregnyl)	Nonpituitary chorionic gonadotropin
There is no prototype for this classification	follitropin alfa (Gonal-F) follitropin beta (Follistim) lutropin alfa (Luveris) menotropins (Pergonal) urofollitropin (Metrodin) urofollitropin purified (Bravelle)	Human Pituitary Gonadotropin
There is no prototype for this classification	cetrorelix (Cetrotide) ganirelix (Antagon)	Gonadotropin-Releasing Hormone (GnRH) Antagonists
clomiphene (Clomid)	There are no related drugs at this time	Ovulation Stimulant

 # FERTILITY AGENTS CLIENT TEACHING

- Continue follow-up care with health care provider if being treated for infertility.
- Teach client to monitor for therapeutic and adverse effects.

 Continue follow-up care with health care provider if being treated for infertility.

- Take exactly as prescribed and follow all directions carefully.
- Follow health care provider's instructions on timing and frequency of coitus during therapy.
- Keep a journal to note physical or emotional changes or related symptoms; take and record basal body temperature.
- Monitor and report rapid increases in weight.
- Contact health care provider if pregnancy is suspected.
- Contact health care provider if experiencing abdominal pain as this could be a sign of an ovarian cyst.

Contact health-care provider if experiencing abdominal pain as this could be a sign of an ovarian cyst.

- Advise client that fertility agents when taken for infertility can result in multiple births.

Clomiphene (Clomid)

- If a dose is missed, take as soon as remembered, or if close to next dose, double the dose.
- If more than one dose is missed, contact the health care provider.
- Report visual changes to health care provider.

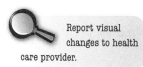

Report visual changes to health care provider.

 ## ACTION

Nonpituitary Chorionic Gonadotropins

Chorionic Gonadotropin

- Similar to luteinizing hormone (LH) in the anterior pituitary gland and acts on the ovary to induce ovulation[2]

Human Pituitary Gonadotropins

- Menotropins (Pergonal), urofollitropin (Metrodin), and urofollitropin purified (Bravelle) are equal to the effects produced by follicle stimulating hormones (FSH) and LH and are obtained from the urine of postmenopausal women.[2]
- Follitropin beta (Follistim) and follitropin alfa (Gonal-F) have FSH effects and are produced by recombinant DNA technology.[3]
- Lutropin alfa (Luveris) has LH effects and is produced by recombinant DNA technology.[3]

Gonaditropin-Releasing Hormone (GnRH) Antagonists

- GnRH antagonists block the endogenous release of LH, which prevents premature ovulation.[2]

Ovulation Stimulants

Clomiphene (Clomid)

- Increases the release of FSH and LH from the anterior pituitary gland, which stimulates ovulation, increases maturation of ovarian follicle, and the development of the corpus luteum.

USE

Nonpituitary Chorionic Gonadotropin

- Hypogonadism, nonobstructive cryptorchidism, and stimulation of ovulation

Human Pituitary Gonadotropins

- Spermatogenesis in men in combination with chorionic gonadotropin, and promotion of follicular stimulation

GnRH Antagonists

- Prevention of premature ovulation

Ovulation Stimulants

Clomiphene (Clomid)

- Treatment of infertility

 ADVERSE EFFECTS AND SIDE EFFECTS

- *Fertility Agents are Pregnancy Category X, except gonadorelin (Factrel) is Pregnancy Category B, and chorionic gonadotropin alpha (Ovidrel), chorionic gonadotropin (Chorex, Pregnyl) are Pregnancy Category C.*
- Fluid retention, flushing, gynecomastia, headache, abdominal pain, nausea, vomiting multiple pregnancies, ovarian hyperstimulation

 INTERACTIONS

All Fertility Agents

- Few interactions

CONTRAINDICATIONS

All Fertility Agents

- Adrenal or thyroid dysfunction
- Hormonally dependent tumors
- Hypersensitivity
- Primary ovarian failure
- Pregnancy
- Ovarian cysts
- Undiagnosed uterine bleeding

 ## NURSING IMPLICATIONS

All Fertility Agents

- Monitor for and report abdominal pain.
- Monitor for hypersensitivity reactions.
- Monitor for ovarian hyperstimulation.
- Monitor weight and report if weight increases quickly.
- Provide support to client and partner throughout treatment.
- Monitor serum estradiol.

Monitor for and report abdominal pain.

Provide support to client and partner throughout treatment.

Monitor serum estradiol.

Nonpituitary Chorionic Gonadotropin

Chorionic Gonadotropin Alfa (Ovidrel)

- Give SC.

Chorionic Gonadotropin (Chorex, Pregnyl)

- Give IM.
- Reconstitute with diluent provided by manufacturer.

Nonpituitary Chorionic Gonadotropins

- Generally indicated for 3 months

- Males for treatment of hyogonadism: inspect genitalia for puberty and monitor testosterone levels.

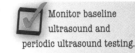

Males for treatment of hyogonadism: inspect genitalia for puberty and monitor testosterone levels.

Human Pituitary Gonadotropins

- Depending on drug, give SC or IM.
- Reconstituted with sodium chloride injection USP
- Monitor baseline ultrasound and periodic ultrasound testing.

Monitor baseline ultrasound and periodic ultrasound testing.

Ovulation Stimulants

Clomiphene (Clomid)

- Give PO and administer at same time daily to maintain drug level.
- Given over 5 days starting on day 5 of the menstrual cycle, repeated until conception occurs or 3 cycles of therapy are completed.
- Monitor for visual disturbances.
- Response to drug usually occurs 5 to 10 days after last day of treatment.

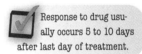

Given over 5 days starting on day 5 of the menstrual cycle, repeated until conception occurs or 3 cycles of therapy are completed.

Response to drug usually occurs 5 to 10 days after last day of treatment.

REFERENCES

1. Karch A. *Focus on Nursing Pharmacolog,* 4th ed. Philadelphia, PA: Wolters Kluwer/Lippincott Williams and Wilkins; 2008:642.

2. Lehne RA. *Pharmacology for Nursing Care*, 6th ed. Philadelphia, PA: Saunders Elsevier; 2007:739.

3. Lehne RA. *Pharmacology for Nursing Care*, 6th ed. Philadelphia, PA: Saunders Elsevier. 2007:740.

PART VIII · QUESTIONS

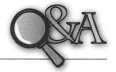

1. In which of the following conditions are estrogens contraindicated ?
   a. Gout
   b. Rheumatoid arthritis
   c. Undiagnosed vaginal bleeding
   d. Hyperthyroidism

2. Which of the following should the nurse include in teaching a client how to apply transdermal estrogen?
   a. For best absorption, place the disc over the breasts or waistline.
   b. The site does not need to be changed with each administration.
   c. Do not reapply disc if it falls off.
   d. Apply disc to an intact and hairless part of the abdomen.

3. How often does the subdermal Norplant system need to be replaced?
   a. Yearly
   b. Every 2 years
   c. Every 3 years
   d. Every 5 years

4. Which of the following should be included in a teaching plan for a client taking progestins?
   a. Instruct client how to do monthly breast self-exams.
   b. Blurred vision and headache are common adverse effects and do not need to be reported.
   c. When using as a contraceptive, take progestin every other day.
   d. If client suspects that she is pregnant, it is safe to continue taking.

5. A client taking the oral contraceptive Ortho-Novum 10/11 reports to the nurse that she has missed 3 consecutive doses. Which action should the nurse instruct the client to take?
   a. Take 3 tablets a day for the next 3 days.
   b. Take 3 tablets a day for the next 3 days and use a second method of birth control.
   c. Discontinue medication and use another form of birth control until menses begin or pregnancy has been ruled out.
   d. Omit skipped doses, resume regular dosing, and use another form of birth control.

6. A client complains of nausea while taking an oral contraceptive. Which of the following interventions should the nurse recommend to the client?

   a. Discontinue oral contraceptive and contact the health care provider.

   b. Take medication with food.

   c. Take medication 30 minutes before eating.

   d. Lie down for 30 minutes after taking.

7. Which of the following should be included in a teaching plan for a client taking alendronate (Fosamax)?

   a. Take alendronate (Fosamax) with food or juice to promote absorption of alendronate.

   b. Lie down for 30 minutes after taking alendronate.

   c. Take with an antacid to minimize gastrointestinal side effects.

   d. Take with 6 to 8 ounces of water and sit up for at least 30 minutes after taking.

8. Of the following, which drug works on estrogen receptors on bone, stimulates estrogen receptors, and blocks estrogen receptors on breast tissue?

   a. Alendronate (Fosamax)

   b. Etidronate (Didronel)

   c. Raloxifene (Evista)

   d. Tiludronate (Skelid)

9. Which of the following is correct concerning intravenous (IV) administration of oxytocin (Pitocin) for the induction of labor? It is administered:

   a. IV push.

   b. By IV bolus.

   c. Via an infusion pump.

   d. Without connection to a Y-site injection to an IV.

10. Which of the following are indications for methylergonovine (Methergine)?

    a. Induction of labor

    b. Prevention or treatment of postpartum hemorrhage caused by uterine atony or subinvolution

    c. Promotion of milk letdown for lactation

    d. Fetal stress testing

11. Nursing care for a client receiving the endocervical gel form of dinoprostone (Prepidil) includes:
    a. Keeping the client supine for 5 to 10 minutes after insertion.
    b. Administering the gel cold.
    c. Administering the drug with the client in a lateral position.
    d. Preventing contact of drug on skin.

12. Uterine relaxants are generally indicated after how many weeks of gestation?
    a. 14 weeks
    b. 16 weeks
    c. 18 weeks
    d. 20 weeks

13. Which of the following must be checked before each dose of parenteral magnesium sulfate?
    a. Temperature
    b. Patellar reflex
    c. Magnesium levels
    d. Urine output

14. Which of the following nursing measures should the nurse include for a client receiving ritodrine (Yutopar).
    a. Place client on her right side
    b. Encourage ambulation
    c. Use sodium chloride for IV infusion
    d. Monitor for hyperglycemia

15. Which of the following adverse effects of fertility agents should be reported immediately to the health care provider?
    a. Abdominal pain
    b. Increased appetite
    c. Hypothermia
    d. Weight loss

16. Of the following, which fertility agent is obtained from the urine of postmenopausal women?
    a. Chorionic gonadotropin (Ovidrel)
    b. Clomiphene (Clomid)
    c. Gonadorelin (Factrel)
    d. Menotropins (Pergonal)

17. Which fertility agent is also used to diagnose hypogonadism in males and females?
    a. Chorionic gonadotropin (Ovidrel)
    b. Clomiphene (Clomid)
    c. Gonadorelin (Factrel)
    d. Menotropins (Pergonal)

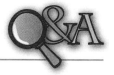

PART VIII · ANSWERS

1. **The correct answer is c.** Estrogens are contraindicated in thromboembolic disease, pregnancy, lactation, undiagnosed vaginal bleeding, hypersensitivity, and estrogen-dependent neoplasms.

2. **The correct answer is d.** The disc should be applied to an intact and hairless part of the abdomen. The site should change with each administration to prevent skin irritation. The site should not be reused for 7 days. The disc can be reapplied if it falls off. The disc should not be placed over the breasts or waistline, and should not be placed where clothing can rub the disc loose.

3. **The correct answer is d.** The subdermal Norplant system slowly releases progestin and needs to be replaced every 5 years.

4. **The correct answer is a.** The client should do monthly breast self-exams and report breast changes or lumps to the health care provider. Blurred vision and headache are not a common adverse effects and could be signs that the client is having a stroke. Progestin when used for contraceptive purposes should be taken daily and the client should stop taking if she suspects that she is pregnant as congenital anomalies have been reported during the first 4 months of pregnancy with its use.

5. **The correct answer is c.** The nurse should instruct the client to discontinue taking Ortho-Novum 10/11 and use another form of birth control until menses begin or pregnancy has been ruled out.

6. **The correct answer is b.** Oral contraceptives can be taken with food to help relieve nausea.

7. **The correct answer is d.** Alendronate (Fosamax) should be taken with a full glass of water at least 30 minutes before first food, beverage, or medication of the day. Antacids, food, orange juice, mineral water, and milk decrease absorption. The client should remain upright for at least 30 minutes after taking to minimize esophageal irritation and facilitate passage to stomach.

8. **The correct answer is c.** Raloxifene (Evista) is a SERM that works on estrogen receptors on bone, stimulates estrogen receptors, and blocks estrogen receptors on breast tissue. Alendronate (Fosamax), etidronate (Didronel), and tiludronate (Skelide) are bisphosphonates.

9. **The correct answer is c.** IV administration of oxytocin (Pitocin) should be via an infusion pump and connected to a Y-site injection to an IV for use during adverse reactions.

10. **The correct answer is b.** Methylergonovine (Methergine) is indicated to prevent or treat postpartum or postabortion hemorrhage caused by uterine atony or subinvolution.

11. **The correct answer is d.** Prevent contact of drug on the skin and make sure that hands are washed thoroughly after administering. The gel should be at room temperature when administering and the client should be supine for at least 15 to 30 minutes after insertion. The client should be in a dorsal position so that the cervix can be visualized with a speculum.

12. **The correct answer is d.** Uterine relaxants are generally indicated after 20 weeks of gestation. Spontaneous labor before 20 weeks is frequently associated with a defective fetus.

13. **The correct answer is b.** The patellar reflex should be checked before each dose of parenteral magnesium sulfate. If the response is absent, no additional doses should be given until the reflex is positive. Magnesium levels, vital signs, and I & O should be monitored periodically throughout therapy.

14. **The correct answer is d.** The client should be monitored for hyperglycemia as this is an adverse effect of ritodrine. The client should be placed on her left side to prevent decreased blood pressure. The client is on bedrest during therapy, and sodium chloride for IV infusion is avoided to prevent the risk of pulmonary edema.

15. **The correct answer is a.** Abdominal pain may indicate hyperstimulation of the ovaries and should be immediately reported to the health care provider. Anorexia and weight gain may occur with use of fertility agents. Hypothermia is not an adverse effect of fertility agents.

16. **The correct answer is d.** Menotropins (Pergonal) is obtained from the urine of postmenopausal women.

17. **The correct answer is c.** Gonadorelin (Factrel), a gonadotropin-releasing hormone, is used to diagnose hypogonadism in males and females.

IX

Male Reproductive System Drugs

Marilyn J. Herbert-Ashton, MS, RN, BC

QUICK LOOK AT THE CHAPTER AHEAD

Androgens are the male sex hormones produced by the testes, ovaries, and adrenal cortex. They stimulate spermatogenesis, development of male secondary sex characteristics, and sexual maturity at puberty. Testosterone is the major endogenous androgen and is the prototype of the androgenic hormones. Androgens also have anabolic effects, which stimulate the formation and maintenance of muscular and skeletal protein. Athletes have used androgens to increase athletic performance, which has led to abuse of androgens. Androgens are considered controlled substances and are classified as Schedule III drugs. They have serious adverse effects such as hepatotoxicity, and their risks outweigh their benefits in increasing athletic performance.

Chemical derivatives of testosterone are known as anabolic steroids. They have a high anabolic activity.

Androgen inhibitors block the effect of endogenous androgens, inhibit the enzyme 5-alpha-reductase, and are called 5-alpha-reductase inhibitors. They are used to stop prostatic growth in benign prostatic hypertrophy (BPH).

Phosphodiesterase inhibitors enhance the effects of nitric oxide, a chemical that relaxes smooth muscle and increases blood flow to the penis during sexual stimulation.

61

Androgens, Androgen Inhibitors, and Phosphodiesterase Inhibitors

TERMS
- ☐ oxandrolone (Oxandrin)
- ☐ sildenafil (Viagra)
- ☐ testosterone (Testoderm, Depo-Testosterone, Androderm)

Table 61-1 Androgens, Androgen Inhibitors, and Phosphodiesterase Inhibitors

Prototype Drug	Related Drugs	Drug Classification
testosterone (Testoderm, Depo-Testosterone, Androderm)	There are no related drugs at this time	Androgens (Natural androgenic hormones)
There is no prototype for this classification	danazol (Danocrin) fluxymesterone (Halotestin) methyltestosterone (Android) testolactone (Teslac)	(Synthetic androgenic hormones)
oxandrolone (Oxandrin)	nandrolone (Durabolin) oxymetholone (Anadrol)	(Anabolic steroids)
There is no prototype for this classification	finasteride (Proscar, Propecia) dutasteride (Avodart)	Androgen Inhibitors (5-alpha-reductase inhibitors)
sildenafil (Viagra)	vardenafil (Levitra) tadalafil (Cialis)	Phosphodiesterase inhibitors

ANDROGENS, ANDROGEN INHIBITORS, AND PHOSPHODIESTERASE INHIBITORS CLIENT TEACHING

All Androgens and Androgen Inhibitors

- Take exactly as prescribed, dose is tapered before being discontinued, and do not discontinue without consulting with health care provider.
- Advise other health care providers (eg, specialist, surgeon, dentist) about medication use before surgery or treatment.
- Continue regular follow-up care with health care provider with periodic laboratory testing.

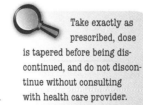

Take exactly as prescribed, dose is tapered before being discontinued, and do not discontinue without consulting with health care provider.

Androgens

- Instruct male clients to report priapism or gynecomastia to health care provider.

- Instruct female clients to report signs of virilism to health care provider.
- Report yellowing of skin (jaundice), hypercalcemia, bleeding, bruising, edema, and weight gain to health care provider.

 Report yellowing of skin (jaundice), hypercalcemia, bleeding, bruising, edema, and weight gain to health care provider.

- Explain the importance of not using androgens for athletic performance and the potential risk of serious adverse effects.

 Explain the importance of not using androgens for athletic performance and the potential risk of serious adverse effects.

- Diabetic clients need to monitor blood sugars for changes as androgens may cause hypoglycemia if taking insulin or oral hypoglycemics.

Transdermal Testosterone

- Apply to clean, dry, hairless area; do not use depilatories.
- May be reapplied after swimming or bathing

 Apply to clean, dry, hairless area; do not use depilatories.

- Testoderm is applied to the scrotum.
- Androderm is applied to abdomen, back, thighs, or upper arms. (Do not apply to scrotum.)
- If female sexual partner develops symptoms of virilization, notify health care provider.

Finasteride (Proscar, Propecia)

- Females who are pregnant or may become pregnant should avoid exposure to semen of client taking drug and should not handle crushed form of drug because of the potential for absorption as finasteride poses a potential risk to a male fetus.[1]

 Females who are pregnant or may become pregnant should avoid exposure to semen of client taking drug and should not handle crushed form of drug because of the potential for absorption as finasteride poses a potential risk to a male fetus.[1]

- May need to take drug for 6 to 12 months to determine if client is responsive to therapy.

- Libido and volume of ejaculate may be decreased during therapy.[1]

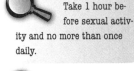

Libido and volume of ejaculate may be decreased during therapy.[1]

Phosphodiesterase Inhibitors

Sildenafil (Viagra), Vardenafil (Levitra), and Tadalafil (Cialis)

- Take 1 hour before sexual activity and no more than once daily.
- Do not take concurrently with nitrates as it could cause fatal hypertension.
- Remind client that these drugs do not protect against sexually transmitted diseases.
- Contact health care provider if erection lasts longer than 4 hours.
- Contact health provider if sudden vision loss occurs.

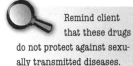

Take 1 hour before sexual activity and no more than once daily.

Remind client that these drugs do not protect against sexually transmitted diseases.

ACTION

Androgens

- Stimulate RNA synthesis, resulting in increased protein production and in natural hormone in males. Stimulate primary sex characteristics and maintenance of secondary sex characteristics, may cause weight gain and increased musculature and strength, and stimulate the production of red blood cells.

Androgen Inhibitors (5-Alpha-Reductase Inhibitors)

- Inhibit the enzyme 5-alpha-reductase, which leads to a decrease in prostate size in men with BPH. Also increases hair growth

Phosphodiesterase Inhibitors

- Enhance nitric oxide effects released during sexual stimulation

℞ USE

Androgens

Testosterone (Testoderm, Depo-Testosterone, Androderm)

- Hypogonadism
- Delayed puberty
- Palliative treatment of androgen-responsive breast cancer
- Danazol (Danocrin) is used to treat endometriosis, fibrocystic breast disease, and hereditary angioedema.
- Testolactone (Teslac) is used to treat prostate cancer and advanced breast cancer in postmenopausal women.
- Fluxymesterone (Halotestin) and methyltestosterone (Android) is used to treat inoperable breast cancer, hypogonadism, and postpartum breast engorgement. Methyltestosterone is also used to treat postpubertal cryptorchidism.
- Oxandrolone (Oxandrin) is used to treat bone pain associated with osteoperosis, promotion of weight gain in debilitated patients, certain cancers, Turner's syndrome, promotion of catabolism related to prolonged glucocorticoid use, and alcoholic hepatitis.
- Nandrolone (Durabolin) is used to treat metastatic breast cancer.
- Oxymetholone (Anadrol) is used to treat various anemias.

Androgen Inhibitors (5-Alpha-Reductase Inhibitors)

- Treatment of BPH and male androgenetic alopecia

Phosphodiesterase Inhibitors

- Used to treat erectile dysfunction

❗ ADVERSE EFFECTS AND SIDE EFFECTS

Androgens

- *Pregnancy category X, although danazol (Danocrin) and testolactone (Teslac) are pregnancy category C.*
- *CV:* Edema

- *CNS:* Headache, depression, insomnia, excitation
- *Endocrine:* Deepening of voice, acne, oily skin, gynecomastia, hirsutism, clitorial enlargement, menstrual irregularities, priapism, and oligospermia
- *F & E:* Hypercalcemia—retention of sodium, chloride, and water
- *GI:* Nausea, vomiting, hepatitis, and appetite changes
- *Hematologic:* Increased serum cholesterol levels and polycythemia

Androgen Inhibitors (5-Alpha-Reductase Inhibitor)

- *Pregnancy category X*
- *GU:* Decreased volume of ejaculate, impotence, and decreased libido

Phosphodiesterase Inhibitors

- *Pregnancy category B*
- *CV:* In clients with preexisting cardiovascular disease, especially those taking nitrates, drug causes severe hypertension and can cause sudden death, cardiovascular collapse, or myocardial infarction.
- *CNS:* Headache
- *Derm:* Flushing
- *GI:* Dyspepsia
- *GU:* Priapism
- *Other:* Sudden vision loss, nonarteritic ischemic neuropathy

INTERACTIONS

Androgens

- Increased anticoagulant activity when taken with oral anticoagulants
- Increased hypoglycemia when taken with antidiabetic agents
- Increased corticosteroid effects when taken with corticosteroids
- Increased risk of hepatoxicity when taken with other hepatoxic agents

Androgen Inhibitors (5-Alpha-Reductase Inhibitors)

- None known

Phosphodiesterase Inhibitors

- Increase risk of severe and potentially fatal hypotenison when taken with nitrates
- Increased risk of hypotension when taken with antihypertensives

CONTRAINDICATIONS

Androgens

- Hypersensitivity
- Pregnancy and lactation
- Hypercalemia
- Male clients with breast or prostate cancer
- Clients with severe cardiac, renal, or hepatic disease
- Genital bleeding

Androgen Inhibitors (5-Alpha-Reductase Inhibitors)

- Hypersensitivity
- Pregnancy
- Concurrent use with phosphodiesterase inhibitor

Phosphodiesterase Inhibitors

- Hypersensitivity
- Concurrent use with organic nitrates
- Concurrent use of alpha blockers with vardenafil (Levitra) and tadalafil (Cialis)

NURSING IMPLICATIONS

Androgens

- Give PO, bucal, SC (implant), IM, or transdermal.
- Monitor I & O, and weight; report changes that may indicate fluid retention.

 Monitor I & O, and weight; report changes that may indicate fluid retention.

- Monitor blood pressure and report changes.
- Monitor hemoglobin and hematacrit periodically throughout therapy.
- Monitor liver function studies and cholesterol levels periodically throughout therapy.
- Monitor calcium levels and alkaline phosphate levels in clients with metastatic cancer.
- Monitor for symptoms of hypercalcemia.
- Women: monitor for symptoms of virilism and report to health care provider; men: monitor for precocious puberty in boys. Bone age determinations should be done every 6 months to assess rate of bone maturation.
- Monitor for symptoms of BPH.
- Monitor PSA levels in clients using transdermal testosterone.
- Give deep IM into gluteal muscle.
- Monitor for adverse effects. (See "Client Teaching" on page 517.)
- Therapeutic effects may take 6 to 12 months.[2]

> Monitor blood pressure and report changes.

> Monitor liver function studies and cholesterol levels periodically throughout therapy.

Androgen Inhibitors (5-Alpha-Reductase Inhibitors)

Finasteride (Proscar, Propecia) and dutastecide (Avodart)

- Give PO.
- Assess for prostatic hypertrophy.
- Monitor PSA before and periodically throughout therapy.

Phosphodiesterase Inhibitors

- Give PO.
- These drugs have no effect in the absence of sexual stimulation.

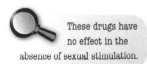

> These drugs have no effect in the absence of sexual stimulation.

REFERENCES

1. Skidmore-Roth L. *Mosby's Nursing Drug Reference.* St. Louis, MO: Mosby Elsevier; 2007:460.

2. Lilley L, Harrington S, Snyder J. *Pharmacology and the Nursing Process*, 5th ed. St. Louis, MO: Mosby; 2007:532.

PART IX · QUESTIONS

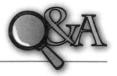

1. Transdermal testosterone (Androderm) can be applied to all of the following sites EXCEPT:
   a. Abdomen.
   b. Back.
   c. Upper arms.
   d. Scrotum.

2. Which of the following drugs is used to treat benign prostatic hypertrophy (BPH)?
   a. Danazol (Danocrine)
   b. Finasteride (Proscar, Propecia)
   c. Fluxymesterone (Halotestin)
   d. Methyltestosterone (Android)

3. Of the following, which agent is contraindicated in clients taking sildenafil (Viagra)?
   a. Aspirin
   b. Nitroglycerin
   c. Saw Palmetto
   d. Vitamin E

4. How soon should sildenafil (Viagra) be taken before intercourse?
   a. 5 minutes
   b. 10 minutes
   c. 15 minutes
   d. 60 minutes

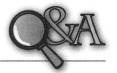

PART IX · ANSWERS

1. **The correct answer is d.** Transdermal testosterone (Androderm) is not applied to the scrotum; transdermal Testoderm is applied to the scrotum.

2. **The correct answer is b.** Finasteride (Proscar, Propecia) is a 5-alpha-reductase inhibitor, used to treat BPH.

3. **The correct answer is b.** Nitroglycerin taken with sildenafil (Viagra) can cause severe hypotension and sudden cardiac death.

4. **The correct answer is d.** Sildenafil (Viagra) should be taken 1 hour before intercourse, and no more than once daily.

X

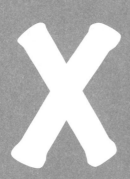

Gastrointestinal System Drugs

Nancy Elaine Clarkson, MEd, RN, BC

QUICK LOOK AT THE CHAPTER AHEAD

Peptic ulcer disease (PUD) involves the eating away of the stomach lining and other nearby areas of the GI tract and is most often caused by the bacteria, Helicobacter pylori (H. pylori).[1] Approximately 10% of the US population experiences PUD at some time.[1]

There are several categories of drugs that are used to aid in the treatment of PUD. The combination of bismuth and antibiotics is used to remove the infection of H. pylori. There are currently three combination drugs that are used for this purpose: **bismuth subsalicylate, metronidazole, and tetracycline (Helidac); amoxicillin, clarithromycin, and lansoprazole (Prevpac); and ranitidine** and **bismuth citrate (Tritec)**. Other groups of drugs used to control the acid produced in the stomach are **Histamine-2 antagonists, proton pump inhibitors, antacids,** and **two miscellaneous drugs.** These drug categories will be discussed in detail.

62

Antiulcer Drugs

TERMS
- ☐ **aluminum hydroxide with magnesium hydroxide (Maalox)**
- ☐ **cimetidine (Tagament)**
- ☐ **omeprazole (Prilosec)**

Table 62-1 Antiulcer Drugs

Prototype Drug	Related Drugs	Drug Classification
cimetidine (Tagament)	famotidine (Pepcid) nizatidine (Axid) ranitidine (Zantac)	Histamine-2 antagonists
omeprazole (Prilosec)	esomeprazole (Nexium) lansoprazole (Prevacid) pantoprazole (Protonix) rabeprazole (Aciphex)	Proton pump inhibitors
aluminum hydroxide with magnesium hydroxide (Maalox)	aluminum carbonate (Basaljel) aluminum hydroxide (Amphojel) calcium carbonate (Tums) magaldrate (Riopan) magnesium hydroxide (Milk of Magnesia) magnesium oxide (Mag-ox) sodium bicarbonate (Bell/Ans)	Antacids
There is no prototype for this classification	misoprostol (Cytotec) sucralfate (Carafate)	Miscellaneous drugs

ANTIULCER DRUGS CLIENT TEACHING

Histamine-2 Antagonists

- Do not breast-feed.
- Report GI bleeding to physician.
- Can take with or without food
- No activities requiring concentration until drug effects are known.
- No smoking, aspirin, nonsteroidal anti-inflammatory drugs (NSAIDs), or alcohol
- Do not abruptly stop drug.

Report GI bleeding to physician.

Proton Pump Inhibitors

Report diarrhea and any urinary changes.

- Do not breast-feed.
- Report diarrhea and any urinary changes.

Antacids

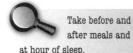

- Take before and after meals and at hour of sleep.
- Shake liquids.
- Do not take other drugs with these drugs; separate by at least 1 hour.
- If on low sodium diet, client must take antacid that is low sodium magaldrate (Riopan).
- Chew tablets and take a full glass of milk or water afterwards.

Take before and after meals and at hour of sleep.

Do not take other drugs with these drugs; separate by at least 1 hour.

If on low sodium diet, client must take antacid that is low sodium magaldrate (Riopan).

Miscellaneous Drugs

Misoprostol (Cytotec)

- Do not breast-feed.
- Do not get pregnant.
- Report menstrual irregularities.
- Don't take magnesium antacids as this increases risk of diarrhea.

Don't take magnesium antacids as this increases risk of diarrhea.

Sucralfate (Carafate)

- Do not breast-feed.
- Prevent constipation via exercise, increased fluids, and fiber in diet.
- Take this drug for 4 to 8 weeks.

℞ ACTION

Histamine-2 Antagonists

- Decrease secretion of gastric acid and formation of pepsin by blocking histamine-2 receptor sites

Proton Pump Inhibitors

- Reduce stomach acid by working on secretory surface receptors to stop the last phase of acid production

Antacids

- Mix with hydrochloric acid to neutralize stomach secretions and prevent transformation of pepsinogen to pepsin

Miscellaneous Drugs

Misoprostol (Cytotec)

- Stops secretion of gastric acid and elevates production of mucus and bicarbonate to preserve the stomach lining

Sucralfate (Carafate)

- Forms a protective covering over ulcer sites and guards against pepsin, bile salts, and acid, which stops further breakdown of the sites

USE

Histamine-2 Antagonists

- Gastroesophageal reflux disease (GERD)
- Heartburn
- Zollinger-Ellison Syndrome and other diseases of hypersecretion of gastric acids
- Stress ulcers
- GI bleeding
- Gastric and duodenal ulcers

Proton Pump Inhibitors

- Short-term treatment for gastric and duodenal ulcers, GERD, esophagitis
- Long-term treatment of hypersecretory diseases
- *H. pylori* infection

Antacids

- Treat and prevent gastritis, GI bleeding, stress ulcers, heartburn, GERD, PUD, esophagitis

Miscellaneous Drugs

Misoprostol (Cytotec)

- Prevention of gastric ulcers from use of NSAIDs.

Sucralfate (Carafate)

- Duodenal ulcer

ADVERSE EFFECTS AND SIDE EFFECTS

Histamine-2 Antagonists

- *Pregnancy category B, except for nizatidine (Axid), which is category C*
- *CNS:* Confusion, hallucinations, drowsiness, headache, dizziness
- *CV:* Hypotension, arrhythmias (both are rare)
- *Derm:* Reversible alopecia, rash, Stevens-Johnson Syndrome
- *F & E:* Elevated creatinine, BUN, serum uric acid
- *GI:* Constipation, diarrhea
- *GU:* Reversible impotence, gynecomastia, galactorrhea
- *Hematologic:* Elevated prothrombin time
- *Other:* Fever, joint pain in clients with arthritis

Proton Pump Inhibitors

- *Pregnancy category B, except for omeprazole (Prilosec), which is category C*
- *CNS:* Tiredness, dizziness, headache, insomnia
- *Derm:* Pruritus, alopecia, rash, dry skin
- *GI:* Dry mouth, nausea, diarrhea, abdominal pain
- *GU:* Blood and/or protein in the urine
- *Resp:* Nasal stuffiness, hoarseness, cough, nosebleed
- *Other:* Fever, back pain

Antacids

- *Pregnancy category C, except for magnesium hydroxide (Milk of Magnesia) and sodium bicarbonate, which are category B. Calcium carbonate (Tums) is not rated.*

- *F & E:* Hypophosphatemia, hypermagnesemia in clients with renal disease
- *GI:* Magnesium antacids cause diarrhea; aluminum antacids cause constipation; acid rebound
- *Other:* Encephalopathy, osteomalacia; aluminum antacids can accumulate in CNS, bone, and blood.

Miscellaneous Drugs

Misoprostol (Cytotec)

- *Pregnancy category X*
- *CNS:* Headache
- *GI:* Constipation, diarrhea, nausea, vomiting, abdominal pain, flatulence
- *GU:* Menstrual irregularities, uterine contractions

Sucralfate (Carafate)

- *Pregnancy category B*
- *CNS:* Insomnia, dizziness
- *Derm:* Rash
- *GI:* Constipation, diarrhea, nausea
- *Other:* Back pain

INTERACTIONS

Histamine-2 Antagonists

- Elevate activity and toxic effects of the following: theophylline (Theo-Dur), warfarin (Coumadin), diazepam (Valium), propranolol (Inderal), phenobarbital, phenytoin (Dilantin), lidocaine (Zylocaine)
- Concurrent use with antacids lessens absorption of histamine-2 antagonists.

Proton Pump Inhibitors

- Concurrent use with warfarin (Coumadin), phenytoin (Dilantin), and diazepam (Valium) may increase levels of these drugs.

Antacids

- Effects of cholinergic drugs are lessened.
- Effects of anticholinergics are elevated.
- Speed up excretion of acidic drugs and slow excretion of alkaline drugs.

Miscellaneous Drugs

Misoprostol (Cytotec)

- Concurrent use with magnesium antacids risks increased diarrhea.

Sucralfate (Carafate)

- Concurrent use with aluminum salts increases risk of aluminum toxicity.
- Absorption of the following drugs is decreased: digoxin (Lanoxin), tetracycline, phenytoin (Dilantin), quinolones.

 CONTRAINDICATIONS

Histamine-2 Antagonists

- Pregnancy
- Lactation
- Allergy to these drugs
- Kidney and liver disease

Proton Pump Inhibitors

- Pregnancy
- Lactation
- Allergy to these drugs

Antacids

- Cautious use in pregnancy and lactation
- Allergy to these drugs
- Electrolyte disorders

* GI obstruction
* Kidney disease

Miscellaneous Drugs

Misoprostol (Cytotec)

* Pregnancy
* Lactation

Sucralfate (Carafate)

* Kidney disease or dialysis
* Allergy to drug components
* Cautious use in pregnancy and lactation

NURSING IMPLICATIONS

Histamine-2 Antagonists

* Give PO, IM, or IV.
* Separate administration with antacids by giving 1 hour before or 2 hours after antacid dosing.
* IV solutions become unstable after 48 hours.
* Client is at risk for vitamin B_{12} deficiency when cimetidine (Tagamet) is taken in divided doses.
* Drug is usually taken for 4 weeks.
* Monitor I & O.
* Assess pulse in initial days of dosing. Slow heart rate needs to be reported to physician.
* Assess blood pressure.
* Elderly can become confused. Stop drug if this occurs.
* Monitor the following blood tests: CBC, liver, and kidney function.
* Assess for adynamic ileus.

 Separate administration with antacids by giving 1 hour before or 2 hours after antacid dosing.

 IV solutions become unstable after 48 hours.

Client is at risk for vitamin B_{12} deficiency when cimetidine (Tagamet) is taken in divided doses.

Assess pulse in initial days of dosing. Slow heart rate needs to be reported to physician.

 Elderly can become confused. Stop drug if this occurs.

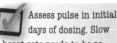

Proton Pump Inhibitors

- Give PO and IV.
- Monitor the following tests: urinalysis, hepatic function.

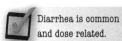
Monitor the following tests: urinalysis, hepatic function.

- Tablets must be taken whole.
- Antacids can be taken with this drug.
- Separate administration by at least 1 hour from other oral drugs.
- Tablets must be thoroughly chewed.
- Monitor serum electrolytes.
- Shake suspensions.
- Monitor client for electrolyte problems.

Monitor serum electrolytes.

Miscellaneous Drugs

Misoprostol (Cytotec)

- Give PO.
- Administer with food to prevent GI distress.
- Diarrhea is common and dose related.

Diarrhea is common and dose related.

Sucralfate (Carafate)

- Give PO.
- Separate administration with antacids by at least a half hour.
- If administering via nasogastric tube, use diluent from pharmacy.
- Binds with many drugs. Consult with pharmacist to determine which drugs can be administered with it.

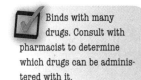
Binds with many drugs. Consult with pharmacist to determine which drugs can be administered with it.

REFERENCE

1. Lehne RA. *Pharmacology for Nursing Care*, 6th ed. Philadelphia, PA: Saunders Elsevier; 2007:891.

The laxatives are a group of drugs that are used to assist in the defecation process. They are able to do a number of things depending on their classification: speed up the passage of feces, soften the stool, or enlarge the volume of the stool. Unfortunately, this is a group of drugs that is often misused by clients as many individuals do not understand the principles of proper bowel function.

63

Laxatives

TERMS
☐ bisacodyl (Dulcolax)
☐ docusate sodium (Colace)
☐ magnesium hydroxide (Milk of Magnesia)
☐ psyllium (Metamucil)

Table 63-1 Laxatives

Prototype Drug	Related Drugs	Drug Classification
magnesium hydroxide (Milk of Magnesia)	magnesium citrate (Citrate of Magnesia) magnesium sulfate (Epsom salts)	Saline laxatives
bisacodyl (Dulcolax)	cascara sagrada (Cascara Sagrada Fluid extract Aromatic) castor oil (Fleet Flavored Castor Oil) senna (Senokot)	Stimulant laxatives
psyllium (Metamucil)	lactulose (Chronulac) polycarbophil (Fibercon)	Bulk-forming laxatives
docusate sodium (Colace)	glycerin (Sani-Supp) mineral oil (Neo-Culrol)	Lubricant laxatives

LAXATIVES CLIENT TEACHING

For All Laxatives

- Bowel function should be maintained with increased fiber in diet, increased fluids, and exercise.

Saline Laxatives

- Do not breast-feed.
- Take at bedtime or in the morning.
- Drink 8 ounces of water after administration to advance drug action.

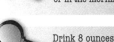

Take at bedtime or in the morning.

Drink 8 ounces of water after administration to advance drug action.

Stimulant Laxatives

- Do not breast-feed.
- Do not chew tablets.
- Take with 8 ounces of water or other liquid.

Do not chew tablets.

Take with 8 ounces of water or other liquid.

Bulk-Forming Laxatives

- Do not breast-feed.
- Add powder to liquid if using standard formulation.
- Add liquid to powder if using effervescent formulation.
- Drink 8 ounces of water after administration.
- Appetite may be diminished if taken before meals.
- Check sodium and sugar content of drug if on restricted diet.

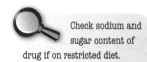

Check sodium and sugar content of drug if on restricted diet.

Lubricant Laxatives

- Do not take with mineral oil.
- Take with 8 ounces of water. Liquid form can be mixed in juice, milk, etc.

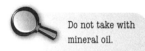

Do not take with mineral oil.

ACTION

Saline Laxatives

- Act in both small and large intestine by elevating the amount of fluid, which causes enhanced pressure in the intestine. This stimulates stretch receptors and speeds up peristalsis, which results in quick emptying of the bowel.

Stimulant Laxatives

- Work on the nerve plexus in the wall of the intestine, which speeds up peristalsis

Bulk-Forming Laxatives

- Cause water to be retained in the stool, which causes distention of the bowel and results in defecation

Lubricant Laxatives

- Covers fecal material, which slows down absorption of water. Stool becomes softened and easier to pass.

USE

Saline Laxatives

- Constipation
- Bowel preparation for GI diagnostic tests
- Evacuation of bowel after GI diagnostic testing

Stimulant Laxatives

- Constipation
- Bowel preparation for diagnostic tests
- Evacuation of bowel after GI diagnostic testing

Bulk-Forming Laxatives

- Constipation
- Lactulose (Chronulac) is used to treat and prevent portal-systemic encephalopathy, which includes hepatic coma.

Lubricant Laxatives

- Softens stool for easy passage without straining

ADVERSE EFFECTS AND SIDE EFFECTS

Saline Laxatives

- *Pregnancy category B, except magnesium sulfate (Epsom salts), which is category A*
- *CNS:* Depression, weakness
- *CV:* Slowed heart beat, low blood pressure, heart block
- *F & E:* Electrolyte imbalance, alkaline urine
- *GI:* Diarrhea, nausea, vomiting, cramps
- *Respiratory:* Respiratory depression
- *Other:* Dehydration, coma

Stimulant Laxatives

* *Pregnancy category C*
* *F & E:* Calcium and potassium imbalance
* *GI:* Diarrhea, nausea, cramping

Bulk-Forming Laxatives

* *Pregnancy category C*
* *GI:* Diarrhea, nausea, vomiting
* *Hematologic:* Eosinophilia

Lubricant Laxatives

* *Pregnancy category C*
* *Derm:* Rash
* *GI:* Diarrhea, nausea, cramps
* *Other:* Irritated throat from liquid preparation

INTERACTIONS

Saline Laxatives

* Retard absorption of tetracyclines, quinolones, isoniazid, digoxin (Lanoxin), dicumarol

Stimulant Laxatives

* Enteric-coated tablets will be dissolved early if given with antacids and abdominal cramps will result.

Bulk-Forming Laxatives

* Interferes with action and absorption of salicylates, digoxin (Lanoxin), antibiotics, warfarin (Coumadin), nitrofurantoin (Furadantin)

Lubricant Laxatives

* Elevates absorption of mineral oil

CONTRAINDICATIONS

Saline Laxatives

* Pregnancy
* Lactation
* Children under 2 years of age
* Kidney disease
* Intestinal obstruction
* Nausea
* Vomiting
* Diarrhea
* Fecal impaction
* Colostomy
* Ileostomy

Stimulant Laxatives

* Intestinal obstruction
* Fecal impaction
* Nausea
* Vomiting
* Abdominal cramps
* Acute abdomen

Bulk-Forming Laxatives

* Appendicitis
* Children under 2 years of age
* Fecal impaction
* Nausea
* Vomiting
* Intestinal or esophageal obstruction

Lubricant Laxatives

* Pregnancy
* Intestinal obstruction
* Kidney disease
* Clients on sodium restriction
* Nausea
* Vomiting
* Structural deformities of rectum or colon

NURSING IMPLICATIONS

Saline Laxatives

* Give PO.
* Suspension formula must be shaken before administration.
* Give on empty stomach.
* Client can become dependent on laxative use so assess need.
* Assess for UTI and urinary stones.
* Monitor serum magnesium.

 Suspension formula must be shaken before administration.

 Client can become dependent on laxative use so assess need.

 Monitor serum magnesium.

Stimulant Laxatives

* Give PO and PR.
* Assess need carefully as client can become dependent on laxative use.
* Clients receiving anticoagulants may have lowered absorption of vitamin K.
* Enteric-coated tablets must be swallowed whole.
* Milk and antacids should be given 1 hour before or 1 hour after administration of these drugs so enteric coating is left intact.

 Assess need carefully as client can become dependent on laxative use.

 Clients receiving anticoagulants may have lowered absorption of vitamin K.

Bulk-Forming Laxatives

- Give PO.
- Monitor elderly for drug aspiration.
- Monitor digoxin (Lanoxin) and warfarin (Coumadin) drug levels.
- Retrosternal pain may indicate drug settled in esophagus.
- Expect drug results 12 to 24 hours after administration.

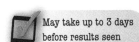
Monitor elderly for drug aspiration.

Lubricant Laxatives

- Give PO and PR.
- May take up to 3 days before results seen
- Stop drug if diarrhea occurs.

May take up to 3 days before results seen

Diarrhea is not a disease of the GI tract but a symptom of a GI system disorder.[1] The antidiarrheals are able to decrease peristalsis, which enables the stool to become more formed and less fluid. These drugs act either locally or systemically. All of these drugs relieve diarrhea but do not cure the underlying cause.

64
Antidiarrheals

TERM
- [ ] diphenoxylate with atropine sulfate (Lomotil)

Table 64-1 Antidiarrheals

Prototype Drug	Related Drugs	Drug Classification
diphenoxylate with atropine sulfate (Lomotil)	bismuth subsalicylate (Pepto-Bismol) difenoxin with atropine sulfate (Motofen) loperamide (Imodium) octreotide (Sandostatin) paregoric (Camphorated opium tincture)	Antidiarrheals

ANTIDIARRHEALS CLIENT TEACHING

For All Antidiarrheals

- Increase fluid intake to 2 to 3 quarts of fluid daily to prevent dehydration.
- Stop drug when diarrhea is gone.
- No activities requiring concentration until drug effects are known
- Drug should be taken only as ordered.
- Do not breast-feed.

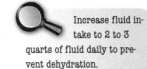

Increase fluid intake to 2 to 3 quarts of fluid daily to prevent dehydration.

For Bismuth Subsalicylate (Pepto-Bismol)

- Use cautiously with other drugs that contain aspirin and salicylates.
- Stools and tongue can turn black.
- Contact physician if diarrhea lasts for more than 2 days.

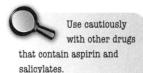

Use cautiously with other drugs that contain aspirin and salicylates.

ACTION

The antidiarrheals act in a number of ways.

- Opiate derivatives (diphenoxylate with atropine [Lomotil], difenoxin with atropine [motofen], and paregoric [camphorated opium tincture]) act directly on the areas of the CNS that control movement of the GI tract.

- Bismuth subsalicylate (Pepto-Bismol) works directly on the GI tract lining to slow movement and reduce inflammation.
- Loperamide (Imodium) acts on GI tract muscles to decrease peristalsis.
- Octreotide (Sandostatin) represses the action of a number of GI enzymes.

 ## USE

- Chronic and acute diarrhea
- Traveler's diarrhea
- Diarrhea that occurs with Acquired Immune Deficiency Syndrome, carcinoid tumors, radiation, and chemotherapy treatments

 ## ADVERSE EFFECTS AND SIDE EFFECTS

- *Pregnancy category B, except for bismuth subsalicylate (Pepto-Bismol), which is category A, and diphenoxylate with atropine (Lomotil) and difenoxin with atropine (Motofen), which are category C*
- *CNS:* Headache, dizziness, fatigue
- *CV:* Tachycardia, arrhythmias
- *Derm:* Rash, itching
- *EENT:* Blurred vision
- *F & E:* Dehydration, fluid and electrolyte imbalance
- *GI:* Constipation, nausea, vomiting, abdominal cramps and distension, paralytic ileus
- *GU:* Urinary retention
- *Resp:* Respiratory depression with opiate derivatives
- *Other:* Dry mouth, physical dependence with opiate derivatives

 ## INTERACTIONS

- Anticholinergics and CNS depressants increase effects of opiate derivative antidiarrheals.

CONTRAINDICATIONS

- Allergy to antidiarrheals
- Pregnancy
- Lactation
- Acute abdomen
- GI obstruction
- Diarrhea from poisoning
- Opiate-derivative antidiarrheals should not be used for chronic diarrhea, due to risk of physical dependence.

 ## NURSING IMPLICATIONS

For All Antidiarrheals

- Give PO, SC, IM, or IV.
- Assess for dehydration and fluid and electrolyte balance.
- Give after each liquid stool.
- Assess consistency and frequency of stools.

> ☑ Assess for dehydration and fluid and electrolyte balance.

Diphenoxylate with Atropine (Lomotil)

- Tablets can be crushed.
- Continue treatment for up to 36 hours before deciding if drug is not effective.

> ☑ Continue treatment for up to 36 hours before deciding if drug is not effective.

Bismuth Subsalicylate (Pepto-Bismol)

- Contains aspirin and should not be given to clients with aspirin allergy
- Tablets must be chewed.
- Shake suspension.
- Drink 8 ounces of liquid after each dose.
- Assess for black tongue and dark stools, which can occur and will go away.

> ☑ Contains aspirin and should not be given to clients with aspirin allergy

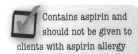

> ☑ Assess for black tongue and dark stools, which can occur and will go away.

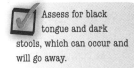

Octreotide (Sandostatin)

- Preferred route is SC.
- Rotate SC sites.
- Administer injections between meals and at hour of sleep.
- If given IM, give injection slowly and have drug come to room temperature before administration.

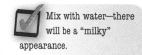

Preferred route is SC.

Paregoric (Camphorated Opium Tincture)

- Mix with water—there will be a "milky" appearance.
- If diarrhea worsens, it may be related to an infection.
- Client may become physically dependent.

Mix with water—there will be a "milky" appearance.

REFERENCE

1. Lehne RA. *Pharmacology for Nursing Care*, 6th ed. Philadelphia, PA: Saunders Elsevier; 2007:916.

The antiemetics are drugs that are used in the treatment and prevention of nausea and vomiting. They come from a variety of drug classifications. In general, these drugs work on the cerebral cortex, chemoreceptor trigger zone (CTZ), vomiting center, or the inner ear to deal with nausea and vomiting.

65

Antiemetics

TERMS
☐ meclizine (Antivert)
☐ metoclopramide (Reglan)
☐ ondansetron (Zofran)
☐ prochlorperazine (Compazine)

Table 65-1 Antiemetics

Prototype Drug	Related Drugs	Drug Classification
prochlorperazine (Compazine)	chlorpromazine (Thorazine) perphenazine (Trilafon) promethazine (Phenergan) thiethylperazine (Torecan)	Phenothiazines
metoclopropamide (Reglan)	There are no related drugs	Prokinetic agent
meclizine (Antivert)	buclizine (Bucladin-S Softab) cyclizine (Marezine) dimenhydrinate (Dramamine) hydroxyzine (Vistaril)	Antihistamines
ondansetron (Zofran)	dolasetron (Anzemet) granisetron (Kytril) palonosetron (Aloxi)	5-HT3 receptor antagonists
There is no prototype drug for this classification	dronabinol (Marinol) trimethobenzamide (Tigan)	Miscellaneous agents

ANTIEMETICS CLIENT TEACHING

For All Antiemetics

- Do not drink alcohol.
- Do not breast-feed.
- Do not get pregnant.
- No activities requiring concentration until drug effects are known.
- Take drug before nausea and vomiting start.

Phenothiazines

- Prochlorperazine (Compazine) may turn urine reddish-brown.

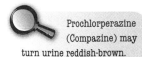

Prochlorperazine (Compazine) may turn urine reddish-brown.

5-HT Receptor Antagonists

- Headache is common side effect and will require pain medication.

Headache is common side effect and will require pain medication.

ACTION

Phenothiazines

- Work directly on the CTZ to prevent or treat nausea and vomiting

Prokinetic Drug

- Desensitizes nerves in the CTZ to substances that cause vomiting

Antihistamines

- Interfere with the action of acetylcholine in the brain

5-HT3 Receptor Antagonists

- Block serotonin receptors in the CTZ and the periphery

Miscellaneous Drugs

Dronabinol (Marinol)

- It is not known how this drug works, but it is believed to act on a "control mechanism" found in the medulla oblongata.

Trimethobenzamide (Tigan)

- Acts directly on the CTZ

USE

Phenothoazines

- Severe nausea and vomiting
- Nausea and vomiting occurring with anesthesia
- Intractable hiccups

Prokinetic Drug

- Prevention of nausea and vomiting associated with cancer chemotherapy

Antihistamines

- Nausea and vomiting associated with motion sickness
- Prevention and treatment of nausea and vomiting associated with anesthesia in obstetrics and general surgery

5-HT3 Receptor Antagonists

- Nausea and vomiting associated with cancer chemotherapy

Miscellaneous Drugs

Dronabinol (Marinol)

- Nausea and vomiting associated with cancer chemotherapy in adults

Trimethobenzamide (Tigan)

- Nausea and vomiting

ADVERSE EFFECTS AND SIDE EFFECTS

Phenothizines

- *Pregnancy category C, except for thiethylperazine (Torecan), which is category X*
- *CNS:* Extrapyramidal reactions, drowsiness, dizziness
- *CV:* Low blood pressure
- *Derm:* Photosensitivity
- *EENT:* Blurred vision
- *Endocrine:* Amenorrhea, galactorrhea
- *GI:* Jaundice
- *Hematologic:* Agranulocytosis, leukopenia

Prokinetic Drug

- *Pregnancy category B*
- *CNS:* Extrapyramidal reactions, fatigue, restlessness, sedation
- *Derm:* Rash

- *Endocrine:* Impotence, amenorrhea, galactorrhea, gynecomastia
- *GI:* Diarrhea, dry mouth
- *Hematologic:* Methemoglobinemia
- *Other:* Periorbital edema

Antihistamines

- *Pregnancy category B, except hydroxyzine (Vistaril) and buclizine (Bucladin-S Softab), which are category C*
- *CNS:* Drowsiness, fatigue
- *EENT:* Blurred vision
- *GI:* Dry mouth

5-HT Receptor Antagonists

- *Pregnancy category B*
- *CNS:* Sedation, headache
- *GI:* Diarrhea
- *Other:* Hypersensitivity

Miscellaneous Drugs

Dronabinol (Marinol)

- *Pregnancy category B*
- *CNS:* Drowsiness
- *CV:* Syncope, high blood pressure, othostatic hypotension, rapid heart beat
- *GI:* Diarrhea, dry mouth
- *Other:* Muscle pain

Trimethobenzamide (Tigan)

- *Pregnancy category C*
- *CNS:* Pseudoparkinsonism
- *CV:* Low blood pressure
- *GI:* Jaundice, hepatitis, diarrhea
- *Other:* Hypersensitivity

INTERACTIONS

For All Antiemetics

- Concurrent use with antihypertensives causes additive hypotension.
- Concurrent use with CNS depressants causes additional CNS depression.
- Concurrent use with anticholinergics causes additional anti-cholinergic effects.

Phenothiazines

- Antiseizure drug dose may need to be increased as seizure threshold is decreased.
- Antidiarrheals and antacids decrease absorption.
- Concurrent use with Kava-kava may elevate risk for dystonic reactions.
- Elevated drug metabolism with phenobarbitol

Prokinetic Drug

- Concurrent use diminishes absorption of digoxin (Lanoxin), tetracycline (Achromycin), lithium (Eskalith), diazepam (Valium), acetaminophen (Tylenol), and aspirin.
- Concurrent use antagonizes effects of ropinirole (Requip), amantadine (Symmetrel), levodopa (Dopar), pergolide (Permax), bromocriptine (Parlodel).
- Increased extrapyramidal reactions when given concurrently with phenothiazines

5-HT3 Receptor Antagonists

- Concurrent use with rifampin (Rifadin) can decrease drug levels.

Miscellaneous Drugs

Dronabinol (Marinol)

- Elevated heart rate when given with atropine and tricyclic antidepressants

CONTRAINDICATIONS

For All Antiemetics

- Any condition where client is experiencing CNS depression
- Pregnancy
- Lactation
- Liver disease
- Severe high or low blood pressure

 ## NURSING IMPLICATIONS

For All Antiemetics

- Parenteral forms should not be mixed with other drugs in a syringe.
- IM administration should be deep into large muscle mass.
- Take 1 half-hour before travel if using to prevent motion sickness.
- Take a half-hour to 1 hour before cancer chemotherapy to prevent associated nausea and vomiting.
- Do not administer to clients who are experiencing CNS depression or who have low blood pressure.
- Drug may mask condition causing nausea and vomiting.
- Z track IM injections

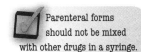
Parenteral forms should not be mixed with other drugs in a syringe.

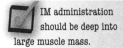
IM administration should be deep into large muscle mass.

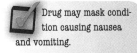
Do not administer to clients who are experiencing CNS depression or who have low blood pressure.

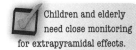
Drug may mask condition causing nausea and vomiting.

Phenothiazines

- Give PO, IM, IV, or PR.
- Monitor CBC
- Children and elderly need close monitoring for extrapyramidal effects.

Children and elderly need close monitoring for extrapyramidal effects.

Prokinetic Drug

- Give PO, IM, or IV.
- Monitor serum electrolytes and aldosterone.
- Children and elderly need close monitoring for extrapyramidal effects.

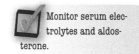
Monitor serum electrolytes and aldosterone.

Antihistamines

- Give PO.
- Give with or without food.

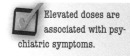
Give with or without food.

5-HT3 Receptor Antagonists

- Give PO, IM, or IV.
- Assess for diarrhea.

Assess for diarrhea.

Miscellaneous Drugs

Dronabinol (Marinol)

- Give PO.
- Drug effects can last for days.
- Elevated doses are associated with psychiatric symptoms.
- Do not stop abruptly.

Elevated doses are associated with psychiatric symptoms.

Trimethobenzamide (Tigan)

- Give PO, IM, or PR.
- Capsule can be opened and mixed with food or liquid.
- Low blood pressure can occur in surgical client receiving IM form of drug.
- Stop drug if fever develops.

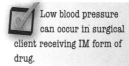
Low blood pressure can occur in surgical client receiving IM form of drug.

PART X • QUESTIONS

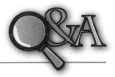

1. All of the following are proton pump inhibitors EXCEPT:
    a. Omeprazole (Prilosec).
    b. Lansoprazole (Prevacid).
    c. Nizatidine (Axid).
    d. Esomeprazole (Nexium).

2. Which age group is particularly sensitive to the effects of histamine-2 antagonists?
    a. Adolescents
    b. Middle-aged adults
    c. Elderly
    d. Young adults

3. Magnesium antacids cause which of the following side effects?
    a. Constipation
    b. Proteinuria
    c. Elevated uric acid level
    d. Diarrhea

4. The nurse is aware of which of the following implications related to misoprostol (Cytotec)?
    a. Give with food
    b. Binds with many drugs
    c. Monitor client for electrolyte problems.
    d. IV solutions are unstable after 48 hours.

5. Which laxatives are considered to be the most natural?
    a. Saline laxatives
    b. Stimulant laxatives
    c. Bulk-forming laxatives
    d. Lubricant laxatives

6. The nurse should observe for which side effect of the saline laxatives?
    a. Potassium imbalance
    b. Alkaline urine
    c. Eosinophilia
    d. Skin rash

7. The nurse should teach the client which of the following about the stimulant laxatives?
   a. Shake the suspension form before taking.
   b. You would not have results from the drug for 3 days.
   c. You should take this at bedtime.
   d. Do not chew the tablet form.

8. A client receiving a bulk-forming laxative tells the nurse he has pain in his chest. The best response for the nurse is:
   a. "Take some Tylenol."
   b. "You may be developing ulcer disease."
   c. "The laxative may be settling in your esophagus."
   d. "You need to take an antacid."

9. Loperamide (Imodium) works by:
   a. Acting on GI muscles.
   b. Stopping action of GI enzymes.
   c. Stimulating areas of the CNS that control GI function.
   d. Decreasing inflammation of the GI tract.

10. Bismuth subsalicylate (Pepto-Bismol) should not be taken by clients who have an allergy to:
   a. Antibiotics.
   b. Warfarin.
   c. Aspirin.
   d. Opiates.

11. A client taking an antidiarrheal should be assessed for which of the following adverse effects?
   a. Appendicitis
   b. Peptic ulcer
   c. Urinary frequency
   d. Dehydration

12. The nurse teaches the client that which of the following is a common side effect of the 5-HT receptor antagonists?
   a. Headache
   b. Constipation
   c. Elevated blood pressure
   d. Blurred vision

13. The nurse should follow all of the guidelines for administration of parenteral antiemetics EXCEPT:
    a. Z track the IM.
    b. Give IM in deltoid site.
    c. Cannot mix with other drugs in a syringe.
    d. IM should be given deeply into tissue.

14. A client who is ordered to take oral trimethobenzamide (Tigan) is unable to swallow the capsule. What should the nurse do?
    a. Ask the physician to order a different medication.
    b. Request the pharmacist to send it in a liquid form.
    c. Give the medication per rectum.
    d. Open the capsule and mix the contents with water.

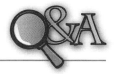

PART X · ANSWERS

1. **The correct answer is c.** Nizatidine (Axid) is a histamine-2 antagonist.

2. **The correct answer is c.** Histamine-2 antagonists can cause confusion in the elderly, and if this occurs, the drug must be stopped.

3. **The correct answer is d.** Magnesium antacids cause diarrhea, while aluminum antacids cause constipation.

4. **The correct answer is a.** Misoprostol (Cytotec) should be given with food to decrease GI irritation.

5. **The correct answer is c.** The bulk-forming laxatives are the most natural as they imitate the process in the body that results in defecation.

6. **The correct answer is b.** Saline laxatives can cause alkaline urine that could lead to the formation of urinary stones.

7. **The correct answer is d.** Enteric-coated tablets must be swallowed whole to keep the enteric coating intact.

8. **The correct answer is c.** A client taking a bulk-forming laxative who complains of retrosternal pain may be experiencing accumulation of the drug in the esophagus. Stop the drug and notify the physician.

9. **The correct answer is a.** Loperamide (Imodium) acts on GI muscles to decrease peristalsis.

10. **The correct answer is c.** Bismuth subsalicylate (Pepto-Bismol) contains aspirin and should not be taken by clients who have aspirin allergy.

11. **The correct answer is d.** Antidiarrheals can cause electrolyte imbalance and dehydration, so the client should be assessed for these problems.

12. **The correct answer is a.** Headache is a common side effect of the 5-HT receptor antagonists, and it usually requires pain medication to relieve it.

13. **The correct answer is b.** IM antiemetics should be given deeply into a large muscle mass.

14. **The correct answer is d.** Trimethobenzamide (Tigan) capsules can be opened and mixed with food or liquid.

XI

Drugs Acting on the Immune System and Antineoplastic Agents

Nancy Elaine Clarkson, MEd, RN, BC

Immunizing agents have been used to protect individuals from infectious diseases for over 200 years.[1] The process of immunization includes giving an antigen to cause an antibody formation for active immunity or a serum from those already immune for passive immunity. The agents that are used consist of vaccines including the toxoids and immune serums (including antitoxins)—collectively called **biologicals.** The immunization of entire populations has proven to be the best defense in disease prevention. While immunization does carry some risk, it is riskier not to immunize people. This chapter will address the vaccines and toxoids together as a group and the immune serums and antitoxins together as another group.

66

Immunizing Agents

Table 66-1 Immunizing Agents

Prototype Drug	Related Drugs	Drug Classification
There is no prototype drug for this classification	hepatitis A vaccine, inactivated (Havrix) hepatitis A vaccine, inactivated, with hepatitis B recombinant vaccine (Twinrix) hepatitis B vaccine (Energix-B) influenza virus vaccine (Fluzone) influenza virus vaccine, intranasal (FluMist) japanese encephalitis vaccine (JE-VAX) measles virus vaccine (Attenuvax) measles, mumps, rubella vaccine (MMR II) measles, mumps, rubella, varicella virus vaccine (ProQuad) measles and rubella virus vaccine, live (M-R-Vax II) mumps virus vaccine (Mumpsvax) poliovirus vaccine, inactivated (Ipol) rabies vaccine (Imovax Rabies) rubella virus vaccine (Meruvax II) rubella and mumps vaccine, live (Biavax II) smallpox vaccine (Dryvax) varicella virus vaccine (Varivax) yellow fever vaccine (Yf-Vax)	Viral vaccines
There is no prototype drug for this classification	BCG (TICE BCG) cholera vaccine haemophilus B conjugate vaccine (ActHIB)	Bacterial vaccines

continues

Table 66-1 Immunizing Agents (continued)

Prototype Drug	Related Drugs	Drug Classification
	haemophilus B vaccine and hepatitis B surface conjugate antigen (Comvax) meningococcal polysaccharide vaccine (Menomune-A/C/Y/W-135) pneumococcal vaccine polyvalent (Pneumovax 23) pneumococcal 7-valent conjugate vaccine (Prevnar) typhoid vaccine (Vivotif Berna Typhim VI)	
There is no prototype drug for this classification	diphtheria and tetanus toxoids, combined, adsorbed (DT) diphtheria and tetanus toxoids and acellular pertussis vaccine, adsorbed (DTaP) diphtheria and tetanus toxoids and acellular pertussis and Haemophilus influenza type B conjugate vaccines (DTaP-Hib) diphtheria and tetanus toxoids and acellular pertussis, adsorbed, and hepatitis B (recombinant) and inactivated, poliovirus vaccine, combined (Pediatrix)	Toxoids
There is no prototype drug for this classification	anti-thymocyte immune globulin (Thymoglobulin) Cytomegalovirus immune globulin (CytoGam) hepatitis B immune globulin (Nabi-HB) immune globulin, intramuscular (BayGam)	Immune Syrums

Table 66-1 Immunizing Agents (continued)

Prototype Drug	Related Drugs	Drug Classification
	immune globulin, intravenous (Gamimune) lymphocyte immune globulin (Atgam) rabies immune globulin (BayRab) respiratory syncytial virus immune globulin (RespiGAM) RHo immune globulin (BayRho-D) RHo immune globulin, microdose (BayRho-D Mini-Dose) tetanus immune globulin (Bay Tet) vaccinia immune globulin IV (VIGIV) varicella zoster immune globulin	
There is no prototype drug for this classification	antivenin black Widow spider antivenin (Antivenin) crotalidae polyvalent immune fab (CroFab)	Antitoxins/Antivenins

IMMUNIZING AGENTS CLIENT TEACHING

For All Vaccines, Toxoids, Immune Serums, and Antitoxins

- Keep a written record of all immunizations for each family member.
- Use acetaminophen (Tylenol) to relieve pain at injection site and fever.

 Keep a written record of all immunizations for each family member.

 Use acetaminophen (Tylenol) to relieve pain at injection site and fever.

* Stay with health care provider at least 30 minutes after receiving immunization.
* If unsure if you have received immunization, it is better to take it than chance getting the disease.
* Make sure children receive required immunizations at correct age intervals.

 Stay with health care provider at least 30 minutes after receiving immunization.

Vaccines and Toxoids

* Women must avoid pregnancy for 3 months after receiving Rubella and Varicella vaccine.
* Must stay away from pregnant women, those with depressed immune systems, and newborns after receiving Varicella vaccine

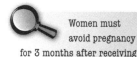 Women must avoid pregnancy for 3 months after receiving Rubella and Varicella vaccine.

ACTION

Vaccines and Toxoids

* Cause active immunity to develop via the antigen-antibody response. A number of vaccines provide life-long protection from disease, while toxoids require additional dosing to keep immunity going.

Immune Serums and Antitoxins

* Cause passive immunity to develop via the antigen-antibody response
* Offer temporary protection to those exposed or already undergoing disease

USE

Vaccines and Toxoids

* Chickenpox
* Cholera
* Diphtheria

- Haemophilus B
- Hepatitis A and B
- Influenza
- Measles
- Meningococcus
- Mumps
- Pertussis
- Pneumococcus
- Polio
- Rabies
- Rubella
- Tetanus
- Tuberculosis
- Typhoid fever
- Yellow fever

Immune Serums and Antitoxins

- Cytomegalovirus infection after kidney transplant
- After exposure to hepatitis A and B, measles, mumps, rubella
- After organ transplant and bone marrow transplant
- Kawasaki's disease
- Immunoglobulin deficiency
- Chronic lymphocytic leukemia
- Aplastic anemia
- Allograft rejection in kidney transplant
- Persons exposed to rabies who were not previously immunized
- Respiratory syncytial virus
- Sensitization to Rh factor
- Varicella zoster
- Snake bite
- Black Widow spider bite
- Tetanus

ADVERSE EFFECTS AND SIDE EFFECTS

Vaccines, Toxoids, Immune Serums, and Antitoxins

- *Pregnancy categories will not be listed as these drugs are contraindicated in pregnancy. The physician needs to ultimately decide whether or not a pregnant client should receive an immunization.*

- *CNS:* Shock, unconsciousness, convulsions, encephalitis, peripheral neuropathy
- *Derm:* Rash, itching
- *Resp:* Dyspnea
- *Other:* Pain and tenderness at site of injection, fever, muscle aches, serum sickness, anaphylaxis

 ## INTERACTIONS

Vaccines, Toxoids, immune Serums, and Antitoxins

- Phenytoin (Dilantin), antineoplastic drugs, corticosteroids, and any immunosuppressant drug will decrease effects of vaccines
- Isoniazid decreases effects of BCG vaccine
- Salicylates given to a child who has received the Varicella vaccine can elevate chance of Reye's syndrome developing.

 ## CONTRAINDICATIONS

Vaccines and Toxoids

- Pregnancy
- Immune deficiency in the body
- Allergy to any parts of the vaccine or toxoid
- Clients who have received blood, blood products, or immune globulin in last 3 months
- Cautious use in acute infection, febrile convulsions, brain injury

Immune Serums and Antitoxins

- Pregnancy
- Allergy to any parts of the serum or antitoxin
- Cautious use in client who already received immune serum and in coagulation disorders

NURSING IMPLICATIONS

For All Vaccines, Toxoids, immune Serums, and Antitoxins

- Always aspirate after injection to prevent mistaken IV administration.
- Never give expired product.
- Use products that are reconstituted within recommended time frame.
- Emergency equipment and drugs must be readily available.
- Client should be observed for one-half hour after receiving injection.

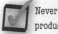
Always aspirate after injection to prevent mistaken IV administration.

Never give expired product.

Use products that are reconstituted within recommended time frame.

Emergency equipment and drugs must be readily available.

Vaccines and Toxoids

- Give SC and IM.
- MMR vaccine must be given within 8 hours of reconstituting. Only use diluent supplied by drug manufacturer.
- Do not administer hepatitis B vaccine in gluteal muscles; give SC to clients who bleed from IM injections.
- If client has symptoms of an acute infection, do not give immunization.

MMR vaccine must be given within 8 hours of reconstituting. Only use diluent supplied by drug manufacturer.

If client has symptoms of an acute infection, do not give immunization.

Immune Serums and Antitoxins

- Give IM and IV.
- Use an 18- to 20-gauge needle and give in gluteal muscle for Human Immune Serum Globulin.

REFERENCE

1. Spratto G, Woods A. *PDR Nurse's Drug Handbook.* Clifton Park, NY: Delmar Learning; 2006:1694.

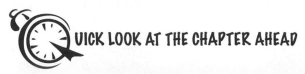

As the name implies, the immunosuppressant agents interfere with the immune response. They are used to prevent rejection in organ transplantation and in the treatment of autoimmune diseases. The older members of the group tend to suppress the entire immune response, and this in turn can leave the client exposed to any number of life-threatening infections as well as increase the risk for cancer. The newer members of the group have been developed to act more specifically on the immune system and have fewer adverse effects.

67

Immunosuppressant
Agents

TERMS
☐ cyclosporine
  (Sandimmune)
☐ muromonab-CD3
  (Orthoclone OKT3)

Table 67-1 Immunosuppressant Agents

Prototype Drug	Related Drugs	Drug Classification
cyclosporine (Sandimmune)	alefacept (Amevive) azathioprine (Imuran) glatiramer acetate (Copaxone) methotrexate (Rheumatrex) mycophenolate (CellCeft) pimecrolimus (Elidel) sirolimus (Rapamune) tacrolimus (Prograf)	T- and B-cell suppressors
muromonab CD3 (Orthoclone OKT3)	adalimubab (Humira) alemtuzmab (Campath) basiliximab (Simulect) bevacizumab (Avastin) cetuximab (Erbitux) daclizumab (Zenapax) efalizumab (Raptiva) erlotinib (Tarceva) gemtuzumab (Mylotarg) ibritumomab (Zevalin) ifliximab (Remicade) natalizumab (Tysabri) omalizumab (Xolair) palivizumab (Synagis) pegaptanib (Macugen) rituximab (Rituxan) trastuzumab (Herceptin)	Monoclonal antibodies

 IMMUNOSUPPRESSANT AGENTS CLIENT TEACHING

For All Immunosuppressant Agents

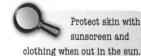

- Protect skin with sunscreen and clothing when out in the sun.
- Notify physician before taking any drugs when taking immunosuppressants.
- Do not become pregnant while on drug therapy.
- You are at high risk for infection, so wash your hands frequently; stay away from individuals who are ill and report sore throat, fever, or any symptoms of feeling unwell to physician.

Protect skin with sunscreen and clothing when out in the sun.

Notify physician before taking any drugs when taking immuno-suppressants.

- All side effects need to be reported immediately to physician.

T- and B-Cell Suppressors

Do not become pregnant while on drug therapy.

- Can take with food
- Do not breast-feed
- Excess hair will go away when you stop taking drug.
- Drugs should be taken on same schedule each day to maintain drug levels.
- Oral solutions should be mixed in glass not plastic and drunk immediately after mixing.

Can take with food

Drugs should be taken on same schedule each day to maintain drug levels.

Monoclonal Antibodies

Do not become pregnant while on drug therapy or for 3 months after ending therapy.

- Do not become pregnant while on drug therapy or for 3 months after ending therapy.
- Notify physician of fever, infection, nausea, vomiting, wheezing, or chest pain.
- Eat small, frequent meals to keep weight stable.

ACTION

T and B Cell Suppressors

- The action is not fully known. These drugs do interfere with the release of T-cell growth factor and interleukins, hamper the activity of helper and suppressor T-cells, and prevent antibody production by B-cells.

Monoclonal Antibodies

- Block specific receptor sites in the immune system. The prototype drug, muromonab-CD3 (Orthoclone OKT3), acts as an antibody to T-cells and inactivates them, thus suppressing the immune system.

USE

T- and B-Cell Suppressors

* Prevention of rejection in kidney, heart, and liver transplants
* Rheumatoid arthritis
* Decreases relapses in multiple sclerosis

Monoclonal Antibodies

* Prevention of rejection in kidney, heart, and liver transplants
* Respiratory syncytial virus (RSV)
* Crohn's disease
* Relapsed follicular B-cell non-Hodgkin's lymphoma
* Breast cancer tumors that over-express HER2 protein
* B-cell chronic lymphocytic leukemia
* Colorectal cancer
* Plaque psoriasis
* Relapsing forms of multiple sclerosis
* Asthma
* Neovascular age-related macular degeneration

 ## ADVERSE EFFECTS AND SIDE EFFECTS

T- and B-Cell Suppressors

* *Pregnancy category C, except for glatiramer acetate (Copaxone), which is category B, and azathioprine (Imuran) and methotrexate (Rheumatrex), which are category D*
* *CNS:* Tremor, headache, seizures, depression, confusion, hallucinations
* *CV:* High blood pressure
* *Derm:* Hirsutism, acne, oily skin
* *EENT:* Tinnitus, hearing loss
* *Endocrine:* Elevated blood glucose, gynecomastia
* *F & E:* Decreased serum bicarbonate, elevated potassium, and magnesium
* *GI:* Nausea, vomiting, diarrhea, gingival hyperplasia, anorexia

- *GU:* Nephrotoxicity
- *Hematologic:* Anemia, leukopenia, thrombocytopenia
- *Resp:* Sinusitis
- *Other:* Sore throat, lymphoma, leg cramps, fever, chills, edema, weight loss

Monoclonal Antibodies

- *Pregnancy category C, except adalimumab (Humira), basiliximab (Simulect), omalizumab (Xolair), and trastuzumab (Herceptin) which are category B, and erlotinib (Tarceva), gemtuzumab (Mylotarg) and infliximab (Remicade), which are category D.*
- *CNS:* Tremor
- *CV:* Elevated heart rate
- *GI:* Diarrhea, nausea, vomiting
- *Resp:* Wheezing, difficulty breathing, chest pain, pulmonary edema
- *Other:* Chills, fever, risk of *Pneumocystis carinii*, Legionella, Crytococcus, Serratia, Cytomegalovirus, Herpes simplex

INTERACTIONS

T- and B-Cell Suppressors

- Drugs that are toxic to the kidney and liver increase the toxicity of T and B cell suppressors.

Monoclonal Antibodies

- Concurrent use with other immunosuppressants greatly elevates immune suppression and can lead to development of cancer and severe infections.

CONTRAINDICATIONS

T-and B-Cell Suppressors

- Lactation
- Pregnancy

- Allergy to these drugs
- Liver or kidney disease

Monoclonal Antibodies

- Overload of fluid
- Allergy to these drugs

NURSING IMPLICATIONS

T- and B-Cell Suppressors

- Give PO and IV.
- IV administration should be slow.
- Monitor client for at least one-half hour after IV administration started.
- Do not give oral form with grapefruit juice.
- Monitor vital signs.
- Monitor I & O.
- Monitor the following blood tests: K, liver, and kidney function.
- If client has psoriasis, monitor the following blood tests: K, magnesium, BUN, CBC, uric acid.
- Assess neurological function on an ongoing basis.

IV administration should be slow.

Monitor client for at least one-half hour after IV administration started.

Assess neurological function on an ongoing basis.

Monoclonal Antibodies

- Give SC, IM, or IV.
- IV form should not be mixed with other drugs.
- Assess client for "first dose response" (chills fever, dyspnea).
- Monitor for fluid overload.
- Do not administer if client's temperature is above 100° F.
- Monitor vital signs.

IV form should not be mixed with other drugs.

Assess client for "first dose response" (chills fever, dyspnea).

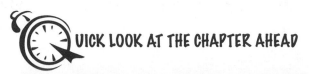

The biologic response modifiers are a group of drugs that can either extend the immune system's ability to rid the body of damaging attackers or help the immune system to function normally. This group is composed of the **interferons, interleukins, hematopoietic agents,** and **colony-stimulating factors.** They are mainly used in the treatment of cancer and in other autoimmune diseases. While these drugs play an important role in the battle against life-altering diseases, they have serious side effects which make it very difficult for clients to deal with.

68

Biologic Response Modifiers

TERMS
- ☐ **interferon alfa-2a (Roferon-A)**
- ☐ **aldesleukin (Proleukin)**
- ☐ **epoetin alfa (Epogen, Procrit)**
- ☐ **filgrastim (Neupogen)**

Table 68-1 Biologic Response Modifiers

Prototype Drug	Related Drugs	Drug Classification
interferon alfa-2a (Roferon-A)	interferon alfa-2b (Intron-A) interferon alfacon-1 (Infergen) interferon alfa-n1 lymphoblastoid (Wellferon) interferon alfa-n3 (Alferon N) interferon beta-1a (Avonex) interferon beta-1b (Betaseron) interferon gamma-1b (Actimmune) peginterferon alfa-2a (Pega sys)	Interferons
aldesleukin (Proleukin)	oprelvekin (Neumega)	Interleukins
epoetin alfa (Epogen; Procrit)	darbepoetin alfa (Aranesp)	Hematopoietic agents
filgrastim (Neupogen)	pegfilgrastim (Neulasta) sargramostim (Leukine)	Colony-stimulating factors

BIOLOGIC RESPONSE MODIFIERS CLIENT TEACHING

For All Biologic Response Modifiers

- Tell all health care providers you are taking one of these drugs.
- Wash hands frequently.
- Avoid crowds and those who are sick.
- Follow-up blood tests and physician visits must be done.

Interferons

- Increase fluid intake.
- Take drug at hour of sleep to decreases common side effects.

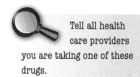

Tell all health care providers you are taking one of these drugs.

Wash hands frequently.

Avoid crowds and those who are sick.

- Keep drug in refrigerator.
- Vial must not be shaken or frozen.
- Learn correct injection technique.
- Use the same brand.
- Do not get pregnant.

Take drug at hour of sleep to decreases common side effects.

Interleukins

- Do not get pregnant.
- No over-the-counter drugs unless approved by physician.

No over-the-counter drugs unless approved by physician.

Hematopoietic Agents

- Do not breast-feed.
- Headache is common.
- Seizures may occur during first 3 months of therapy, so no activities that require concentration
- Go to all check-ups.

Seizures may occur during first 3 months of therapy, so no activities that require concentration

Colony-Stimulating Factors

- Do not breast-feed.
- Tell physician if you have bone pain, so you will be given pain medication.

Tell physician if you have bone pain, so you will be given pain medication.

℞ ACTION

Interferons

- Prevent reproduction and growth of cancer cells and viruses

Interleukins

- Stop growth of cancer cells by extending the activity and numbers of lymphocytes

Hematopoietic Agents

- Enhance the creation of red blood cells in the bone marrow

Colony-Stimulating Factors

- Enhance the creation of red blood cells, platelets, and white blood cells by attaching to receptor sites on cells in the bone marrow

 # USE

Interferons

- Multiple sclerosis
- Chronic hepatitis B and C
- Malignant melanoma
- Genital warts
- AIDS-related Kaposi's sarcoma in adults
- Hairy cell leukemia in adults
- Chronic myelogenous leukemia

Interleukins

- Kidney cell carcinoma
- Prevention of severe thrombocytopenia in nonmyeloid cancers

Hematopoietic Agents

- Anemia that occurs in chronic renal failure and cancer chemotherapy

Colony-Stimulating Factors

- Chronic neutropenia
- Mobilization of stem cells for collection
- Stop infection in clients with neutropenia from cancer chemotherapy
- Enhancement of bone marrow function after bone marrow transplant

ADVERSE EFFECTS AND SIDE EFFECTS

Interferons

- *Pregnancy category C*
- *CNS:* Sleepiness, psychosis, seizures, hallucinations, confusion, irritability
- *CV:* Orthostatic hypotension, rapid heart beat, EKG changes, cyanosis
- *GI:* Dry mouth, anorexia, nausea, vomiting, diarrhea, elevated hepatic function tests
- *GU:* Elevated creatinine and BUN, proteinuria
- *Hematological:* Thrombocytopenia, neutropenia

Interleukins

- *Pregnancy category C*
- *CNS:* Headache, fatigue
- *CV:* myocardial infarction (MI,) congestive heart failure, arrhythmias
- *Derm:* Rash
- *GI:* Toxic to liver
- *Hematologic:* Eosinophilia
- *Resp:* Respiratory distress
- *Other:* Capillary leak syndrome, fever, chills, muscle aches

Hematopoietic Agents

- *Pregnancy category C*
- *CNS:* Seizures, dizziness, headache, weakness
- *CV:* Chest pain, edema, high blood pressure
- *GI:* Diarrhea, nausea, vomiting

Colony-Stimulating Factors

- *Pregnancy category C*
- *CNS:* Headache
- *CV:* Edema, high blood pressure
- *Derm:* Rash, hair loss

- *GI:* Diarrhea, nausea, vomiting, anorexia
- *Hematologic:* Blood dyscrasias
- *Resp:* Sore throat, dyspnea, cough
- *Other:* Bone pain, fever

INTERACTIONS

Interferons

- Use with Interleukins risks possibility of kidney failure
- Additional myleosuppression with antineoplastics
- Elevated levels of theophylline (Theo-Dur) if given together
- Concurrent use with antivirals can cause blood disorders.
- Concurrent use with vinblastine (Velban) elevates risk of neurotoxicity.

Interleukins

- Corticosteroids decrease effects of interleukins.
- Concurrent use with the following increases effects of Interleukins: antineoplastics, NSAIDs, opioid analgesics, antihypertensives, aminoglycosides.

Hematopoietic Agents

- None

Colony-Stimulating Factors

- Antagonistic effect when given with myelosuppressive antineoplastic agents.

CONTRAINDICATIONS

Interferons

- Allergy to drug components and mouse immunoglobulin
- Children under 18 years of age
- Lactation
- Pregnancy

Interleukins

- Lactation
- Pregnancy
- Allergy to any drug components

Hematopoietic Agents

- Lactation
- Allergy to drug components
- Uncontrolled hypertension

Colony-Stimulating Factors

- Myeloid cancers
- Antineoplastic agents
- *Escherichia coli (E. coli)*

 NURSING IMPLICATIONS

Interferons

- Give SC or IM.
- SC administration should be given at same time each day.
- Monitor I & O.
- Expect flu-like syndrome 2 to 6 hours after one dose, which decreases with ongoing therapy.
- Elderly more likely to be cardiotoxic.
- Vital signs
- No activities requiring concentration until drug effects are known
- Assess for oral *Candida albicans.*
- Monitor lab tests: CBC, platelets, liver, and kidney function.
- Assess for bleeding.

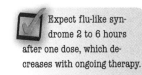
Expect flu-like syndrome 2 to 6 hours after one dose, which decreases with ongoing therapy.

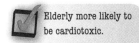
Elderly more likely to be cardiotoxic.

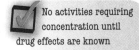
No activities requiring concentration until drug effects are known

Interleukins

- Give SC or IV.
- Do not shake vial when mixing drug.

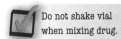
Do not shake vial when mixing drug.

- IV form is compatible with D5W.
- Must be used within 48 hours of reconstitution
- No in-line filters for IV use
- Monitor for infection and cardiac function.
- Monitor lab tests: CBC, electrolytes, kidney, and liver function.

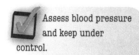
Monitor for infection and cardiac function.

Hematopoietic Agents

- Give SC or IV.
- Do not shake vial.
- IV form is given as a bolus over 1 minute.
- Assess blood pressure and keep under control.
- Monitor hematocrit and inform physician if elevating quickly. Risk for seizures increases during this time.
- Assess neurological status and for thrombotic events.
- Monitor lab tests: platelets, CBC, kidney function, electrolytes, activated partial prothromboplastine time.

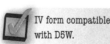
Assess blood pressure and keep under control.

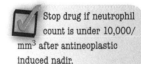
Monitor hematocrit and inform physician if elevating quickly. Risk for seizures increases during this time.

Colony-Stimulating Factors

- Give SC or IV.
- Solution in vial can stay at room temperature for 6 hours and then must be discarded.
- IV form is compatible with D5W.
- Check temperature every 4 hours.
- Assess bone pain.
- MI and arrhythmias are seen in clients with history of heart disease.
- Stop drug if neutrophil count is under 10,000/mm^3 after antineoplastic induced nadir.
- Monitor lab tests: platelets, CBC, WBC.

IV form compatible with D5W.

Stop drug if neutrophil count is under 10,000/mm^3 after antineoplastic induced nadir.

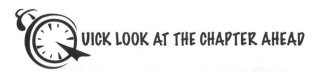
The antineoplastic agents are one of the treatment options for cancer along with surgery and radiation therapy. These drugs work in the reproductive cycle of the cell. Some are active during a particular phase of the cell cycle and are called cell cycle specific, while others act at any point in the cell cycle and are called cell cycle nonspecific. Both malignant and normal cells are affected by the antineoplastic agents. This accounts for their harmful effects on hair follicles, bone marrow, and the gastrointestinal system.

The cytoprotectant agents are a small group of drugs that assist in lessening the harsh and sometimes life-threatening adverse effects of the antineoplastic agents. Some of them work with specific anticancer drugs and others have a generalized effect on the body. This group of drugs will not be discussed in detail, but the reader should be familiar with the names of the drugs included in Table 69-1.

69

Antineoplastic Agents

TERMS
- ☐ cyclophosphamide (Cytoxan)
- ☐ fluorouracil (Adrucil)
- ☐ doxorubicin (Adriamycin)
- ☐ vincristine (Oncovin)
- ☐ tamoxifen (Nolvadex)

Table 69-1 Antineoplastic Agents

Prototype Drug	Related Drugs	Drug Classification
cyclophosphamide (Cytoxan)	busulfan (Myleran) carboplatin (Paraplatin) carmustine (BiCNU) chlorambucil (Leukeran) cisplatin (Platinol-AQ) ifosfamide (Ifex) lomustine (CeeNu) mechlorethamine (Mustargen) melphalan (Alkeran) oxaliplatin (Eloxatin) streptozocin (Zanosar) thiotepa (Thioplex)	Alkylating agents
fluorouracil (Adrucil)	capecitabine (Xeloda) cladribine (Leustatin) clofarabine (Clolar) cytarabine (Ara-C) floxuridine (FUDR) fludarabine (Fludara) mercaptopurine (Purinethol) methotrexate (Folex) pemetrexed (Alimta) pentostatin (Nipent) tioguanine (Lanvis)	Antimetabolites
doxorubicin (Adriamycin)	bleomycin (Blenoxane) dactinomycin (Cosmegen) daunorubicin (DaunoXome) epirubicin (Ellence) idarubicin (Idamycin) mitomycin (Mutamycin) mitoxantrone (Novantrone) plicamycin (Mithracin) valrubicin (Valstar)	Antibiotics
vincristine (Oncovin)	docetaxel (Taxotere) etoposide (Toposar) paclitaxel (Taxol) teniposide (Vumon) vinblastine (Velban) vinorelbine (Navelbine)	Plant alkaloids

continues

Table 69-1 Antineoplastic Agents (continued)

Prototype Drug	Related Drugs	Drug Classification

tamoxifen (Nolvadex)	anastrozole (Arimidex)
	bicalutamide (Casodex)
	estramustine (Emcyt)
	exemestane (Aromasine)
	flutamide (Eulexin)
	fulvestrant (Faslodex)
	goserelin (Zoladex)
	letrozole (Femara)
	leuprolide (Lupron)
	megestrol (Megace)
	nilutamide (Nilandron)
	testolactone (Teslac)
	toremifene (Fareston)
	triptorelin pamoate
	  (Trelstar Depot)
		Hormones and
		  hormone modulators

There is no prototype drug for this classification	asparaginase (Elspar) hydroxyurea (Hydrea) procarbazine (Matulane)	Miscellaneous agents
There is no prototype drug for this classification	amifostine (Ethyol) dexrazoxane (Zinecard) leucovorin (Wellcovorin) mesna (Mesnex) rasburicase (Elitek)	Cytoprotectant agents

ANTINEOPLASTIC AGENTS CLIENT TEACHING

For All Antineoplastics

- Do not become pregnant.
- Do not breast-feed.
- All health care providers need to know you are taking an antineoplastic agent.
- If hair loss occurs, it will be temporary.
- Use soft-bristled toothbrush.
- Inspect mouth daily for sores.
- Avoid crowds and those who are ill.
- Wash hands frequently.
- Attend all physician visits and get blood tests done as ordered.

If hair loss occurs, it will be temporary.

Inspect mouth daily for sores.

Avoid crowds and those who are ill.

- Eat a nutritious diet.
- Do not alter dosing.
- Report all side effects.
- No OTC drugs unless approved by physician.

Alkylating Agents

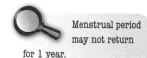

Menstrual period may not return for 1 year.

- Menstrual period may not return for 1 year.
- If unable to take dose, physician must be notified.
- Report bloody urine.

Antimetabolites

Stay out of the sun.

- Stay out of the sun.
- Problems with balance and ambulation must be reported to physician.

Antibiotics

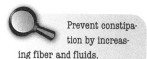

If taking doxorubicin (Adriamycin), urine will be red for up to 2 days after receiving drug.

- If taking doxorubicin (Adriamycin), urine will be red for up to 2 days after receiving drug.

Plant Alkaloids

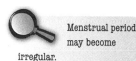

Prevent constipation by increasing fiber and fluids.

- Prevent constipation by increasing fiber and fluids.

Hormones and Hormone Modulators

Menstrual period may become irregular.

- Stay out of the sun.
- Menstrual period may become irregular.

Miscellaneous Agents

Asparaginase (Elspar)

- No activities requiring concentration
- Toxic effects will be experienced.

Hydroxyurea (Hydrea)

- Toxic effects will be experienced.

Procarbazine (Matulane)

- No foods high in tyramines
- No alcohol
- No activities requiring concentration
- Stay out of the sun.
- Report any signs of bleeding.

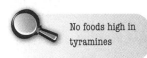

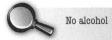

 ACTION

Alkylating Agents

- Interfere with processes that affect DNA, causing the cell to die. They are cell cycle nonspecific.

Antimetabolites

- Interfere with creation of DNA or help produce faulty DNA. They act in the S phase of the cell cycle.

Antibiotics

- Attach to DNA, which impedes copying of DNA and RNA. They are cell cycle nonspecific.

Plant Alkaloids

- Bring about cell death by preventing cell division or interfering with DNA synthesis. They are cell cycle specific.

Hormones and Hormone Modulators

- Stop cancer growth in hormone-dependent tissues by preventing protein synthesis

Miscellaneous Agents

Asparaginase (Elspar)

* Removes an amino acid needed in the synthesis of DNA

Hydroxyurea (Hydrea)

* Prevents formation of DNA by hindering the presence of the nucleoside, thymidine

Procarbazine (Matulane)

* Action is unknown. This drug acts in the S phase of cell cycle.

 USE

Alkylating Agents

* Cancer of the breast, uterus, bladder, pancreas, ovary, lung, brain, and testicle
* Multiple myeloma
* Hodgkin's disease
* Leukemia
* Lymphoma
* Antimetabolites
* Leukemia
* GI and breast cancer
* Basal cell carcinoma
* Psoriasis
* Rheumatoid arthritis

Antibiotics

* Cancer of bladder, testicle, pancreas, stomach
* Leukemia
* Multiple sclerosis
* Bone pain in prostate cancer
* Kaposi's sarcoma
* Lymphoma

Plant Alkaloids

- Cancer of lung, testicle, ovary, breast
- Leukemia
- Sarcoma
- Lymphoma
- Hodgkin's disease

Hormones and Hormone Modulators

- Cancer of breast, prostate

Miscellaneous Agents

Asparaginase (Elspar)

- Acute lymphocytic leukemia

Hydroxyurea (Hydrea)

- Sickle cell anemia
- Squamous cell carcinoma of head and neck
- Myelocytic leukemia
- Melanoma
- Cancer of ovary

Procarbazine (Matulane)

- Hodgkin's disease

ADVERSE EFFECTS AND SIDE EFFECTS

Alkylating Agents

- *Pregnancy category D, except for cyclophosphamide (Cytoxan) and streptozocin (Zanosar), which are category C*
- *CNS:* Dizziness
- *Derm:* Hair loss, increased pigmentation in skin and nails, facial flushing
- *F & E:* Decreased sodium, increased uric acid, decreased potassium

- *GI:* Anorexia, nausea, vomiting
- *GU:* Kidney toxicity, hemorrhagic cystitis
- *Hematologic:* Neutropenia
- *Resp:* Pneumonitis, pulmonary emboli
- *Other:* Fatigue, increased perspiration

Antimetabolites

- *Pregnancy category D*
- *CNS:* Euphoria
- *CV:* Angina
- *Derm*: Hair loss, photosensitivity, systemic lupus erythematosus-like dermatitis, erythema
- *GI:* Diarrhea, nausea, vomiting, stomatitis
- *Hematologic:* Thrombocytopenia, anemia, leukopenia
- *Other:* Edema of legs, face, eyes and tongue; hypersensitivity reaction; topical application can cause itching, burning, pain, swelling, and scarring

Antibiotics

- *Pregnancy category D, except for dactinomycin (Cosmegen), plicamycin (Mithracin), and valubicin (Valstar), which are category C*
- *CNS:* Sleepiness
- *CV:* Irreversible cardiac damage
- *Derm:* Hair loss, increased pigmentation of buccal mucosa, tongue and nails, facial flushing with quick IV administration, and rash; extravasation from IV administration can cause severe tissue damage from cellulitis to tissue necrosis.
- *F & E:* Increased uric acid
- *GI:* Diarrhea, stomatitis, nausea, vomiting, anorexia
- *GU:* Blood in the urine
- *Hematologic:* Anemia, leukopenia, severe myelosuppression
- *Other:* Tearing, fever

Plant Alkaloids

- *Pregnancy category D, except for paclitaxel (Taxol), which is category X*

- *CNS:* Paresthesias of feet and hands, peripheral neuropathy, seizures, headache
- *CV:* High or low blood pressure
- *Derm:* Hair loss
- *EENT:* Double vision, intolerance to light, blindness
- *F & E:* Increased potassium and uric acid
- *GI:* Constipation, paralytic ileus in children, stomatitis, nausea, vomiting, anorexia
- *GU:* Dysuria, polyuria, urine retention
- *Resp:* Bronchospasm
- *Other:* Fever, weight loss

Hormones and Hormone Modulators

- *The following are pregnancy category C: nilutamide (Nilandron) and testolactone (Teslac); the following are pregnancy category D: anastrozole (Arimidex), exemestane (Aromasine), flutamide (Eulexin), fulvestrant (Faslodex), letrozole (Femara), tamoxifen (Nolvadex), and toremifene (Fareston); the following are pregnancy category X: bicalutamide (Casodex), estramustine (Emcyt), goserelin (Zoladex), leuprolide (Lupron), megestrol (Megace), and triptorelin pamoate (Trelstar Depot).*
- *CNS:* Headache, dizziness, sleepiness, confusion
- *CV:* Thrombosis
- *Derm:* Rash, photosensitivity, hair loss
- *EENT:* Blurred vision, retinopathy
- *F & E:* Increased calcium
- *GI:* Anorexia, nausea, vomiting
- *GU:* Menstrual changes, leaking of milk from breasts
- *Hematologic:* Thrombocytopenia, leukopenia
- *Resp:* Shortness of breath
- *Other:* Hot flashes, bone pain, increased weight

Miscellaneous Agents

Asparaginase (Elspar)

- *Pregnancy category C*
- *CNS:* Agitation, confusion, hallucinations, depression
- *Endocrine:* Elevated blood glucose
- *F & E:* Increased uric acid, decreased calcium and albumin

- *GI:* Pancreatitis, nausea, vomiting, anorexia
- *GU:* Kidney failure
- *Hematologic:* Leukopenia, decreased fibrinogen, platelets and clotting factors
- *Other:* Infection, allergic reaction, weight loss, increased sweating

Hydroxyurea (Hydrea)

- *Pregnancy category D*
- *Derm:* Rash, red face
- *F & E:* Increased uric acid
- *GI:* Nausea, vomiting, diarrhea
- *GU:* Kidney dysfunction; increased BUN and creatinine
- *Hematologic:* Decreased bone marrow function
- *Other:* Fever, chills

Procarbazine (Matulane)

- *Pregnancy category D*
- *CNS:* Seizures, paresthesias, headache, dizziness, hallucinations
- *CV:* Low blood pressure, elevated heart rate
- *Derm:* Hair loss, flushing, itching, dermatitis, increased pigmentation, photosensitivity
- *Endocrine:* Growth of breast tissue in males
- *GI:* Nausea, vomiting
- *GU:* Shrinking of testicles
- *Hematologic:* Decreased bone marrow function
- *Resp:* Cough, pleural effusion
- *Other:* Fever, chills, increased perspiration

INTERACTIONS

Alkylating Agents

- Do not give with other drugs that are toxic to liver and kidneys as there is an additive effect.

Antimetabolites

- Any drug that has similar toxicities to this group will result in additive toxicities.

Antibiotics

- Any drug that has similar toxicities to this group will result in additive toxicities.

Plant Alkaloids

- Any drug with hepatic toxicity will have an additive effect.

Hormone and Hormone Modulators

- Elevated chance of bleeding if taken with anticoagulants

Miscellaneous Agents

Asparaginase (Elspar)

- Concurrent use with corticosteroids and vincristine (Oncovin) increases toxicity.
- Concurrent use with insulin and sulfonylureas decreases effects of these drugs.

Hydroxyurea (Hydrea)

- No interactions

Procarbazine (Matulane)

- Any drug with CNS depressant effect will have an additive depressant effect.
- Hypertensive crisis may occur with ephedrine (Efedon), sympathomimetics, MAOI, tricyclic antidepressants (TCAs), and foods containing tyramine.

CONTRAINDICATIONS

For All Antineoplastic Agents

- Pregnancy
- Lactation
- Allergy to any of these drugs
- Bone marrow depression

Alkylating Agents

* Liver or kidney disorder
* Antimetabolites
* GI disease
* Liver or kidney disorder

Antibiotics

* GI, liver, pulmonary, cardiac, or kidney disease

Plant Alkaloids

* GI, kidney, or liver disease

Hormones and Hormone Modulators

* Liver or kidney disease
* Toremifene (Fareston) cannot be given when calcium is elevated.

Miscellaneous Agents

Asparaginase (Elspar)

* Pancreatitis
* Chickenpox
* Herpes

Hydroxyurea (Hydrea)

* There are no contraindications for this drug.

Procarbazine (Matulane)

* Alcohol
* Foods containing tyramines

NURSING IMPLICATIONS

For All Antineoplastic Agents

* Use safe handling precautions if preparing IV form.

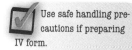

Use safe handling precautions if preparing IV form.

- Monitor lab tests: CBC, kidney, and liver function
- Monitor I & O.
- Weigh client.
- Prevent infection.

Alkylating Agents

- Give PO or IV.
- Administer PO form without food.
- Give antiemetic for nausea/vomiting.
- Report all side effects.
- Monitor lab tests: platelets, serum electrolytes.
- Leukopenia is side effect to be most concerned about. Blood count reconverts to normal 7 to 10 days after drug is stopped.
- Granulocyte count less than 1000 is considered a medical crisis.

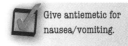

Give antiemetic for nausea/vomiting.

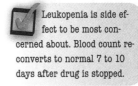

Leukopenia is side effect to be most concerned about. Blood count reconverts to normal 7 to 10 days after drug is stopped.

Antimetabolites

- Give PO, IM, topical, or IV.
- Wear gloves for topical application.
- Assess client's mouth.
- Stop drug if client is confused or disoriented.
- If WBC is less than 3500/mm^3, client will need to be put in protective isolation.

Stop drug if client is confused or disoriented.

If WBC is less than 3500/mm^3, client will need to be put in protective isolation.

Antibiotics

- Give SC, IM, IV, or intravesically.
- Assess IV site and terminate infusion if there is burning or discomfort at site.
- Assess oral mucous membranes.
- Frequent oral hygiene
- Assess heart function before, during, and after therapy.
- No rectal temperatures or medications

Assess oral mucous membranes.

Assess heart function before, during, and after therapy.

Plant Alkaloids

- Give IV.
- No rectal temperatures or medications
- Assess walking.
- Peripheral neuropathy and paresthesias are often seen in children and stop after 6 weeks of treatment.

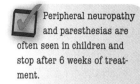

Peripheral neuropathy and paresthesias are often seen in children and stop after 6 weeks of treatment.

Hormones and Hormone Modulators

- Give PO or SC.
- Pain indicates cancer is responding to drug.
- Medicate with analgesics as needed.
- Effects of drug may take 4 to 10 weeks to occur.

Effects of drug may take 4 to 10 weeks to occur.

Miscellaneous Agents

Asparaginase (Elspar)

- Give IV.
- Skin test is done before IV administration.
- IV administration requires continuous monitoring by health care provider.
- Allergic reactions typically happen 30 to 60 minutes after IV dose.
- Assess for neurotoxic reaction (levels of consciousness change) in initial days of therapy.
- Diabetics need close assessment of glucose levels.
- Monitor lab tests: serum uric acid, ammonia, amylase, and calcium; coagulation studies.
- Toxicity is seen more in adults than children.

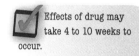

Skin test is done before IV administration.

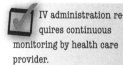

IV administration requires continuous monitoring by health care provider.

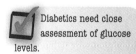

Diabetics need close assessment of glucose levels.

Hydroxyurea (Hydrea)

- Give PO.
- Contents of capsules can be mixed with water if client is unable to swallow capsule.
- Monitor lab tests: platelet count.

- If client's uric acid level is elevated, increase daily fluid intake to 2 to 3 L/day.
- Stop drug if WBC and platelet levels drop.

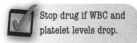

Stop drug if WBC and platelet levels drop.

Procarbazine (Matulane)

- Give PO.
- Stop drug if WBC count and platelet levels drop.
- Monitor lab tests: platelets.
- Nausea and vomiting are common, and tolerance will occur after initial week of therapy.
- Assess for CNS effects and report to physician.

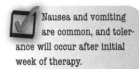

Nausea and vomiting are common, and tolerance will occur after initial week of therapy.

PART XI · QUESTIONS

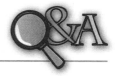

1. What can happen to a child who has taken aspirin just after receiving the varicella vaccine?
    a. Nothing, the child will be fine.
    b. Reye's syndrome may develop.
    c. Respiratory distress may occur.
    d. Increased bleeding time.

2. Vaccines, toxoids, immune serums, and antitoxins are contraindicated in:
    a. Pregnancy
    b. Coagulation disorders
    c. Brain injury
    d. Febrile convulsions

3. Which of the following side effects may occur after receiving a vaccine?
    a. Vomiting
    b. Headache
    c. Pain at injection site
    d. Heart palpitations

4. The monoclonal antibodies are used to treat all of the following EXCEPT:
    a. Crohn's Disease.
    b. Plaque psoriasis.
    c. Rheumatoid arthritis.
    d. Asthma.

5. The T and B suppressors are used in all the following EXCEPT:
    a. Multiple sclerosis
    b. Rheumatoid arthritis
    c. Prevention of organ transplant rejection
    d. Crohn's disease

6. An important concept that the nurse must teach the client receiving an immunosuppressant agent is
   a. Daily weights are a must.
   b. Infection is a major concern.
   c. It is okay to become pregnant.
   d. These drugs are compatible with most other drugs.

7. Interferons are used to treat:
   a. Multiple sclerosis.
   b. Kidney cancer.
   c. Anemia.
   d. Neutropenia.

8. Which statement about the Interleukins is true?
   a. They act on receptor sites in the bone marrow.
   b. They are pregnancy category C drugs.
   c. They cause seizures.
   d. They have no drug interactions.

9. The nurse knows which of the following about the colony-stimulating factors?
   a. They are compatible with D5W.
   b. The oral route is preferred.
   c. Neurological assessment must be done daily.
   d. A flu-like syndrome can develop.

10. The antineoplastic agents affect normal and abnormal cells all over the body. That is the reason effects of these drug are routinely seen in all the following EXCEPT:
    a. Bone marrow.
    b. Hair follicles.
    c. Cardiac.
    d. Gastrointestinal system.

11. Which antineoplastic hormone is contraindicated if the client has an elevated calcium level?
    a. Tamoxifen (Nolvadex)
    b. Testolactone (Teslac)
    c. Toremifene (Fareston)
    d. Leuprolide (Lupron)

12. Which side effect of the alkylating agents should the nurse be most concerned about?
    a. Leukopenia
    b. Pulmonary emboli
    c. Hemorrhagic cystitis
    d. Dizziness

13. The nurse knows that teaching about the plant alkaloids has been successful when the client states the following:
    a. "I will stay out of the sun."
    b. "I won't eat aged cheese."
    c. "I will increase the fiber in my diet."
    d. "I know my urine will turn red."

14. All antineoplastic agents are contraindicated when the client has
    a. Pulmonary disease.
    b. Cardiac disease.
    c. Pancreatitis.
    d. Bone marrow depression.

PART XI • ANSWERS

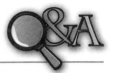

1. **The correct answer is b.** If salicylates are given to a child who has just received the varicella vaccine, Reye's syndrome may develop.

2. **The correct answer is a.** Vaccines, toxoids, immune serums, and antitoxins are contraindicated in pregnancy as there may be harmful effects to the fetus.

3. **The correct answer is c.** Pain and tenderness at the injection site are common side effects after receiving a vaccine.

4. **The correct answer is c.** The monoclonal antibodies are used to treat prevention of rejection in organ transplants, respiratory syncytial virus, Crohn's Disease, relapsed follicular B-cell non-Hodgkin's lymphoma, breast cancer tumors that overexpress HER2 protein, B-cell chronic lymphocytic leukemia, colorectal cancer, plaque psoriasis, relapsing forms of multiple sclerosis, asthma, and neovascular age-related macular degeneration.

5. **The correct answer is d.** The T and B suppressors are not used in Crohn's disease. The monoclonal antibodies are used for that illness.

6. **The correct answer is b.** It is imperative for the nurse to teach the client on immunosuppressant agents that he or she is at high risk for infection and must wash hands frequently, stay away from those who are ill, and report sore throat, fever, and other symptoms of feeling unwell to the physician.

7. **The correct answer is a.** Interferons are used to treat multiple sclerosis, genital warts, hepatitis B and C, malignant melanoma, AIDS-related Kaposi's sarcoma in adults, and chronic myelogenous leukemia.

8. **The correct answer is b.** The Interleukins are pregnancy category C drugs. The other answers are false.

9. **The correct answer is a.** The colony-stimulating factors are compatible with D5W. The other answers are incorrect.

10. **The correct answer is c.** The antineoplastic agents affect normal and abnormal cells in the bone marrow causing anemia and infection; hair follicles causing alopecia; and gastrointestinal system causing nausea and vomiting.

11. **The correct answer is c.** Toremifene (Fareston) is contraindicated in clients with elevated calcium levels.

12. **The correct answer is a.** Leukopenia is a major decrease in white blood cells, and this could lead to a massive infection that could be fatal.

13. **The correct answer is c.** Plant alkaloids can cause constipation, and the client must increase fluids and fiber while taking them.

14. **The correct answer is d.** Antineoplastic agents can further depress bone marrow function and are contraindicated when the client has this.

XII

Herbal Remedies

Marilyn J. Herbert-Ashton, MS, RN, BC

70

Common Herbal Remedies

The use of herbal remedies continues to increase. Just because these remedies may come from plant sources, does not mean they are safe. Companies manufacturing herbal remedies are not regulated by the US Food and Drug Administration (FDA), which means that there is no way to know if they are pure, potent, or effective. However, in 2003 the FDA proposed expanded oversight to regulate labeling, manufacturing, and safety of dietary supplements.

According to a survey conducted in 2001, up to 72% of individuals using a complementary therapy and being seen by a physician did not disclose at least one type of complementary therapy to their physician. Three-fifths of those who did not disclose to their physician stated that "the doctor never asked."[1,2]

In 1997, approximately 15 million adults were using herbal remedies and vitamins, in addition to their prescription medications.[3,4] It is imperative that the nurse become more knowledgable about herbal remedies, assess client use when interviewing clients, and become more familiar with herbal-drug interactions.

Herbs are available in many forms, including balms, extracts, essential oils, salves, lozenges, capsules, tablets, teas, or infusions.

Table 70–1 has popular herbals including their use(s), side effects, herb-drug interactions, and select nursing considerations.

COMMON HERBAL REMEDIES CLIENT TEACHING

- Advise health care provider, dentist, and specialists if taking herbal remedies.
- Consult with health care provider before taking herbal remedies if taking prescription or over-the-counter drugs, have diabetes mellitus, hypertension, pregnant, lactating, cardiovascular disease, bleeding disorders, thyroid disease, glaucoma, benign prosatic hypertrophy (BPH), epilepsy, psychiatric disorders, or a history of cerebral vascular accident (CVA).[5]
- Take exactly as prescribed and notify health care provider if adverse reactions occur.
- Purchase herbal remedies that have labels that include the herb name, the name and address of the manufacturer, batch number, and expiration date.[6]

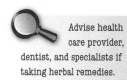

Advise health care provider, dentist, and specialists if taking herbal remedies.

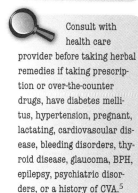

Consult with health care provider before taking herbal remedies if taking prescription or over-the-counter drugs, have diabetes mellitus, hypertension, pregnant, lactating, cardiovascular disease, bleeding disorders, thyroid disease, glaucoma, BPH, epilepsy, psychiatric disorders, or a history of CVA.[5]

Take exactly as prescribed and notify health care provider if adverse reactions occur.

Purchase herbal remedies that have labels that include the herb name, the name and address of the manufacturer, batch number, and expiration date.[6]

Table 70-1 Herbs at a Glance

Herb/Uses	Side Effects	Herb-Drug Interactions	Select Nursing Considerations
Black cohosh *Uses:* Relief of menopausal symptoms, menstrual cramps, and premenstrual syndrome	Nausea, diarrhea, dizziness, nervous system and visual disturbances, decreased heart rate, perspiration, spontaneous abortion	Potentiates the effects of antihypertensives, leading to hypotension; potentiates the hypoglycemic effects of insulin and oral hypoglycemics.	Contraindicated in pregnancy (may cause spontaneous abortion). Tell clients not to use in place of estrogen replacement therapy. Monitor blood pressure in clients taking antihypertensives.
Echinacea *Uses:* Treatment and prevention of colds, flu, other upper respiratory infections, and urinary tract and other mild infections. Topical echinacea, used for treatment of psoriasis, burns, eczema, and wounds.	Allergic reaction, nausea, vomiting, fever; hepatotoxicity when used for longer than 8 weeks	Decreases the effects of cyclosporine (Neoral, Sandimmune), methotrexate (Amethopterin, Folex PFS, Rheumatrex), anabolic steroids, and other cancer chemotherapeutic and immunosuppressant drugs. With extended use, increases the risk of liver toxicity when used with other hepatotoxic drugs, such as ketoconazole (Nizoral).	Contraindicated in clients with human immunodeficiency virus (HIV) infection, tuberculosis, and autoimmune diseases, such as lupus or multiple sclerosis. Tell clients not to use for longer than 8 weeks to prevent over-stimulation of the immune system. Assess for signs and symptoms of liver toxicity such as jaundice, brown urine, clay colored stools, changes in liver function tests.
Ephedra (ma-huang) *Uses:* Treatment of colds, flu, asthma, bronchospasm, congestion, and bronchitis. Dieters use as an appetite suppressant, also used as a	Heart attack, seizures, stroke, kidney stones, dizziness, motor restlessness, tremors, irritability, insomnia, headache, anorexia, nausea, vomiting,	Increases the effects of theophyline, decongestants, monoamine oxidase inhibitors (MAOIs), caffeine, and other CNS stimulants. Increases blood glucose levels. Can cause cardiac arrythmias when administered	Should not be taken by clients with heart disease, hypertension, glaucoma, hyperthyroidism, diabetes mellitus, prostate enlargement, or psychiatric or seizure disorders because of sympathetic nervous system

central nervous system (CNS) and cardiovascular stimulant.	flushing, tingling, tachycardia, increased blood pressure and blood glucose levels, weight loss, death	with cardiac glycosides or halothane.	effects. Contraindicated in pregnancy (may cause uterine contractions). Should not be used with OTC products containing ephedra alkaloids Note: Products containing more than 10 mg/dose are banned in the United States. Stroke, MI, and death have occurred with high doses.
Feverfew Uses: Treatment of migraine, suppress inflammation, fever, GI upset, and stimulate menstruation.	Nausea, vomiting, diarrhea, abdominal pain	Increases the risk of bleeding with antiplatelet drugs and anticoagulants	• Avoid chewing feverfew. • If allergic to ragweed, may also be allergic to feverfew.
Garlic Uses: Treatment of hypertension, hypercholesterolemia, atherosclerosis, colds, flu, gastrointestinal (GI) disturbances, rheumatism, asthma, diabetes mellitus; cancer prevention	Allergic reaction, headache myalgia, fatigue, halitosis, GI upset, diarrhea, nausea, vomiting; enhances bleeding	Increases the effects of anticoagulant, antiplatelet, and thrombolytic drugs, including abciximab (ReoPro), anegrelide HCL (Agrylin), clopidogrel bisulfate (Plavix) dipyridamole (Persantine), sulfinpyrazone (Anturane), ticlodipine HCL (Ticlid), tirofiban HCL (Aggrastat), warfarin sodium (Coumadin), and aspirin, increasing the risk of bleeding.	Teach clients to recognize signs and symptoms of bleeding, such as bruising and tarry stools. Tell clients not to substitute garlic for diabetes medications, antihypertensives, or cholesterol-reducing drugs.

continues

Table 70-1 Herbs at a Glance (continued)

Herb/Uses	Side Effects	Herb-Drug Interactions	Select Nursing Considerations
Ginger *Uses*: Treatment of motion nausea, and vomiting (except in pregnancy), GI discomfort, flatulence, anorexia, arthritis, and other inflammatory conditions	Allergic reaction, dermatitis; large overdoses can cause CNS depression and cardiac arrhythmias; enhances bleeding	Increases the effects of anticoagulant and antiplatelet drugs. Decreases the effects of antihypertensives	Should be taken when nausea and vomiting are anticipated. Teach clients to recognize signs and symptoms of bleeding. Not indicated for morning sickness. Monitor blood pressure in clients taking antihypertensives. Contraindicated in clients with bleeding disorders.
Gingko biloba *Uses*: Treatment of dementia, cerebrovascular insufficiency, intermittent claudication, macular degeneration, vertigo, tinnitus. Improvement of memory and cognition	Allergic reaction, headache, nausea, vomiting, diarrhea, dizziness, palpitations, skin reaction, decreased fertility; enhances bleeding	Potentiates the effects of anticoagulant, antiplatelet, and thrombolytic drugs. Increases the effects of MAOIs	Teach clients to recognize signs and symptoms of bleeding.
Ginseng *Uses*: To improve physical and mental stamina, enhance athletic performance, treat erectile dysfunction, protect the heart, and lower blood pressure	Chest pain, nausea, vomiting, diarrhea, palpitations, hypertension, insomnia, pruritus, Stevens-Johnson syndrome, nervousness; enhances bleeding	Increases the effects of antidiabetic agents and insulin, causing hypoglycemia. Increases the effects of MAOIs, corticosteroids, and caffeine. Increases the risk of bleeding when used with antiplatelet agents of nonsteroidal anti-inflammatory drugs	Teach clients to recognize signs and symptoms of bleeding. Limit use to 3 weeks. Watch for ginseng abuse syndrome (insomnia, hypertension, edema, diarrhea, hypertonia) in clients also using other stimulants. Caffeine intake should be limited.

Kava kava *Uses:* Treatment of anxiety, restlessness, tension, nervousness	Liver damage and toxicity, jaundice, visual problems, dilated pupils, hangover, sedation, extrapyramidal effects (dyskinesia, torticollis, exacerbation of the symptoms of Parkinson's disease)	Increased risk of liver toxicity when used with other hepatotoxic drugs. Increases the sedative effects of benzodiazepines, alcohol, and other CNS depressants. Coma has occurred when used with alprazolam (Xanax). Antagonizes levodopa (Dopar, Larodopa, L-Dopa)	Contraindicated in liver disease. Assess for signs and symptoms of hepatotoxicity. Tell clients not to drink alcohol, take other CNS depressants, or perform activities that require mental alertness when taking the herb. Limit use to 3 months or less to avoid psychological dependence. Should not be used by clients with Parkinson's disease because it antagonizes dopamine.
Saw palmetto *Uses:* To relieve symptoms of benign prostatic hypertrophy, to manage urinary tract infection, and as a mild diuretic	GI upset, nausea, abdominal pain, hypertension, headache urinary retention, back pain	Reduces the absorption of iron. Decreases the effectiveness of hormone therapy, oral contraceptives (OCs), and adrenergic drugs	Tell men that the herb can cause false-positive prostate-specific antigen test results. Warn women that taking the herb can prevent birth control pills from working. Contraindicated in pregnancy due to its hormonal effects.
St. John's wort *Uses:* Treatment of depression, anxiety, nervous unrest, excitability, neuralgia, and mood disturbances associated with menopause	Insomnia, vivid dreams, restlessness, anxiety, agitation, irritability, GI upset, fatigue, dizziness, headache, allergic reaction, confusion, dry mouth	Increases the adverse effects of antidepressants. Can cause serotonin syndrome (sweating, tremor, flushing, confusion, agitation) when taken with selective serotonin reuptake inhibitors (SSRIs). Increased risk of skin reactions when taken with	Explain that the herb can take up to 6 weeks to work. Assess for suicidal ideation and worsening of depression. Tell clients not to take the herb with other antidepressants. Tell clients taking the herb with warfarin to advise the health care team if they

continues

Table 70-1 Herbs at a Glance (continued)

Herb/Uses	Side Effects	Herb-Drug Interactions	Select Nursing Considerations
St. John's wort (continued)		other photosensitive drugs, such as tetracycline, thiazides, or sulfonamides. Decreases the absorption of iron. Reduces serum levels of digoxin (Lanoxin), cyclosporine, indinavir sulfate (Crixivan), amitriptyline HCL (Elavil), nortriptyline HCL (Aventyl, Pamelor), warfarin, and theophyline. Causes breakthrough bleeding when used with OCs. Reduces barbiturate-induced sleep times and prolongs narcotic-induced sleep times	plan to discontinue the herb's use. Such discontinuation can cause a surge in warfarin levels. Instruct clients to avoid sun exposure. Make sure clients with HIV know that the herb can reduce the effectiveness of certain protease inhibitors.
Valerian root Uses: Treatment of insomnia, anxiety, agitation, restlessness	Allergic reaction, daytime drowsiness, dizziness, and depression	May increase the sedative effects of barbiturates	Tell clients not to drink alcohol, take other CNS depressants, or operate heavy machinery when taking this herb.

Reprinted with permission from RN Magazine. Getting a handle on herbals. *RN-: Traveling Nursing Today.* 2002; September:20–21.

NURSING IMPLICATIONS FOR HERBAL REMEDIES

- Take an herbal history and ask about the use of "natural remedies" including herbal teas, infusions, balms, extracts, essential oils, salves, lozenges, capsules, or tablets.
- Children and alcoholics should avoid using tinctures and extracts due to their alcohol content.
- Assess for plant or flower allergies, as some herbs come from plant or flower sources.
- Clients scheduled for surgery should stop taking herbals 2 to 3 weeks before surgery, and if that is not possible, ask client to bring herbal in its original container for the anesthesiologist to see.[7]

REFERENCES

1. Eisenberg DM, Kessler RC, et al. Perceptions about complementary therapies relative to conventional therapies among adults who use both: results from a national survey. *Ann Intern Med.* 2001;35(5):344.

2. Herbert-Ashton MJ. Getting a handle on herbals. *RN: Traveling Nurse Today.* 2002;Sept:16–17.

3. Eisenberg DM, Davis RB, et al. Trends in alternative medicine use in the United States, 1990–1997. *JAMA.* 1998; 280(18):1569.

4. Herbert-Ashton MJ. Getting a handle on herbals. *RN: Traveling Nurse Today.* 2002;Sept:16.

5. Cupp MJ. Herbal remedies: adverse effects and drug interactions. *American Family Physician.* 1999; March 1. Available at: www.aafp.org/afp/990301ap/1239.html. Accessed July 17, 2003.

6. McKenry LM, Tessier E, Hogan M. *Mosby's Pharmacology in Nursing,* 22nd ed. St. Louis, MO: Mosby Elsevier; 2006:230–231.

7. American Society of Anesthesiologists. Anesthesiologists warn: if you're taking herbal products, tell your doctor before surgery. Available at: http://www.asahq.org/PublicEducation/herbal.html. Accessed May 28, 2002.

PART XII • QUESTIONS

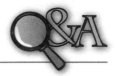

1. Which of the following herbs may be used to provide relief of menopause symptoms?
    a. Black cohosh
    b. Ginger
    c. Kava Kava
    d. Valerian root

2. Which of the following herbs may be used to relieve symptoms of BPH?
    a. Black cohosh
    b. Saw palmetto
    c. St. John's wort
    d. Valerian

3. Side effects of echinacea may include:
    a. Allergic reaction.
    b. Hypothermia.
    c. Urinary retention.
    d. Chest pain.

4. Of the following, which herb increases the sedative effects of barbiturates?
    a. Ephedra (ma-huang)
    b. Ginseng
    c. Saw palmetto
    d. Valerian root

5. Which of the following herbs may take up to 6 weeks to work?
    a. Echinacea
    b. Ginkgo biloba
    c. Kava Kava
    d. St. John's wort

PART XII · ANSWERS

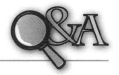

1. **The correct answer is a.** Black cohosh may be used to provide relief of menopause symptoms.

2. **The correct answer is b.** Saw palmetto may be used to relieve symptoms of BPH.

3. **The correct answer is a.** Side effects of echinacea may include allergic reactions. Echinacea is from the asteraceae family, which includes sunflowers, daisies, and ragweed. Clients allergic to asteraceae may be allergic to echinacea.

4. **The correct answer is d.** Valerian root increases the sedative effects of barbiturates.

5. **The correct answer is d.** St. John's wort, when used in the treatment of depression or anxiety, may take up 6 weeks to work.

Appendix I
Vitamins

Appendix I Vitamins

Vitamin	Use	Adverse Effects and Side Effects	Nursing Implications
Fat-Soluble Vitamins (A, D, E, K)			
A Retinol (Aquasol A)	Growth and development of bones, vision, mucous membrane, and skin	Usually few adverse side effects: headache, increased intracranial pressure, lethargy, nausea, vomiting	Contraindicated in clients with hypersensitivity, and oral malabsorption syndromes. If unable to take PO, IM administration available. Take with food. Monitor for hypervitaminosis and discontinue if overdose occurs. Store in light-resistant container.
D Calcitriol (Rocaltrol dihydroxy-vitamin D_3) • calcifediol (D_3) (Calderal) • ergocalciferal (D_2) (Calciferal, Drisdol) • dihydrotachysterol (DHT, D_2) (DHT, Hytakerol)	Prevents and treats rickets; promotes absorption and metabolism of calcium, phosphorus, and magnesium; controls parathyroid hormone (PTH) levels	Usually few adverse side effects; anorexia, fatigue, headache, convulsions, hematuria, renal failure, hypertension, pruritus, muscle pain, decreased bone growth, nausea, vomiting	Available PO, IM. Contraindicated in hypersensitivity, renal dysfunction, hypercalcemia or hyperphosphatemia. Avoid magnesium-containing antacids and laxatives. Can take without regard to food. Give deep IM. Monitor Vitamin D levels and for adverse effects. Encourage sunlight unless contraindicated.
E (d-alpha tocopherol, Aquavit E, others)	Antioxidant; assists body's use of vitamin A	Usually few adverse side effects: fatigue, headache, nausea, diarrhea, weakness, blurred vision	Available PO, IM. Contraindicated in hypersensitivity. Take before or after meals. Store in a light-resistant container. May increase action of anticoagulants
K phytonadione (Aqua-Mephyton)	Antidote for oral anti-coagulants, blood clotting as it affects factors II, VII, IX, and X, found in the liver; in newborns, used to prevent hemorrhage disease	Usually nontoxic: headache, nausea, rash, urticaria, decreased liver function tests	Available PO, SC, IM, avoid IV use if possible. Contraindicated in clients with hypersensitivity, severe liver disease, and last few weeks of pregnancy. Keep drug away from light. Can take without regard to food. Avoid alcohol, aspirin, and ibuprofen while taking, and report bleeding to health care provider.

Minerals decrease absorption of fat-soluble vitamins, avoid concurrent use.

Appendix I Vitamins

Vitamin	Use	Adverse Effects and Side Effects	Nursing Implications
Water-Soluble Vitamins (Ascorbic Acid and B-Complex)			
C Ascorbic Acid	Antioxidant, prevention and treatment of scurvy wound healing and tissue repair, promotes collagen formation, and iron absorption	Usually nontoxic. Mega-doses: abdominal discomfort, headache, formation of renal stones, nausea, vomiting, diarrhea	Large doses may decrease effects of anticoagulants. When discontinuing, if taking large doses of vitamin C, taper doses to prevent rebound scurvy. Available PO, SC, IM, IV
B_{12} Cyanocobalamin	Essential for RBCs, metabolism of body cells, growth and metabolism of carbohydrates (CHO), fats, and proteins. Treatment of B_{12} deficiency and pernicious anemia	Usually nontoxic. Large doses: prorates, diarrhea, fever, hypokalemia, flushing, CHF	Contraindicated in clients with hypersensitivity, optic nerve atrophy. Available PO, SC, IM, intranasal. Give with food. Clients with gastric, ileal resections, small bowel disease, or malabsorption require parental use. Lifelong need for B_{12} therapy after gastrectomy or ileal resection
B_9 Folic acid	Prevention and treatment of megablastic anemia, promotes fetal development during pregnancy	Fever, rash	Available PO, SC, IM (deep), IV. Contraindicated in uncorrected pernicious anemia. Urine may turn an intense yellow color. Monitor folic acid levels, reticulocyte levels, hemoglobin, and hematocrit throughout therapy.
B_3 Niacin	Treatment and prevention of pellagra, adjunct in some hyperlipidemias	GI upset, hepatoxicity, blurred vision, flushing, prorates	Available PO. Contraindicated in clients with hypersensitivity. Administered with food. Long-term and high-dose therapy, monitor hepatic function, glucose, and uric acid levels.
B_6 Pyridoxine	Treatment and prevention of pyridoxine deficiency, neuropathy, and management of isonizid overdose	Large doses: lethargy, flushing, paresthesias, pain at injection site	Available PO, IM, IV. Parental form, avoid exposure to light.

continues

Appendix I Vitamins

Vitamin	Use	Adverse Effects and Side Effects	Nursing Implications
Water-Soluble Vitamins (Ascorbic Acid and B-Complex)			
B_2 Riboflavin	Treatment and prevention of riboflavin deficiency	Large doses: yellow urine discoloration	Avoid alcohol during therapy, as riboflavin absorption can be impaired.
B_1 Thiamine	Treatment of beriberi, prevention of Wernicke's encephalopathy, supplement for cirrhosis, alcoholism, or clients with GI disease	Usually in large doses or IV use, otherwise uncommon. Vascular collapse, hypotension, angioedema, respiratory distress, restlessness	Contraindicated in clients with hypersensitivity. Available PO, IV, IM, IV. Monitor site for redness and induration

Appendix II
Minerals

Appendix II Minerals

Name	Use	Adverse Effects and Side Effects	Nursing Implications
Calcium	Treatment for hypoglycemia; dietary supplement in lactation and pregnancy; assists cardiac contraction in cardiac arrest; decreases gastric acid	Bleeding kidney dysfunction, urinary stones, metabolic alkalosis, nausea, vomiting, constipation, anorexia	Assess serum calcium levels; taking with OTC drugs that contain calcium can increase calcium level in body; administer with food; do not give with milk or dairy products; decreased absorption if given with high fiber foods
Iron	Prevention or treatment for low iron level; iron deficiency anemia; supplemental epoetin therapy	Constipation, heartburn, nausea, anorexia, diarrhea, black stools	Best to give on an empty stomach but can give with food to decrease gastric upset; liquid form should be taken via a straw to prevent staining of teeth; assess hemoglobin and reticulocyte levels; assess bowel movements as constipation is common. For IM use Z-tracr method (deep IM).
Magnesium	Treatment for deficiency; anticonvulsant in preeclampsia and eclampsia	Hypermagnesia: hypothermia, heart block, respiratory distress, loss of tendon reflexes, CNS depression	Explain to client that diarrhea can occur; if taken with OTC drugs that contain magnesium can increase magnesium level in body.
Phosphorus	Treats deficiency states	Confusion, diarrhea, muscle cramps	Separate administration of phosphorus from antacids by 2 hours. Do not give to client on a potassium or sodium restricted diet. Assess potassium level. Excessive diarrhea must be reported to physician.
Zinc	Treats deficiency states; common cold; rheumatoid arthritis	Nausea, vomiting, diarrhea	Do not give with high fiber foods, phosphates, or calcium; can give with food, check OTC drugs for zinc levels to avoid overdose.

Appendix III
Pregnancy Categories

CATEGORY A

- No risk to fetus based on human research.

CATEGORY B

- Research in animals shows no risk to fetus, but no human research has been done .

CATEGORY C

- If benefit of drug outweighs risk, then drug is given. Animal research shows fetal risk, but no human research to rule out risk, or there is no human or animal research.

CATEGORY D

- Human research shows fetal risk. If situation is life-threatening, benefit may outweigh risk.

CATEGORY X

- Use in humans is contraindicated.

CATEGORY UK

- Unknown, unclassified

Bibliography

BIBLIOGRAPHY

Abrams AC. *Clinical Drug Therapy Rationales for Nursing Practice,* 8th ed. Philadelphia, PA: Lippincott; 2006.

Aschenbrenner D, Venable S. *Drug Therapy in Nursing.* Philadelphia, PA: Lippincott; 2006.

Broyles BC, Reiss B, Evans M. *Pharmacological Aspects of Nursing Care.* 7th ed. Albany, NY: Delmar-Thompson; 2007.

Foster S, Tyler VE. *Tyler's Honest Herbal,* 4th ed. New York, NY: Hawthorne Press; 1999.

Gruenwald J. *PDR for Herbal Medicines,* 3rd ed. Montvale, NJ: Medical Economics; 2004.

Herbert-Ashton, M. Getting a handle on herbals. *RN TNT.* 2002;Sept:16–24.

Karch A. *Focus on Nursing Pharmacology,* 4th ed. Philadelphia, PA: Wolters Kluwer/Lippincott, Williams & Wilkins; 2008.

Karch A. *Lippincott's Nursing Drug Guide.* Philadelphia, PA: Lippincott, Williams & Wilkins; 2007.

Kee JL, Hayes ER, McCuistion LE. *Pharmacology: A Nursing Process Approach,* 5th ed. St. Louis, MO: Saunders Elsevier; 2006.

Lehne RA. *Pharmacology for Nursing Care,* 6th ed. Philadelphia, PA: Saunders, Elsevier; 2007.

Lilley L, Harrington S, Snyder J. *Pharmacology and the Nursing Process,* 5th ed. St. Louis, MO: Mosby; 2007.

McKenry LM, Tessier E, Hogan M. *Mosby's Pharmacology in Nursing,* 22nd ed. St. Louis, MO: Mosby Elsevier; 2006.

Nursing Herbal Medicine Handbook, 3rd ed. Philadelphia, PA: Lippincott, Williams & Wilkens; 2005.

Skidmore-Roth L. *Mosby's Nursing Drug Reference.* St. Louis, MO; Mosby Elsevier; 2007.

Spratto G, Woods A. *PDR Nurse's Drug Handbook.* Clifton Park, NY: Thompson Delmar Learning; 2006.

Youngkin E, Sawin K, Kissinger J, Israel D. *Pharmacotherapeutics: a Primary Care Clinical Guide.* Upper Saddle River, NJ: Pearson/ Prentice Hall; 2005.

Drug Index

Subject Index

Water damage
noted
12/29/16
RC